MAJOR PROBLEMS IN INTERNAL MEDICINE

Published

MAJOR PROBLEMS IN INTERNAL MEDICINE

In Preparation

Potts: Disorders of Calcium Metabolism
Havel and Kane: Diagnosis and Treatment of Hyperlipidemias
Siltzbach: Sarcoidosis
Scheinberg and Sternlieb: Wilson's Disease and Copper Metabolism
Atkins and Bodel: Fever
Lieber and De Carli: Medical Aspects of Alcoholism
Merrill: Glomerulonephritis
Goldberg: The Scientific Basis and Practical Use of Diuretics
Kilbourne: Influenza
Deykin: Diseases of the Platelets
Cohen: Amyloidosis
Salmon: Multiple Myeloma
Weinstein: Infective Endocarditis
Sasahara: Pulmonary Embolism
Smith: Renal Lithiasis
Swartz: Meningitis
Sparling: Venereal Diseases
Brooks: Diseases of the Exocrine Pancreas
McLees: Critical Care
Engel: Psychosocial Problems in Medical Practice
Utz: Systemic Mycotic Infections
Solomon and Chopra: Graves Disease and Hyperthyroidism

NEIL H. RASKIN, M.D.

Professor of Neurology
School of Medicine
University of California
San Francisco, California

OTTO APPENZELLER, M.D., Ph.D.

Professor of Neurology and Medicine
University of New Mexico
School of Medicine
Albuquerque, New Mexico

HEADACHE

VOLUME

XIX

IN THE SERIES
MAJOR PROBLEMS IN INTERNAL MEDICINE
Lloyd H. Smith, Jr., M.D., Editor

W. B. SAUNDERS COMPANY • PHILADELPHIA • LONDON • TORONTO

W. B. Saunders Company: West Washington Square
Philadelphia, PA   19105

1 St. Anne's Road
Eastbourne, East Sussex BN21, 3UN, England

1 Goldthorne Avenue
Toronto, Ontario M8Z 5T9, Canada

Library of Congress Cataloging in Publication Data

Raskin, Neil H

Headache.

(Major problems in internal medicine; v. 19)
1. Headache.   I. Appenzeller, Otto, joint author.
II. Title.   III. Series. [DNLM: 1. Headache. W1
MA492T v. 19 / W342 R225h]

RC392.R37   616.8'57   79-66042
ISBN 0-7216-7467-4

HEADACHE   ISBN   0-7216-7467-4

Last digit is the print number: 9   8   7   6   5   4   3

FOREWORD

It has been estimated that approximately one in three of all Americans suffer from severe headaches at least at some stage of life. Headache may be the most common symptom of malaise in human experience. Nostrums for its alleviation are hawked with cheerful exuberance via the tyranny of radio and television, with a cacophony not infrequently creating the very symptoms which they are designed to alleviate. More than 30 million pounds of aspirin are ingested annually in the United States, most of it to relieve headache. The parenchyma of the brain itself is stated to be insensitive to pain. Unfortunately this does not hold true for its surrounding structures, including blood vessels and the cranial muscles. The mechanisms of pain in headache are still imperfectly understood, as witness the morass of theories which still obscures our understanding of the pathogenesis of migraine, for example.

Most headaches obviously do not require professional attention and are just as well left to the home remedies and mild analgesics which are promoted with such puerile panegyrics. There are, however, at least two general considerations which complicate this cavalier attitude toward headache:

1) Headache may be the nonspecific but early harbinger of serious illness. As an example, it is the most frequent first sign of a brain tumor. Accelerated hypertension, uremia, pituitary tumor or meningitis may present with headache. The list is alarmingly long and the chances for misdiagnosis (or simple failure to consider an underlying cause) are constantly present. Both the patient and the physician must sort out the important from the trivial and the stakes are high that this be done accurately.

2) Recurrent headaches may be the cause of severe disability as well as of discomfort. Medical experience, most of it empirical, has evolved different forms of treatment which may be relatively specific for certain syndromes. Although the pathogenesis of migraine, representing both genetic and environmental factors, is not clearly defined, drugs are available which can both reduce the number of attacks and

reduce the severity of a given attack. The considerable specificity in this response requires that the correct diagnosis of migraine must be sorted out from other forms of headache. Furthermore, optimal treatment of a migrainous patient (or for that matter of a patient with tension headaches) requires a skillful trial of the available modalities individualized to the particular patient. Temporal arteritis requires even more specific therapy, i.e. glucocorticoids, for the relief of symptoms and prevention of complications. Headache is therefore not in itself sufficient diagnosis either for prognosis or as a guide to treatment.

In this monograph Drs. Raskin and Appenzeller have written an authoritative review of the pathogenesis, differential diagnosis and treatment of the various forms of headache now recognized in clinical practice. This is information of interest to the general internist and is not the exclusive domain of the neurologist. The importance of headache both as a symptom and as a signal justifies the inclusion of such a comprehensive review in *Major Problems in Internal Medicine*.

LLOYD H. SMITH, JR., M.D.

PREFACE

"Sanctus, sanctus, Dominus, Deus, Sabaoth. Say this thing every day for thy head against headache; after repeating it place thy spittle upon thy palm and put it on thy temples and at the back of thy head and say the Pater thrice thereupon and draw a cross with thy spittle on the top of thy head and on thy head also draw the form of the letter U."

Irish manuscript, 8th century*

Until relatively recently the advice offered above was probably about as effective as many alternatives for the amelioration of headache; this in large measure was a reflection of both the paucity and low productivity of headache research, which for many years lagged far behind the spectacular strides that were being made in many other areas of medicine. However, the past fifteen years have seen the emergence of headache as a serious and important scientific problem, and substantial advances have been made in the treatment of the commonest headache disorders, although the rate of therapeutic progress generally has exceeded that of the deciphering of headache mechanisms. This gap has been narrowed during the past few years, and for the participants in this effort and for close observers on the sidelines it has been an exciting and gratifying time; undertaking the writing of this book is a product of the enthusiasm generated by the authors' involvement in this field for these past several years.

Much of the new information regarding the regulation of the cerebral vasculature, pain modulation, and the biology of central serotonergic circuits has been published in diverse areas of the scientific literature; we therefore felt it would be valuable to collect these observations and place them into a context relevant to headache disorders in a single volume so that all physicians may keep abreast of this revitalized subject.

---

*Friedman, A.P. (1972): The headache in history, literature and legend. Bull. N.Y. Acad. Med. 48:661–681.

vii

This volume presents thorough reviews of those headache disorders most commonly encountered by physicians rather than an
encyclopedic coverage of the subject. The emphasis is upon recurring
head pain that is not attributable to an underlying structural abnormality. Special effort has been made to present the available data
that pertain not only to mechanisms of headache but to the descriptive clinical features and details of therapy as well.

Some liberties have been taken in speculation, perhaps more so
than in other monographs of this series. However, we have tried to do
no more than extrapolate from experimental data and base such conclusions on sound biological principles. In the absence of controlled
experiments, we have permitted ourselves occasionally to draw from
our own experience. Some readers may be intolerant to our exercise
of this prerogative, especially when citing our own data, but this is not
an apology. The scientific method can and should be extended to
observations made clinically as well as to those made at the laboratory
bench; the validity of experiential information depends upon the
observer's appreciation of the 95 per cent confidence limits of his
normative data. These are, at present, difficult to quantify and communicate in a manner that would satisfy the usual criterion of validity
of biological evidence—that there is a probability of less than 5 per
cent that the observation occurred fortuitously. We should very much
like to assure our readers of our awareness of these principles.

Interest in headache has been revived during this past decade or
so by a rigorous attitude toward the subject, fostered largely by the
approach of Dr. James W. Lance and his colleagues in Sydney,
Australia, as denoted by our many citations of their work.

Finally, we should like to acknowledge for their many helpful
suggestions and review of the manuscript, Véronique Raskin, and
Drs. Michael Aminoff, Donald Palatucci, and Howard Fields.

NEIL H. RASKIN, M.D.
OTTO APPENZELLER, M.D., Ph.D.

CONTENTS

CHAPTER 1

HEADACHE: AN OVERVIEW

Headache is a common symptom of our time. References to headache in the literature of the past 3,000 years suggest that it has always been with us (Friedman, 1972). Sigmund Freud, Thomas Jefferson, Ulysses S. Grant and Charles Darwin were among the more well-known individuals who suffered from "sick headache." Currently, 5 to 10 per cent of the population seek intermittent medical aid for the relief of disabling headache, and over 40 per cent of North Americans have experienced severe headache at some point in their lives (Ziegler et al, 1977). The symptom of headache is therefore a public health problem worthy of serious attention and study. Until recently, however, little attention was directed toward this problem, probably because of the widely held view (unsupported by evidence) that the primary mechanism of the commonest headache types was psychologic in nature. Although it continues to be clear that anxiety, worry and stress are common trigger factors for headache, the hypothesis that has aroused interest in the scientific community is that headache may be the manifestation of a lowered biologic threshold to a large variety of stimuli. The nature of that threshold and the mechanisms by which headache may be triggered are of some interest, and will be critically surveyed in this monograph. Recent lines of evidence drawn from diverse biologic fields of interest suggest the possibility that *altered reactivity of brain stem serotonergic neurons and the regulation of the synaptic turnover of serotonin may be important to the mechanism of recurring headache,* and these data will be examined in some detail.

The traditional classification of the commonest recurring headaches into tension and migraine types is open to challenge. There is a consensus among physicians who have studied migraine patients that the classic description of migraine as hemicranial pulsatile pain, associated with vomiting and preceded by a characteristic vis-

1

ual aura, is not a frequent form of this disorder (Selby and Lance, 1960). Moreover, contraction of muscles of the neck and scalp occurs in migraine headache as well as in tension headache (Pózniak-Patewicz, 1976; Bakal and Kaganov, 1977); cervical muscle contraction has even been reported to be a frequent aura in migraine (Pearce, 1977). Furthermore many patients with headaches that conform to the muscle contraction pattern (occipitofrontal, constricting, nonrhythmic, constant daily pain) have received relief from pharmacologic agents that probably are vasoactive and not myoactive (Lance, Curran and Anthony, 1965). A seemingly heretical hypothesis now being tested is that the immediate mechanism of headache in most patients, including those currently classified as tension headache sufferers, is instability in the regulation of arterial tone. It is essential to note, however, that the earlier classifications of headache represented a point of view of careful and perceptive physicians; the evidence from which inferences were drawn, however, was sparse.

PAIN

To place the subject of head pain into context, we must briefly consider the subject of pain in general. One of the greatest achievements of medicine is the alleviation of pain, which began with the use of opiates hundreds of years ago, and received more recent impetus with the introduction of anesthesia. The treatment of pain has been empiric, and has not really stemmed from an understanding of its mechanisms. In the last few years, however, we have gained some insight into how pain is perceived.

The transmission and modulation of pain appear to depend on discrete neural pathways. Information derived from specific peripheral pain receptors, nociceptors, is processed at spinal cord, brain stem and thalamocortical levels, although the ultimate cortical receiving region is not known. Serotonin has been implicated as an inhibitory transmitter in the brain stem pain modulating system (Basbaum and Fields, 1978).

The most comprehensive and comprehensible idea of how pain is perceived is expressed in the gate-control theory of pain (Melzack and Wall, 1965). The theory proposes that a neural network in the dorsal horn of the spinal cord may increase or decrease the flow of information from the peripheral primary afferent terminals to central pain transmission neurons. This "gating" mechanism, therefore, modulates somatic information before it evokes pain perception. The *degree* to which the gate affects sensory transmission is determined by both peripheral and descending influences. Neural areas responsible for pain perception are activated when the level of activity in pain transmission neurons exceeds a critical level. The presence or absence of pain, then, is determined by a balance between the incoming afferent impulses and central influences upon the gate; thus, a lesion (anatomic or biochemical) that impairs the normal descending or segmental inhibitory influences could open the gate, resulting in pain. Psychologic factors such as attention, past experience and state of mind may also influence pain perception through the same mechanism (Melzack, 1973).

The most common type of pain is that which results from activation of peripheral nociceptors in the presence of a normally functioning nervous system, as in the pain arising from scalded skin or appendicitis. Another type of pain is the result of injury to the central or peripheral nervous system, and may occur without activation of peripheral receptors. At present it is not entirely clear which types of headache originate centrally and/or peripherally. Headache may arise from dysfunction, displacement or encroachment on pain-sensitive cranial structures, and these, for the most part, are vascular. The proximal portion of the cerebral arteries and the large veins and venous sinuses are the most important pain-sensitive structures (Ray and Wolff, 1940). Other structures, such as the meninges, upper cervical nerve roots and scalp muscles, may also be involved in the genesis of head pain, but the brain itself, most of the meninges, the ventricular linings and the choroid plexuses are pain-insensitive structures. The blood vessels are innervated by branches of the trigeminal, glossopharyngeal and vagal nerves and the upper sensory roots of the spinal cord. The sensitivity of larger arteries with their dense sensory innervation contrasts with the insensitivity of smaller arterioles within the brain, which are sparsely innervated (Purves, 1978).

The traditional view of the origin of headache is that it is peripheral. The pulsation and stretching of arterial walls, or the contraction of skeletal muscle, has been thought to stimulate peripheral receptors in these tissues, resulting in the perception of pain. However, people who habitually frown, clench their teeth or experience anxiety commonly exhibit muscle contraction about the head and neck, but only a small minority complain of headache; likewise, vigorous physical exercise or a hot bath produces arterial vasodilatation, but only rarely does headache ensue. Moreover, many of the vasoactive drugs effective in the treatment of patients with chronic recurring headache have prominent effects on the central nervous system (CNS), and minor or unknown effects peripherally (see Chapter 4). Thus, both vasodilatation and muscle contraction, although resulting in pain at times, may be epiphenomena of a central headache-generating mechanism.

Sicuteri and his colleagues (1974) have proposed that migraine may be a genetic disorder of the brain stem pain modulation system in which the turnover of neurotransmitters, serotonin in particular, may be defective; they have supported this hypothesis with data derived from pharmacologic experiments with laboratory animals and human subjects, using agents that either deplete or replete monamine stores within the CNS. There are also other data that support the hypothesis that brain stem serotonergic neuronal activity is important to the pathophysiology of migraine, and these are reviewed in Chapter 4. These ideas focus on the role of the CNS, the brain stem in particular, in pain modulation. This is an area about which exciting new information has been gathered in recent years.

BRAIN STEM MODULATION OF PAIN

There are discrete brain stem sites that, when electrically stimulated, are capable of suppressing pain transmission; profound analgesia is produced by electrical stimulation in the midbrain periaqueductal gray and in periventricular thalamic sites (Fields and Basbaum, 1978). Direct microinjection of opiates into some of these sites also results in analgesia, and these loci correspond generally to the distribution of endogenous opiate-like peptides, which have been named "endorphins" (Simon and Hiller, 1978). Stimulation-induced analgesia is accompanied by a significant elevation of cerebrospinal fluid (CSF) endorphin-like immunoreactivity in human subjects (Akil et al, 1978; Hosobuchi et al, 1979), and evidence has recently been advanced that endorphin release mediates placebo analgesia for dental postoperative pain (Levine et al, 1978). Moreover, lesions or microinjection of an opiate antagonist at midbrain sites blocks the analgesia produced by systemically administered opiates.

The production of analgesia by systemic opiates probably occurs through an action upon a brain stem system that is "normally" activated by endorphins. A pathway to the spinal cord is required for both opiate- and stimulation-induced analgesia (Mayer and Price, 1976), and the termination of this pathway is in proximity to pain-transmitting neurons of the dorsal horn. This system may well approximate the endogenous mechanism of analgesia and pain perception, but the data bearing on this question are incomplete. Nevertheless, these results are compatible with the concept of a neural pathway that may increase pain threshold by releasing an endogenous compound. Based on the observation that the analgesic effect of morphine is lessened in laboratory animals depleted of serotonin (Harvey and Lints, 1965; Tenen, 1967), Sicuteri (1978) has suggested that abnormalities in endorphin turnover may explain many of the phenomena that occur during migraine attacks; this is an interesting possibility which is, at present, highly speculative.

ACUTE AND CHRONIC PAIN

The behavioral accompaniments of acute pain — perspiration, crying, agitation and writhing — are sometimes believed to be "objective" indicators of pain severity, regardless of the source or chronicity of pain; however, the process of adaptation occurs with pain as well as with other sensations. When pain lasts weeks and months, patients manage to endure it and to function within limits, either through distraction, stoicism or pharmacologic palliation. Sometimes they may appear to be untroubled, in no distress. This process of adaptation that renders discomfort less socially visible sometimes results in doubt, on the physician's part, that a patient is experiencing pain. This is due to a lack of appreciation of an important difference between acute and chronic pain. The assessment of pain severity must be accomplished by talking to patients in addition to examining them; inquiries into functional limitations, loss of pleasurable activities, interference with sleep and the degree of relief obtained from various analgesics are essential in order to obtain data requisite to an estimate of pain severity. Patients who say they are in pain probably should be believed until clear evidence of malingering is obtained. Placebo responsiveness is irrelevant to any of these issues; relief of pain with placebo occurs in one-third of patients (Beecher, 1955), but there is no evidence that placebo responders have lower pain levels than nonresponders (Levine et al, 1978).

REGULATION OF CEREBRAL BLOOD VESSELS

The prominent role of alteration in tone of cerebral arteries as the commonest mechanism of headaches that arise in a variety of circumstances prompts this brief review of the regulatory mechanisms of the cerebral circulation. In general, although the intracranial pressure and blood viscosity exert effects on the circulation of the brain, under most physiologic circumstances, regulation resides in the intrinsic tone of the cerebral vessels which is subject to both metabolic and neurogenic control.

VASCULAR ANATOMY

Each cerebral hemisphere is supplied by the ipsilateral internal carotid artery, whereas the structures contained in the posterior fossa are supplied by the basilar artery. These main arteries communicate with each other in a system of anastomoses, the circle of Willis, at the base of the brain. Under normal conditions little communication occurs between the arterial sources of the circle of

Willis, since the pressure in the contributing vessels is approximately the same (McDonald and Potter, 1951). However, it is known that communication does occur in emergencies, since after ligation of an internal carotid artery the pressure distal to the ligature is maintained at one-half its previous value by contributions through the circle of Willis (Sweet and Bennett, 1948). The capillary supply to the brain is abundant, although less than to other organs such as the heart. There is an average of 1,000 capillaries per mm^2 in cerebral cortex and 300 per mm^2 in white matter, compared to 5,000 capillaries per mm^2 in the myocardium (Dunning and Wolff, 1937). Blood flow loses its laterality to some extent in the cerebral venous system, since the superior and inferior sagittal sinuses receive blood from both cerebral hemispheres. There is unilateral venous drainage from the inferolateral aspects of the hemispheres via the ipsilateral lateral sinus to the internal jugular vein and the superior and inferior petrosal sinuses that flow into the ipsilateral jugular bulb.

Cerebral arteries are richly innervated by adrenergic fibers that originate in the superior cervical and stellate ganglia (Edvinsson, 1975). The internal carotid artery and its branches are more densely innervated than the vertebral artery and its branches; large arteries are innervated more abundantly than small ones. There is no evidence of cholinergic innervation of cerebral resistance vessels, although cholinergic innervation of the carotid artery and its branches and of pial arteries has been demonstrated (Purves, 1978). In addition to the perivascular sympathetic innervation, there is evidence for a central adrenergic pathway to cerebral vessels, originating in the medulla and coursing through the cerebral parenchyma (Swanson and Hartman, 1975). The functional contributions of the central and peripheral innervation to the regulation of vascular tone are unclear. Only minimal alterations in cerebral blood flow (CBF) occur after sympathetic stimulation or denervation *in vivo* (Heistad and Marcus, 1978).

BLOOD PRESSURE

When the mean arterial pressure is reduced below 60 to 70 mm Hg in normotensive individuals it assumes a determinant role in regulating CBF; in hypertensive patients, this lower limit may be as high as 130 mm Hg (Lassen, 1974). When the pressure head is at or above normal values, the cerebral circulation is regulated by changes in cerebrovascular resistance (Sokoloff and Kety, 1960). The maintenance of a constant CBF despite wide variations in cerebral perfusion pressure is called "autoregulation." There is an upper as well as a lower limit to autoregulation of CBF (Strandgaard et al, 1973); this is quite variable among individuals and is higher in hypertensive subjects. The venous pressure, which in most instances represents the intracranial pressure, is an important factor in regulating CBF only when the intracranial pressure exceeds the mean arterial pressure, and in opposing the effects of gravity on the cerebral circulation, by balancing hydrostatic effects on the arterial pressure head. Under most conditions, including cardiac decompensation (Novack et al, 1953), the venous pressure plays a minor role in the regulation of CBF. The most important single factor in determining the cerebrovascular resistance is the narrowing or dilatation of cerebral arteries, especially the arterioles. The variables that operate to alter these vascular dimensions include metabolic and neural factors.

METABOLIC FACTORS

Alterations in the carbon dioxide content of blood profoundly influence the CBF. Hyperventilation, resulting in hypocapnia, produces a marked decrease of CBF, whereas hypercapnia causes intense cerebral vasodilatation so that CBF may double (Lassen, 1968). Endogenous metabolic alterations in brain tissue pH are countered by this remarkably sensitive system in which CBF meets the metabolic demands of the brain. The effects of changes in oxygen tension are the reverse of those of carbon dioxide, but are much less in magnitude; moderate changes in arterial oxygen tension have only a minimal influence on CBF. Measurable CBF increases are not seen until the pO_2 is below 50 mm Hg (Kogure et al, 1970); this is also the level at which lactic acidosis occurs in brain. High concentrations of oxygen exert a mild vasoconstricting effect on the cerebral circulation (Sokoloff, 1959).

NEURAL FACTORS

Purves (1978) has recently summarized the evidence favoring a neural influence in the regulation of cerebral vessels. At present it is difficult to assign a precise role to neurogenic factors; it has been argued that the dense network of adrenergic and cholinergic nerves surrounding cerebral arteries is similar to those in other vascular beds, and probably subserves similar functions, although experiments devised to demonstrate this have fallen short of the mark. There is no question that stimulation of portions of the hypothalamus results in dilatation or constriction of pial arteries, and that autoregulation may be abolished during stimulation of the fastigial nucleus in the cerebellum (Purves, 1978). Thus, powerful dilator and constrictor influences reside within the CNS. These central pathways may provide the basis for the responses of cerebral blood vessels to external stimuli such as temperature change (Stoica et al, 1973) or, perhaps, to internal stimuli that may produce the condition called "migraine."

VASCULAR HEADACHES

Migraine and muscle-contraction, or tension, headache are the diagnoses made in most patients who complain of headache (Table 1–1), but there are numerous conditions and circumstances that result in headache. For the vast majority of these, there is evidence that vasodilatation of intra- and/or extracranial arteries or erratic modulation of vasomotor tone is important to the pain mechanism. These vascular headaches of identifiable causation have sometimes been called "nonmigrainous" in contradistinction to vascular headaches "of the migraine type," which, at our present state of knowledge, are idiopathic. Clinically, vascular headaches are often pulsatile in quality when severe, and are often intensified by motion of the head, physical exertion, coughing or straining, or a change in posture (Kunkle, 1959). Occasionally, transient flashes of light or star figures also accompany nonmigrainous vascular headaches, so that there may be uncertainty in the diagnosis of migraine in vascular headaches of recent onset unless a pathognomonic fortification spectrum precedes the appearance of headache (see Chapter 2). Several examples of these nonmigrainous vascular headaches are described in the following section, illustrating the variety of mechanisms through which vasomotor instability may arise.

CEREBROVASCULAR OCCLUSIVE DISORDERS

Pain receptors within the walls of large pain-sensitive arteries are probably mechanistically important in the headache that accompanies cerebrovascular diseases. The supratentorial vessels and dura are innervated by branches of the first division of the trigeminal nerve, so that pain from these areas is usually referred to the forehead, eye and temple (Feindel et al, 1960). Below the tentorium, pain is commonly referred to the occiput, the ear and the retroauricular area; the pain-sensitive structures in the posterior fossa are innervated by the upper three cervical nerve roots and the 9th and 10th cranial nerves (Kimmel, 1961).

Headache occurs in association with *transient ischemic attacks* (TIAs) in 25 to 40 per cent of patients (Medina et al, 1975); it is the presenting complaint in one-third of those with headache (Grindal and Toole, 1974). Angiographic data regarding localization of occlusion or presence of extracranial collateral dilatation do not correlate with the presence or absence of headache. Head pain most commonly begins in association with other neurologic symptoms or following the resolution of an attack; less frequently, headache heralds the onset of a TIA. It is reported as pulsatile in about one-third of patients and is usually brief, lasting about two hours, but occasionally may be prolonged, lasting several days. It is commonly accentuated by stooping or straining (Bradshaw and McQuaid, 1963). Among patients with TIAs in the carotid artery distribution, headache is often unilateral and frontal or orbital, but also may be holocephalic or occipital. Among patients with TIAs in the vertebrobasilar artery distribution, headache is primarily occipital or nuchal in location, although about one-third of these patients report headache that is either generalized, bifrontal or biparietal. Of five cases of transient monocular blindness, Grindal and Toole (1974) found that four had ipsilateral frontal or orbital pain following the visual disturbance.

Because many patients with transient monocular blindness report bright lines, sparkles, light flashes and color (Fisher, 1971), the distinction between this disorder and migraine sometimes may be difficult. A simple clinical observation can be very helpful in sorting out this differential diagnostic problem. The visual hallucinations that occur during migraine attacks are almost always produced by ischemia of the occipital cortex, and therefore persist when the eyes are closed; on the other hand, in carotid artery disease, the visual phenomena result from an alteration in blood flow to the retina, and are almost always obliterated when the eyes are closed (Murphey, 1973). Studies of regional CBF in patients with TIAs and headache have been carried out during attacks, and compared with that of patients with TIAs without headache (Mathew et al, 1976). Reduced regional cerebral perfusion was common to each group of patients, but no hemodynamic differences were detected. These findings render it unlikely that increased blood flow through dilated

TABLE 1-1. THE FINAL DIAGNOSIS IN PATIENTS
ATTENDING TWO HEADACHE CLINICS

Diagnosis	1,152 PATIENTS[°] Percentage	Diagnosis	200 PATIENTS[°°] Percentage
Migraine	53	Migraine	44.5
Tension headache	41	Depression	14.5
Cluster headache	1	Tension headache	11.5
Brain tumor	<1	Cluster headache	8
Disorders of cervical spine	5	Post-traumatic syndrome	8
and sinuses; systemic and		Eye disorders	5
psychiatric disorders		Brain tumor	3
		Cervical spondylosis	2.5
		Temporal arteritis	2
		Sinusitis	1

[°]Lance, Curran and Anthony, 1965.
[°°]Carroll, 1971.

arterial channels is the mechanism of headache in these patients. Cerebral dysautoregulation has been implicated in the pathogenesis of TIAs (Naritomi et al, 1979); headache may be an expression of the quantitative impairment of the regulation of arterial tone.

According to Fisher (1968), the processes of cerebral arteriosclerosis and of cerebral infarction are painless. The strongest support for this argument stems from the observation that small infarctions that result from occlusion of small penetrating arteries are rarely associated with headache. With occlusion of the larger arteries, the internal carotid and middle cerebral, headache occurs in about 25 per cent of patients, usually unilateral, and frontal or frontotemporal in location. Among patients with an occluded posterior cerebral artery, headache arises in 70 per cent, most of whom report occipital headache. Headache usually begins at the onset of neurologic deficit, almost always starts to subside after the peak neurologic deficit occurs, and is only rarely present two days later. Headache accompanying embolic infarction is invariably ipsilateral to the involved artery; focal arterial distention may be important in this instance.

POST-ENDARTERECTOMY HEADACHE

An intense vascular headache, usually ipsilateral to the operated carotid artery, may appear soon after carotid endarterectomy (Pearce, 1976). There is usually a headache-free interval of 36 to 72 hours after which a syndrome begins that may be very similar to migraine. Focal neurologic symptoms may precede the headache, which is usually anterior in location, pounding in quality and of brief duration, usually lasting one to three hours. Nausea often accompanies the syndrome, which may be triggered by a rapid postural change, the ingestion of alcohol or exposure to glare. The focal symptoms are usually referable to the cerebral hemisphere ipsilateral to the endarterectomy site. The condition is ultimately benign and self-limited, but may persist for several months. Carotid angiography performed at the time of a severe headache showed a normal carotid arterial circulation (Leviton et al, 1975). Messert and Black (1978) have shown that this disorder is not at all uncommon; headache appearing two days after carotid endarterectomy occurred in 21 of 50 consecutive patients who underwent the procedure. Of these 21, 10 developed holocephalic, poorly characterized headache of variable intensity, and 11 developed severe headache with a prominent retrobulbar component ipsilateral to the surgical site, five of whom had strictly hemicranial pain.

In view of the manipulation of the common carotid artery, its adventitia and the carotid sinus, it is perhaps surprising that headache does not occur more often after endarterectomy. The mechanism of the latent interval and the syndrome itself is not clear. The sudden distention of arterial walls previously protected by stenosis is a sound explanation, but does not take into account the latent interval. A disturbance of cerebral arterial autoregulation has been suggested by Leviton et al (1975), but measurement of autoregulation has not yet been performed in this patient population. Autoregulation, the ability to maintain blood flow despite changing perfusion pressure, is defective both in cerebrovascular occlusive disease (Agnoli et al, 1968) and during classic migraine attacks (Simard and Paulson, 1973; Sakai and Meyer, 1978). The restoration of normal pressure to a low pressure bed may further stress cerebral vasoregulation, resulting in vasomotor instability, a cardinal abnormality that appears to underlie the syndrome of migraine.

SYSTEMIC LUPUS ERYTHEMATOSUS

Headache occurs in 45 per cent of patients with systemic lupus erythematosus (SLE). The presence of renal disease, hypertension, corticosteroid therapy or CNS involvement does not correlate with the occurrence of headache (Atkinson and Appenzeller, 1975). The clinical features of the headache attacks are often indistinguishable from those of migraine and, although commonly associated with systemic exacerbations of SLE, headache not infrequently occurs without clinical or serologic evidence of SLE activity (Brandt and Lessell, 1978). Abnormalities of the CSF arise no more often in patients with headache than in those without it. For some, but by no means all of these individuals, the institution or elevation in dosage of corticosteroids results in abatement of headache attacks. The vasoactive migraine drugs have been disappointing in this disorder; fortunately, the duration of the headache sieges tends to be self-limited, so that analgesic support until they stop is reasonable.

Pathologic studies of the brain in SLE have not shown a pathognomonic vascular lesion comparable to the wire loop lesions of the kidney or onion-skin lesions of splenic blood vessels. Occlusive lesions of cerebral capillaries and small arterioles result in microinfarction and occasional hemorrhage, but inflammatory cell infiltrates within arterial walls are not present (Johnson and Richardson, 1969). This noninflammatory involvement of small, poorly innervated intracerebral vessels is not likely to be causally related to headache in this disorder; this is supported by the frequent occurrence of headache without CNS involvement. By contrast, temporal, or giant cell, arteritis is an inflammatory disease affecting large, densely innervated arteries, in which headache is a dominant symptom in most patients. This latter disorder will be discussed in detail in Chapter 9.

PHEOCHROMOCYTOMA

Paroxysmal throbbing headache, often wakening patients from sleep, occurs in 80 per cent of those with pheochromocytoma. Perspiration, palpitation, pallor, nausea and tremor often arise in association with headache. Head pain crescendoes within minutes, then subsides over several minutes. This brief duration is an important diagnostic feature of the headache attacks that are the manifestation of this disorder; in 50 per cent of patients headache lasts less than 15 minutes, and in 70 per cent less than one hour (Thomas et al, 1966). Coughing, sneezing, bending and straining commonly aggravate the pain; standing upright is almost always more comfortable than the supine position. Headaches are usually bilateral, commonly bifrontal, but may affect any part of the head. In patients with bladder pheochromocytoma, micturition may be a specific precipitating factor; in others, exertion, defecation, straining, bending, turning in bed, temperature change and emotional excitement may trigger headache attacks. In only 10 per cent of patients is headache the sole complaint.

Paroxysms of hypertension very often accompany headache in this disorder; measurements taken during headache range from 200/100 to 300/160 mm Hg. However, comparable elevations are also seen in those who do not have headache. Patients with sustained hypertension are far less likely to experience headache than those with paroxysmal elevations of blood pressure. Attempts to relate the occurrence and severity of headache to the type of catecholamine secreted by the tumor have not been successful (Lance and Hinterberger, 1976).

The infusion of norepinephrine into patients susceptible to migraine abolishes or reduces the intensity of headache when the systolic blood pressure is elevated 10 to 40 mm Hg (Ostfeld and Wolff, 1955); however, when infusion is carried out more vigorously, and blood pressure is elevated 40 to 60 mm Hg, vascular headache is intensified. Therefore, the pressor and vasoconstrictor effects of norepinephrine and epinephrine may be competitive factors in the mechanism of headache in pheochromocytoma. In those patients who sustain primarily pressor effects, headache may occur rapidly and remain throughout the paroxysm; in others, intracranial vasoconstriction may prevent headache from developing or terminate it quickly despite the maintenance of hypertension. The sudden rise of blood pressure that may occur in pheochromocytoma is comparable to that of violent exercise, sexual excitement or intense anger, circumstances known to trigger vascular headache on occasion.

COITAL HEADACHE

Hippocrates noted that "immoderate venery" may result in headache (Adams, 1848). Although the anxiety of illicit encounters at times may be accountable for headache, sudden excruciating, throbbing, occipital headache, sometimes accompanied by vomiting and usually occurring during the periorgasmic period, is not likely to be psychogenic in origin. In a few of these patients, headache commences and evolves slowly concurrent with mounting excitement, and some have reported the onset of headache one to two hours after the occurrence of orgasm (Lance, 1976). In some patients, headache occurs fairly regularly with sexual activity, although in most it develops unpredictably and infrequently, and correlates poorly with the level of sexual excitement and the physical exertion expended at these times. Men are afflicted much more commonly than women; the age at onset ranges from the second through the fifth decades of life.

If sexual activity is terminated at the onset of headache, the latter generally subsides in minutes or within one to two hours. If orgasm is achieved, headache usually persists for from several minutes to four hours. A few patients have noted that headache was strictly limited to the upright position, resembling the low pressure headache that may occur after lumbar puncture; in these instances, a low CSF pressure of less than 20 mm H_2O was found (Paulson and Klawans, 1974). This much less common form of this disorder may be due to an arachnoid membrane tear acquired during the physical stress of coitus.

Many of these patients report previous occurrences of migrainous headaches (Martin, 1974), and ergotamine tartrate administration before sexual activity may block the development of headache. No underlying structural lesions in this syndrome have been identified with neuroradiologic procedures. Congenital aneurysms sometimes may rupture during intercourse, and this is the major differential diagnostic possibility in these patients, particularly after the first episode. Although it can be regarded as a "benign" disorder, transient, cerebral ischemic symptoms have been noted occasionally in association with headache. One patient was cured of coital cephalalgia after the removal of an obstructive lesion of the abdominal aorta (Staunton and Moore, 1978). An abnormal pressor response to treadmill exercise was evoked in this patient, as well as in two subjects with symptoms of intermittent limb claudication and in two normal subjects when the circulation to the lower limbs was occluded.

The syndrome itself resembles that of pheochromocytoma, and a similar vascular pressor mechanism, perhaps evoked by buttock and/or leg exertion, may account for it. Masters and Johnson (1966) found that the heart rate during orgasm increased to 110 to 180 per minute, and the blood pressure rose by 40 to 100 mm Hg systolic and 20 to 50 mm Hg diastolic, data comparable to the alterations found with pheochromocytoma. However, the reason why headache occurs on one occasion and not the next, or two hours after orgasm, is unexplained. In patients with migraine, responsiveness to trigger factors is also inconstant; episodic susceptibility to trigger factors that result in vasomotor instability is part of a broader problem, solution of which probably depends on the identification of the central vasomotor regulatory mechanism.

Essential Hypertension

Although paroxysmal hypertension is a sufficient mechanism of vascular headache, the relationship between chronic hypertension and headache remains unsettled. For many years an occipital headache, present on awakening and disappearing as the day wears on, was regarded as the characteristic symptomatic expression of essential hypertension (Platt, 1950). However, the available data suggest that hypertension *per se* is an uncommon cause of headache (Waters, 1971); when hypertension and migraine coexist, however, reduction in blood pressure may lead to a reduction in frequency and severity of headache (Walker, 1959; Traub and Korczyn, 1978).

The mechanisms by which hypertension may be a precipitant of vascular headache apparently vary. For example, Stewart (1955) found that headache was significantly more frequent among patients who knew that they were hypertensive than among those who did not know; this suggests that the anxiety generated by knowledge of the diagnosis is an important factor. It seems clear that waking headache, not particularly occipital, is significantly more common in untreated hypertensive patients than in treated hypertensive patients or control subjects (Bulpitt et al, 1976). Moreover, headache improves more often when the systolic blood pressure is reduced by 60 mm Hg than when it is reduced by 35 mm Hg. The belief of physicians and patients that hypertension and headache are related, and the reduction in anxiety that accompanies the success of antihypertensive therapy, may account for these findings. Others (Badran et al, 1970) have found that headache is statistically more common in hypertensive patients only when the diastolic pressure exceeds 140 mm Hg.

In chronically hypertensive patients, the relationship between CBF and mean arterial pressure is altered in that the range of blood pressure over which autoregulatory responses maintain CBF constant is higher (Strandgaard et al, 1973). There is evidence that this phenomenon occurs primarily at the level of the small resistance cerebral arteries (Stromberg and Fox, 1972). This shift in cerebral autoregulation may be due to damaged small arterial walls; it is also possible that it is a CNS response to hypertension. Antihypertensive drugs have been shown to modify the autoregulatory shift toward normal in most treated patients (Strandgaard, 1976). Since the shift is quite variable among hypertensive patients, this compensatory vascular response may be causally related to hypertensive headache, although there are no data that support this possibility.

ALTITUDE HEADACHE

The ease and speed with which large numbers of people are now able to reach previously remote high mountain regions probably accounts for the increasing incidence of altitude illness. Acute mountain sickness has been known since 1569 when the Jesuit Jose de Acosta described his own symptoms while working in Peru (Appenzeller, 1972). Riding a donkey at an elevation of about 17,500 feet, he experienced severe pounding headache, nausea, dimness of vision, breathlessness, palpitation, anorexia and, later, sleeplessness. Headache is one of the most prominent and potentially disabling symptoms of all forms of mountain sickness, and there is evidence that intracranial and extracranial vasodilatation, triggered by hypoxia and/or lowered barometric pressure, is important in its genesis.

The three major clinical manifestations of altitude illness are acute mountain sickness (described above), high altitude pulmonary edema and cerebral edema. Headache is prominent in all three syndromes and the boundaries between them are not clearly drawn. They often occur together, and probably represent different responses to the common stimulus of hypoxia. Altitude illness is unusual below 8,000 feet, and appears with increasing frequency at higher elevations. At simulated altitudes of 14,000 to 15,000 feet, 28 out of 30 subjects developed headache (King and Robinson, 1972). The headache is throbbing and usually generalized, with lateralization in about 25 per cent of patients. It is aggravated by exertion, coughing and head jolting, and by lying down. Transient relief is afforded by compression of the superficial temporal arteries and by the Valsalva maneuver; the effectiveness of the latter procedure is probably via a reduction in pulse amplitude of intracranial arteries. Ergotamine tartrate is effective, to a degree, in relieving headache in this setting (Carson et al, 1969). It also is often alleviated by the ingestion of cold fluids. Oxygen inhalation remarkably improves all aspects of altitude illness during the early stages, but is of less and less benefit as the syndrome progresses (Houston, 1976, Hultgren, 1979).

Although there are differences of opinion regarding the protective role of prior acclimatization to developing altitude illness, the balance of the evidence to date is that previous altitude exposure is not protective (Houston, 1976). Some people develop headache regularly above a certain altitude, and some have become ill on several occasions, but many others who have one experience with altitude illness continue climbing without recurrence.

Retinal hemorrhages commonly accompany the appearance of headache (Hackett and Rennie, 1976), and papilledema occasionally has been noted. Lumbar puncture was carried out in 34 patients during acute mountain sickness, and showed an increase in CSF pressure of 60 to 210 mm H_2O above the values found after recovery; in one subject a biopsy revealed cerebral edema (Singh et al, 1969).

There is usually a latency of six to 96 hours after arrival at higher altitude before symptoms appear. Hypoxia appears to be a primary factor, but probably produces illness through secondary or tertiary changes, perhaps by interfering with neuronal sodium and potassium membrane gradients (Fishman, 1975). Moreover, since the rate-limiting enzyme that catalyzes the synthesis of brain serotonin is oxygen-dependent (Costa and Meek, 1974), hypoxia results in a lowering of neuronal serotonin that may also be important to the mechanism of headache (see Chapter 4). It is also possible that lowered barometric pressure augments the effects of hypoxia in the generation of this illness. When people are exposed to low barometric pressures equivalent to altitudes of greater than 25,000 feet, and the oxygen content of inspired air is maintained constant, a vascular headache syndrome indistinguishable from migraine frequently appears in addition to joint pains, breathing difficulty and syncope (Engel et al, 1944; Whitten, 1946).

The syndrome is usually alleviated immediately by descent, and slow ascent reduces the severity of all forms of the illness. Acetazolamide, taken for two days before and during ascent to altitude, has been shown to be protective (Hackett and Rennie, 1976).

HANGOVER

In addition to headache, other symptoms such as malaise, fatigue, nausea, lightheadedness, pallor, tremor and hyperexcitability occur in varying admixtures several hours after the imbibition of alcohol has ceased, at a time when tissue levels of alcohol are very low or zero (Himwich, 1956). Headache is a common but not constant feature of the syndrome; it is usually generalized, commonly throbbing, and worsened by postural change, coughing and rapid movement of the head. The syndrome usually lasts five to ten hours, long after all alcohol has been metabolized (Goldberg, 1961). Alterations of electrolyte and water balance induced by alcohol correlate poorly with hangover symptoms (Flynn, 1959). The immediate lessening of symptoms (but ultimately prolonging the syndrome) after drinking alcohol has led to the suggestion that the hangover state may be a mild withdrawal symptom.

Many social drinkers believe that there are differences in both the intoxication and the hangover that result from drinking different alcoholic beverages. Many beverages contain a great number of substances, called "congeners," in addition to ethanol and water, and data indicate that high congener beverages such as cognac and bourbon are more likely to result in hangover than a low congener beverage such as vodka (Damrau and Liddy, 1960; Murphree et al, 1967); however, there is little doubt that ethanol or its metabolites is the major cause of hangover. The most pharmacologically active congeners are the aldehydes, methanol and the fusel alcohols; the minute levels of the aldehydes and methanol in alcoholic beverages have been used as an argument against their implication in the consequences of drinking alcohol. The fusel alcohols consist of various aliphatic and aromatic alcohols formed during fermentation, and include isobutyl, isoamyl, amyl and n-propyl alcohols. They are rapidly metabolized and assessments of a variety of physiologic functions have shown no more than modest effects that could be attributed to these compounds (Wallgren and Barry, 1970). How or whether these substances alter the metabolic consequences of alcohol oxidation has not been carefully studied.

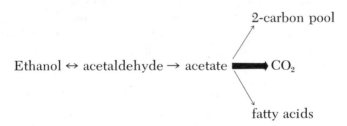

The schema above illustrates the steps involved in the metabolism of ethyl alcohol (Hawkins and Kalant, 1972). The velocity of the first reaction catalyzed by alcohol dehydrogenase (ADH) is slower than the subsequent ones, and therefore is rate-limiting. The equilibrium of the ADH reaction lies far to the left; oxidation of ethanol proceeds because acetaldehyde is continuously removed by the irreversible reaction catalyzed by an aldehyde dehydrogenase. There is a net accumulation of reduced nicotinamide adenine dinucleotide in the liver as a result of ethanol oxidation, and this probably accounts for the mild lactic acidosis that accompanies alcohol ingestion (Isselbacher, 1977). Only a small percentage of ingested ethanol is excreted in the urine, expired air or perspiration; over 90 per cent of ethanol oxidation occurs in the liver. Ethanol is a distinctive pharmacologic agent in that the kinetics of its turnover can be described as zero-order — i.e., regardless of its tissue concentration (above 2 to 3 mM) its rate of decay is constant because liver ADH is saturated at low concentrations of ethanol.

Predictably, blood levels of acetaldehyde and acetate do not vary regardless of the degree of alcoholic intoxication produced (Raskin, 1975). Delayed clearance of the metabolic products of ethanol oxidation has long been suspected in the genesis of the hangover state, and Ogata et al (1966) found elevated blood levels of pyruvate, but not of lactate or acetaldehyde, in subjects with hangover symptoms. The widespread anecdotal observation made by pilots that the inhalation of 100 per cent oxygen effectively ameliorates hangover symptoms (Raskin, unpublished) is consistent with the idea that delayed metabolic restitution of the altered redox state that accompanies alcohol ingestion may bear on the mechanism of hangover. The observations that both alcoholemia (McQueen et al, 1978) and lactic acidosis interfere with cerebral autoregulation (Lassen, 1966) provide a rationale for the vascular headache that accompanies the other symptoms of hangover; similarly, the lactic acidosis that follows major motor seizures (Orringer et al, 1977) may bear on the mechanism of the symptoms that occur during the postictal state, which include vascular headache.

Alcohol dehydrogenase is present in cerebral tissue (Raskin and Sokoloff, 1968) and, although contributing little to the over-all metabolism of an ethanol load, variation in the oxidation of ethanol at cellular sites in the brain may have important effects on neuronal function, and bear on the mechanism of hangover. The depression of brain serotonin turnover by a high blood alcohol level (Hunt and Majchrowicz, 1974; Myers and Melchior, 1978) may also be relevant because of the implication of serotonin in migraine (see Chapters 3 and 4). The vasodilator property of alcohol (Gillespie, 1967) may be important in the precipitation of migraine and cluster headaches, a phenomenon that usually occurs within 40 minutes after the ingestion of an alcoholic beverage. However, it seems unlikely that this pharmacologic action is mechanistically important to a disorder that commences after alcohol has been completely metabolized.

As appears to be true for so many common ailments, there are remarkably few studies bearing on the hangover problem. The performance of experiments that very often must take place on Sunday mornings may be an important factor in perpetuating our ignorance.

ICE CREAM HEADACHE

A brief, sometimes intense midfrontal pain occurs in many people when cold foods or liquids contact the roof of the oropharynx (Raskin and Knittle, 1976). It is less often bitemporal or bimaxillary, and occasionally is occipital in location; the quality of pain is only rarely pulsatile and its duration is usually seconds. Wolff (1943–1944) found that the application of crushed ice to the roof of the mouth produced frontal pain, and to the posterior pharynx, retroauricular headache. Ice in the stomach and esophagus did not produce headache. Ice cream headache occurs in over 90 per cent of patients with migraine, most of whom experience it frequently as an intense pain, often requiring precautions in the ingestion of cold foods. Among normal headache-free subjects, 30 per cent recall ice cream headache at some point in their lives, almost always as an infrequent and mild phenomenon.

Evidence suggests that reflexive vasospasm may be an important mechanism of ice cream headache. Wolf and Hardy (1941) immersed volunteers' hands into cold water and induced a reproducible patterned response. A deep, aching sensation occurred, reaching a maximum in 60 seconds regardless of the strength of stimulus used. These authors found that the pain was not influenced by prior ischemia and did not show the phenomenon of spatial summation, since exposure of one finger to cold caused pain of equal intensity to that experienced when the whole hand was exposed. Moreover, the amplitude of pulsation of the digital artery varied inversely with the intensity of cold pain reported; vasopressin injections, resulting in vasoconstriction, augmented the intensity of cold pain. Local exposure to cold produced pain in many parts of the body; when the vertex of the head was dipped in cold water, pain occurred at the vertex, reached a peak in 60 seconds, and then subsided. Pain spread rapidly to the occiput and temples, and appeared to be more intense than that reported for the hand under similar conditions.

The vascular reaction to cold in patients with erratic vasomotor regulation (migraine) may be excessive. Ice cream headache may be no more than an epitome of the migraine mechanism, and suggests that the latter is a disorder of thresholds to a variety of stimuli. We probably are all capable of experiencing a vascular headache, given an appropriately intense stimulus. Some have thresholds so low that the ordinary stimuli of daily life trigger headache, and this condition aptly describes the nature of migraine. Other probably analogous "threshold" vascular headaches include those resulting from fever, the inhalation of organic solvents, exposure to glare and the ingestion of certain foods; the latter will be discussed in detail in the next section.

FOOD- OR BEVERAGE-PROVOKED HEADACHES

Common foods capable of inducing headache in certain patients include alcoholic beverages, citrus fruits, chocolate and dairy products (Hanington and Harper, 1968; Moffett et al 1974). These reactions have often been ascribed to an allergy to food, but there has been no compelling evidence to support this hypothesis. There is evidence (see Chapter 3) that implicates tyramine and phenylethylamine, principally in cheese and chocolate respectively, as chemicals contained in foodstuffs that may trigger headache. Other headache-inducing chemicals identified to date include sodium chloride (Brainard, 1976), sodium nitrite (Henderson and Raskin, 1972) and monosodium glutamate (Schaumburg et al, 1969). Undoubtedly, there are many other chemicals yet to be identified that, when contained in or added to foodstuffs, may trigger headache. Our rather sparse knowledge of the chemical constituents of food has retarded progress in a potentially important public health area.

"Hot-dog" headache. Many patients experience varying degrees of headache shortly after eating frankfurters or other cured meat products. There is evidence that implicates the nitrite content of these foodstuffs as the cause of such headaches. The headache is usually bitemporal or bifrontal, of pulsatile quality in about 50 per cent of patients, and is sometimes accompanied by facial flushing. These patients are sensitive to sodium nitrite in amounts of 0.5 to 1.0 mg (Henderson and Raskin, 1972). The observation that nitrite impurities in rock salt caused red patches in cured meat led to the deliberate use of fixed concentrations of salt and nitrate to produce a more uniformly colored product. Eventually it became clear that the coloring agent was not sodium nitrate, but sodium nitrite, which is formed in meat by the bacterial and chemical reduction of nitrate; nitrites have been generally substituted for nitrates in the curing process. Nitrite and its decomposition product, nitric oxide, react with myoglobin and hemoglobin to form the red compounds nitrosomyoglobin and nitrosohemoglobin (Halliday, 1967). Government regulations limit the nitrite levels reached during the treatment of cured meats to 200 ppm (200 mg per kg of meat); cooking and storage lead to a reduction in the nitrite contents, so that the range of nitrite concentrations in cured meat is approximately 50 to 130 ppm.

Chinese restaurant syndrome. About 30 per cent of people who eat Chinese food report adverse reactions (Reif-Lehrer, 1977; Kerr et al, 1977). Headache and tightness around the face are the most commonly reported symptoms, but many also report dizziness, diarrhea, nausea and abdominal cramps. Monosodium glutamate (MSG), the chemical precipitant of these symptoms (Schaumburg et al, 1969), is one of the active ingredients in soy sauce and is used as a food additive for its flavor-enhancing properties, more so by some Chinese chefs than others. Pure MSG, injected intravenously, produces a stereotyped sequence of symptoms that begins with a burning or scorching sensation of the chest which spreads to the neck, shoulder, upper limbs and abdomen. This is followed by a sensation of pressure over the chest, and finally by tightness and pressure over the cheeks, at times radiating to the retro-orbital areas.

Orally administered MSG produces symptoms in about 20 minutes; the oral threshold range for minimal symptoms is 1.5 to 12 gm. Oral MSG thresholds of 3 gm or less are usually found in subjects who report symptoms after eating Chinese food. A 200-ml portion of won ton soup, a commonly implicated foodstuff, contains about 3 gm of MSG. The previous ingestion of food delays absorption of MSG, so that susceptible individuals may be protected from experiencing symptoms. Plasma glutamate levels after glutamate ingestion are not different in MSG-sensitive and -nonsensitive persons (Kenney and Tidball, 1972). In laboratory animals fed glutamate, brain glutamate levels do not change, but brain glutamine levels increase (Reif-Lehrer, 1976). Glutamate is present in large amounts in the body and is synthesized in the brain and retina; how its ingestion produces symptoms is not clear. It has been suggested that glutamate-induced release of acetylcholine may explain the syndrome (Ghadimi et al, 1971).

In general, people who experience headache after ingesting one or more foodstuffs are very likely to develop spontaneous unprovoked migraine headaches also (Hanington and Harper, 1968). Chemical thresholds to nitrite, tyramine (Ghose et al, 1977), MSG and probably many other chemicals are lower in some individuals, resulting in a susceptibility to vascular headache and other symptoms under certain conditions. These chemicals have variable actions on arterial walls, rendering simple direct vasodilatation an unlikely mode of action. Indeed, the diverse pharmacologic properties of these compounds suggests that there is a common secondary humoral mediator or central locus of action. The latter would appear to be more consistent with the other observations that have been made regarding the mechanism of other vascular headaches already discussed in this chapter.

Rapid modifications of brain serotonin levels occur after the ingestion of a variety of foodstuffs (Fernstrom, 1978). For neurons of the CNS, the first step in the synthesis of serotonin is uptake from the plasma of the amino acid tryptophan, which is derived primarily from the diet (Costa and Meek, 1974). An active uptake process facilitates the entry of tryptophan into brain so that other amino acids may compete with tryptophan for entry into neurons, with a resultant lowering of the serotonin level. It is possible, although unsupported by evidence, that central serotonergic neuronal activity can be modulated in this manner by many chemicals contained in foods, and may account for the phenomenology of "dietary migraine."

VITAMIN A-INDUCED HEADACHE

It has been known that violent headaches may result from the ingestion of large quantities of vitamin A since Rodahl and Moore (1943) found polar bear liver to contain approximately 15,000 IU of vitamin A per gm, thus identifying the agent responsible for the illness described by Arctic explorers over 100 years ago.

Headache is the predominant symptom of acute hypervitaminosis A; it is often violent and usually is located frontally and retroorbitally. Nausea, abdominal pain, vertigo and sluggishness often accompany the headache, and usually appear four to eight hours after the ingestion of vitamin A. Two million units of vitamin A in a single dose given to four adults produced dull headaches in all four, and no other symptoms (Gerber et al 1954). Chronic hypervitaminosis A has been reported in patients who have ingested at least 50,000 IU of vitamin A daily for weeks to months; the principal symptoms are joint pain, fatigue, alopecia, fissuring of the lips, hepatomegaly and headache (Stimson, 1961). Children more often than adults may develop increased intracranial pressure as a manifestation of vitamin A intoxication (Muenter et al, 1971).

It has recently become clear that the total plasma vitamin A level may be normal in patients with unequivocal chronic hypervitaminosis A (Smith and Goodman, 1976). This underlines the importance of inquiring about patients' vitamin intakes that may explain their symptoms. Over a two-year period, six patients have been encountered who reported daily bifrontal or bitemporal pulsating headache; their symptoms began days to weeks after 25,000 IU of vitamin A ingestion was initiated on a daily basis. In all six patients, plasma vitamin A levels were in the normal range; headache completely subsided several days to weeks after vitamin A intake ceased (Raskin, unpublished observations).

Retinyl palmitate is the vitamin A ester contained in proprietary vitamin preparations. After intestinal absorption, vitamin A is taken up and stored in the liver. It is mobilized from the liver as the free alcohol, retinol, and is transported to other tissues in the plasma, bound to its carrier, retinol-binding protein. Of the vitamin A in plasma, about 5 per cent is in the form of retinyl esters, and the remainder is in the form of bound retinol (Smith and Goodman, 1976). Toxicity to vitamin A appears to be due to an increase in the circulating levels of free retinyl esters that occurs when the capacity of plasma retinol-binding protein is exceeded. This increment may not be detectable by measuring total plasma vitamin A. Unbound vitamin A produces instability of biologic membranes, perhaps because of its capacity to release lysosomal enzymes (Dingle, 1968). It is possible that headache caused by vitamin A ingestion is related to that triggered by cheese, chocolate and ethyl alcohol via a common mechanism. However, the latency of days to weeks before headache commences, and the delay of days to weeks before headache subsides, is more consistent with a direct and specific effect of vitamin A than with a lowered biologic threshold mechanism.

REFERENCES

Adams, F. (1848): The Genuine Works of Hippocrates. Sydenham Society, London, p. 94.

Agnoli, A., Fieschi, C., Bozzoa, L. et al (1968): Autoregulation of cerebral blood flow. Studies during drug-induced hypertension in normal subjects and in patients with cerebrovascular disease. Circulation 38:800–812.

Akil, H., Richardson, D. E., Hughes, J. and Barchas, J. D. (1978): Enkephalin-like material elevated in ventricular cerebrospinal fluid of pain patients after analgetic focal stimulation. Science 201:463–465.

Appenzeller, O. (1972): Altitude headache. Headache 12:126–129.

Atkinson, R. A. and Appenzeller, O. (1975): Headache in small vessel disease of the brain: a study of patients with systemic lupus erythematosus. Headache 15:198–201.

Badran, R. H. A., Weir, R. J. and McGuiness, J. B. (1970): Hypertension and headache. Scott. Med. J. 15:48–51.

Bakal, D. A. and Kaganov, J. A. (1977): Muscle contraction and migraine headache: psychophysiologic comparison. Headache 17:208–215.

Basbaum, A. I. and Fields, H. L. (1978): Endogenous pain control mechanisms: review and hypothesis. Ann. Neurol. 4:451–462.

Beecher, H. (1955): The powerful placebo. J.A.M.A. 159:1602–1606.

Beesou, D. P. and Perl, E. R. (1969): Response of cutaneous sensory units and unmyelinated fibers to noxious stimuli. J. Neurophysiol. 32:1025–1043.

Bradshaw, P. and McQuaid, P. (1963): The syndrome of vertebrobasilar insufficiency. Q. J. Med. 32:279–296.

Brainard, J. B. (1976): Salt load as a trigger for migraine. Minn. Med. 59:232–233.

Brandt, K. D. and Lessell, S. (1978): Migrainous phenomena in systemic lupus erythematosus. Arthritis Rheum. 21:7–16.

Bulpitt, C. J., Dollery, C. T. and Carne, S. (1976): Change in symptoms of hypertensive patients after referral to hospital clinic. Br. Heart J. 38:121–128.

Carroll, J. D. (1971): Diagnostic problems in a migraine clinic. In Background to Migraine, 4th Migraine Symposium, ed. J. N. Cumings. Springer-Verlag, New York, pp. 14–24.

Carson, R. P., Evans, W. O., Shields, J. L. and Hanson, J. P. (1969): Symptomatology, pathophysiology, and treatment of acute mountain sickness. Fed. Proc. 28:1085–1091.

Costa, E. and Meek, J. (1974): Regulation of the biosynthesis of catecholamines and serotonin in the CNS. Annu. Rev. Pharmacol. 14:491–511.

Damrau, F. and Liddy, E. (1960): Hangovers and whisky congeners. Comparison of whisky with vodka. J. Natl. Med. Assoc. 52:262–265.

Dingle, J. T. (1968): Vacuoles, vesicles, and lysosomes. Br. Med. Bull. 24:141–145.

Dunning, H. S. and Wolff, H. G. (1937): The relative vascularity of various parts of the central and peripheral nervous system of the cat and its relation to function. J. Comp. Neurol. 67:433–450.

Edvinsson, L. (1975): Neurogenic mechanisms in the cerebrovascular bed. Acta Physiol. Scand. (suppl.) 427:5–35.

Engel, G. L., Webb, J. P., Ferris, E. B. et al (1944): A migraine-like syndrome complicating decompression sickness. War Med. 5:304–314.

Feindel, W., Penfield, W. and McNaughton, F. (1960): The tentorial nerves and localization of intracranial pain in man. Neurology 10:555–563.

Fernstrom, J. D. (1978): Brain serotonin and nutrition. In Serotonin in Health and Disease, Vol. 3, ed. W. B. Essman. Spectrum, New York, pp. 1–49.

Fields, H. L. and Basbaum, A. I. (1978): Brainstem control of spinal pain-transmission neurons. Annu. Rev. Physiol. 40:217–248.

Fisher, C. M. (1968): Headache in cerebrovascular disease. In Handbook of Clinical Neurology, Vol. 5, eds. P. J. Vinken and G. W. Bruyn. John Wiley & Sons, New York, pp. 124–156.

Fisher, C. M. (1971): Cerebral ischemia — less familiar types. Clin. Neurosurg. 18:267–335.

Fishman, R. A. (1975): Brain edema. N. Engl. J. Med. 293:706–711.

Flynn, P. A. (1959): Water and electrolyte balance after alcohol ingestion. Q. J. Stud. Alcohol 20:128–129.

Friedman, A. P. (1972): The headache in history, literature and legend. Bull. N. Y. Acad. Med. 48:661–681.

Gerber, A., Raab, A. P. and Sobel, A. E. (1954): Vitamin A poisoning in adults. Am. J. Med. 16:729–745.

Ghadimi, H., Kumar, S. and Abaci, F. (1971): Studies on monosodium glutamate ingestion. Biochem. Med. 5:447–456.

Ghose, K., Coppen, A. and Carroll, D. (1977): Intravenous tyramine response in migraine before and during treatment with indoramin. Br. Med. J. 1:1191–1193.

Gillespie, J. A. (1967): Vasodilator properties of alcohol. Br. Med. J. 1:274–277.

Goldberg, L. (1961): Alcohol, tranquilizers and hangover. Q. J. Stud. Alcohol (suppl.) 1:37–58.

Grindal, A. B. and Toole, J. F. (1974): Headache and transient ischemic attacks. Stroke 5:603–606.

Hackett, P. H. and Rennie, D. (1976): The incidence, importance and prophylaxis of acute mountain sickness. Lancet 2:1149–1155.

Halliday, D. (1967): Curing of pig meat. Process. Biochem. 2:32–34.

Hanington, E. and Harper, A. M. (1968): The role of tyramine in the aetiology of migraine, and related studies on the cerebral and extracerebral circulations. Headache 8:84–97.

Harvey, J. A. and Lints, C. E. (1965): Lesions in the medial forebrain bundle: delayed effects on sensitivity to electric shock. Science 148:250–252.

Hawkins, R. D. and Kalant, H. (1972): The metabolism of ethanol and its metabolic effects. Pharmacol. Rev. 24:67–157.

Heistad, D. D. and Marcus, M. L. (1978): Evidence that neural mechanisms do not have important effects on cerebral blood flow. Circ. Res. 42:295–302.

Henderson, W. R. and Raskin, N. H. (1972): "Hot dog" headache: individual susceptibility to nitrite. Lancet 2:1162–1163.

Himwich, H. E. (1956): Alcohol and brain physiology. In Alcoholism, ed. G. N. Thompson. Charles C Thomas, Springfield, Ill., pp. 291–408.

Hosobuchi, Y., Rossier, J., Bloom, F. E., and Guillemin, R. (1979): Stimulation of human periaqueductal gray for pain relief increases immunoreactive β-endorphin in ventricular fluid. Science 203:279–281.

Houston, C. S. (1976): High altitude illness. J.A.M.A. 236:2193–2195.

Hultgren, H. N. (1979): High altitude medical problems. West. J. Med. 131:8–23.

Hunt, W. A. and Majchrowicz, E. (1974): Turnover rates and steady-state levels of brain serotonin in alcohol-dependent rats. Brain Res. 72:181–184.

Isselbacher, K. J. (1977): Metabolic and hepatic effects of alcohol. N. Engl. J. Med. 296:612–616.

Johnson, R. T. and Richardson, E. P. (1969): The neurological manifestations of systemic lupus erythematosus. Medicine 47:337–369.

Kenney, R. A. and Tidball, C. S. (1972): Human susceptibility to oral monosodium L-glutamate. Am. J. Clin. Nutr. 25:140–146.

Kerr, G. R., Wu-Lee, M., El-Lozy, M. et al. (1977): Objectivity of food symptomatology questionnaires. J. Am. Diet. Assoc. 71:263–268.

Kimmel, D. L. (1961): Innervation of spinal dura mater and dura mater of the posterior cranial fossa. Neurology 11:800–809.

King, A. B. and Robinson, S. M. (1972): Vascular headache of acute mountain sickness. Aerospace Med. 43:849–851.

Kogure, K., Scheinberg, P., Reinmuth, O. M. et al (1970): Mechanisms of cerebral vasodilatation in hypoxia. J. Appl. Physiol. 29:223–229.

Kunkle, E. C. (1959): Diagnostic principles and methods. In Headache: Diagnosis and Treatment, eds. A. P. Friedman and H. H. Merritt. F. A. Davis Co., Philadelphia, pp. 23–32.

Lance, J. W. (1976): Headaches related to sexual activity. J. Neurol. Neurosurg. Psychiatry 39:1226–1230.

Lance, J. W., Curran, D. A., and Anthony, M. (1965): Investigations into the mechanism and treatment of chronic headache. Med. J. Australia 2:909–914.

Lance, J. W. and Hinterberger, H. (1976): Symptoms of pheochromocytoma, with particular reference to headache correlated with catecholamine production. Arch. Neurol. 33:281–288.

Lassen, N. A. (1966): Luxury-perfusion syndrome and its possible relation to acute metabolic acidosis localized within the brain. Lancet 2:1113–1115.

Lassen, N. A. (1968): Brain extracellular pH: main factor controlling cerebral blood flow. Scand. J. Clin. Lab. Invest. 22:247–251.

Lassen, N. A. (1974): Control of cerebral circulation in health and disease. Circ. Res. 34:749–760.

Levine, J. D., Gordon, N. C. and Fields, H. L. (1978): The mechanism of placebo analgesia. Lancet 2:654–657.

Leviton, A., Caplan, L. and Salzman, E. (1975): Severe headache after carotid endarterectomy. Headache 15:207–210.

Martin, E. A. (1974): Headache during sexual intercourse. Ir. J. Med. Sci. 143:342–345.

Masters, M. H. and Johnson, V. E. (1966): Human Sexual Response. Little Brown & Co., Boston, pp. 278–294.

Mathew, N. T., Hrastnik, F. and Meyer, J. S. (1976): Regional cerebral blood flow in the diagnosis of vascular headache. Headache 15:252–260.

Mayer, D. J. and Price, D. D. (1976): Central nervous system mechanisms of analgesia. Pain 2:379–404.

McDonald, D. A. and Potter, J. M. (1951): The distribution of blood to the brain. J. Physiol. 114:356–371.

McQueen, J. D., Sklar, F. K., and Posey, J. B. (1978): Autoregulation of blood flow during alcohol infusion. J. Stud. Alcohol 39:1477–1487.

Medina, J. L., Diamond, S., and Rubino, F. A. (1975): Headaches in patients with transient ischemic attacks. Headache 15:194–197.

Melzack, R. (1973): The Puzzle of Pain. Basic Books, Inc., New York.

Melzack, R. and Wall, P. D. (1965): Pain mechanisms: a new theory. Science 150:971–979.

Messert, B. and Black, J. A. (1978): Cluster headache, hemicrania and other head pains: morbidity of carotid endarterectomy. Stroke 9:559–562.

Moffett, A. M., Swash, M., and Scott, D. F. (1974): Effect of chocolate in migraine: a double blind study. J. Neurol. Neurosurg. Psychiatry 37:445–448.

Muenter, M. D., Perry, H. O. and Ludwig, J. (1971): Chronic vitamin A intoxication in adults: hepatic, neurologic and dermatologic complications. Am. J. Med. 50:129–136.

Murphey, F. (1973): The scotomata of carotid artery disease as I remember them. J. Neurosurg. 39:390–393.

Murphree, H. B., Greenberg, L. A. and Carroll, R. B. (1967): Neuropharmacological effects of substances other than ethanol in alcoholic beverages. Fed. Proc. 26:1468–1473.

Myers, R. D. and Melchior, C. L. (1978): Alcohol and alcoholism: role of serotonin. In Serotonin in Health and Disease, Vol. 2, ed. W. B. Essman. Spectrum, New York, pp. 373–430.

Naritomi, H., Sakai, F. and Meyer, J. S. (1979): Pathogenesis of transient ischemic attacks within the vertebrobasilar arterial system. Arch. Neurol. 36:121–128.

Novack, P., Goluboff, B., Bortin, L., Soffe, A. and Shenkin, H. A. (1953): Studies of the cerebral circulation and metabolism in congestive heart failure. Circulation 7:724–731.

Ogata, S., Hosoi, T., Saji, H. et al (1966): Studies on acute alcohol intoxication. Especially concerning its relation to the carbohydrate metabolism. Jap. J. Stud. Alcohol 1:67–79.

Orringer, C. E., Eustace, J. C., Wunsch, C. D., and Gardner, L. B. (1977): Natural history of lactic acidosis after grand-mal seizures. N. Engl. J. Med. 297:796–799.

Ostfeld, A.M. and Wolff, H. G. (1955): Arterenol (norepinephrine) and vascular headache of the migraine type. Arch. Neurol. Psychiatry 14:131–136.

Paulson, G. W. and Klawans, H. L. (1974): Benign orgasmic cephalgia. Headache 13:181–187.

Pearce, J. (1976): Headache after carotid endarterectomy. Br. Med. J. 2:85–86.

Pearce, J. (1977): Migraine: a psychosomatic disorder. Headache 17:125–128.

Platt, R. (1950): Hypertension. Br. Med. J. 1:951–953.

Poźniak-Patewicz, E. (1976): "Cephalgic" spasm of head and neck muscles. Headache 14:261–266.

Purves, M. J. (1978): Do vasomotor nerves significantly regulate cerebral blood flow? Circ. Res. 43:485–493.

Raskin, N.H. (1975): Alcoholism or acetaldehydism? N. Engl. J. Med. 292:422–423.

Raskin, N. H. and Knittle, S. C. (1976): Ice cream headache and orthostatic symptoms in patients with migraine. Headache 16:222–225.

Raskin, N.H. and Sokoloff, L. (1968): Brain alcohol dehydrogenase. Science 162:131–132.

Ray, B. S. and Wolff, H. G. (1940): Experimental studies on headache. Pain-sensitive structures of the head and their significance in headace. Arch. Surg. 41:813–856.

Reif-Lehrer, L. (1976): Possible significance of adverse reactions to glutamate in humans. Fed. Proc. 35:2205–2212.

Reif-Lehrer, L. (1977): A questionnaire study of the prevalence of Chinese restaurant syndrome. Fed. Proc. 36:1617–1623.

Rodahl, K. and Moore, T. (1943): Vitamin A content and toxicity of bear and seal liver. Biochem. J. 37:166–168.

Sakai, F. and Meyer, J. S. (1978): Regional cerebral hemodynamics during migraine and cluster headache measured by the Xe[133] inhalation method. Headache 18:122–132.

Schaumburg, H. H., Byck, R., Gerstl, R. and Mashman, J. H. (1969): Monosodium L-glutamate: its pharmacology and role in the Chinese restaurant syndrome. Science 163:826–828.

Schiller, F. (1975): The migraine tradition. Bull. Hist. Med. 49:1–19.

Selby, G. and Lance, J. W. (1960): Observations on 500 cases of migraine and allied vascular headache. J. Neurol. Neurosurg. Psychiatry 23:23–32.

Sicuteri, F. (1978): Endorphins, opiate receptors and migraine headache. Headache 17:253–256.

Sicuteri, F., Anselmi, B. and Fanciullacci, M. (1974): The serotonin theory of migraine. In Advances in Neurology, Vol. 4, ed. J. J. Bonica. Raven Press, New York, pp. 383–394.

Simard, D. and Paulson, O. B. (1973): Cerebral vasomotor paralysis during migraine attack. Arch. Neurol. 29:207–209.

Simon, E. J. and Hiller, J. M. (1978): The opiate receptors. Annu. Rev. Pharmacol. Toxicol. 18:371–394.

Singh, I. I., Khanna, P. K., Srivastava, M. C. et al (1969): Acute mountain sickness. N. Engl. J. Med. 280:175–184.

Smith, F. R. and Goodman, D. S. (1976): Vitamin A transport in human vitamin A toxicity. N. Engl. J. Med. 294:805–808.

Smith, I., Kellow, A. H. and Hanington, E. (1970): A clinical and biochemical correlation between tyramine and migraine headache. Headache 10:43–52.

Sokoloff, L. (1959): The action of drugs on the cerebral circulation. Pharmacol. Rev. 11:1–85.

Sokoloff, L. and Kety, S. S. (1960): Regulation of cerebral circulation. Physiol. Rev. 40:38–44.

Staunton, H. P. and Moore, J. (1978): Coital cephalgia and ischaemic muscular work of the lower limbs. J. Neurol. Neurosurg. Psychiatry 41:930–933.

Stewart, I. M. G. (1955): Headache and hypertension. Lancet 1:1261–1266.

Stimson, W. H. (1961): Vitamin A intoxication in adults. N. Engl. J. Med. 265:369–373.

Stoica, E., Meyer, J. S., Kawamura, Y. et al (1973): Central neurogenic control of cerebral circulation. Neurology 23:687–698.

Strandgaard, S. (1976): Autoregulation of cerebral blood flow in hypertensive patients. The moderating influence of prolonged antihypertensive treatment on the tolerance to acute, drug induced hypotension. Circulation 53:720–727.

Strandgaard, S., Olesen, J., Skinhøj, E. et al (1973): Autoregulation of brain circulation in severe arterial hypertension. Br. Med. J. 1:507–510.

Stromberg, D. D. and Fox, J. R. (1972): Pressure in the pial arterial microcirculation of the cat during changes in systemic arterial blood pressure. Circ. Res. 31:229–239.

Swanson, L. W. and Hartman, B. K. (1975): The central adrenergic system. J. Comp. Neurol. 163:467–506.

Sweet, W. H. and Bennett, H. S. (1948): Changes in internal carotid pressure during carotid and jugular occlusion and their clinical significance. J. Neurosurg. 5:178–195.

Tenen, S. S. (1967): The effects of p-chlorophenylalanine, a serotonin depletor, on avoidance, acquisition, pain sensitivity and related behaviour in the rat. Psychopharmacologia 10:204–219.

Thomas, J. E., Rooke, E. D. and Kvale, W. F. (1966): The neurologist's experience with pheochromocytoma. J. A. M. A. 197:754–758.

Traub, Y. M. and Korczyn, A. D. (1978): Headache in patients with hypertension. Headache 17:245–247.

Walker, C. H. (1959): Migraine and its relationship to hypertension. Br. Med. J. 2:1430–1433.

Wallgren, H. and Barry, H. (1970): Drug actions in relation to alcohol effects. In Actions of Alcohol, Vol. 2. Elsevier, New York, pp. 621–714.

Waters, W. E. (1971): Headache and blood pressure in the community. Br. Med. J. 1:142–143.

Whitten, R. H. (1946): Scotoma as a complication of decompression sickness. Arch. Ophthalmol. 36:220–224.

Wolf, S. and Hardy, J. D. (1941): Studies on pain. Observations on pain due to local cooling and on factors involved in the "cold pressor" effect. J. Clin. Invest. 20:521–533.

Wolff, H. G. (1943–44): Some observations on pain. Harvey Lect. 39:39–95.

Ziegler, D. K., Hassanein, R. S. and Couch, J. R. (1977): Characteristics of life headache histories in a nonclinic population. Neurology 27:265–269.

CHAPTER 2

MIGRAINE: CLINICAL ASPECTS

Headache has afflicted man since the beginning of recorded time. Migraine was the first headache syndrome to be differentiated, probably because of its sometimes dramatic features of blinding headaches and vomiting. Although descriptions of migraine may be found in the writings of over 3,000 years ago, Aretaeus of Cappadocia, who lived during the 2nd century A.D., is generally regarded as the first to recognize migraine because of his clear description of the disorder. He reported as *heterocrania* a paroxysmal headache disorder that occurred on one side of the head and then the other, recurred at regular intervals, was associated with vomiting and photophobia, and was ameliorated by dark surroundings (Critchley, 1967). About 50 years later Galen (A.D. 131 to 201), focusing on the unilateral localization, introduced the term *hemicrania* (derived from the Greek "hemikranios"), which the Romans translated into Latin as *hemicranium* and later corrupted into low Latin as *hemigranea* and *migranea*. The Old English translation of the term was *megrim* or *mygrame*. The French translation, *migraine*, gained acceptance in the 18th century and has prevailed ever since; the term *migraineur*, derived from the French *migraineux*, denoting a migraine sufferer, is now also in common usage. The passage of time has proved this to be an unfortunate and misleading designation for a condition manifested by lateralized headache in less than 60 per cent of those affected (Olesen, 1978). Furthermore, undue emphasis on the dramatic features of migraine has often led to the incorrect conclusion that periodic headache lacking such features is not migrainous in mechanism.

Galen's conjecture that migraine was caused by the dispatch

of noxious vapors and fluids from extracerebral organs, especially the gallbladder, was widely accepted, and inhibited medical thinking about migraine for some 1,400 years. During the 17th century, scientific thought on migraine began once more with a debate as to whether migraine was primarily vascular or neurogenic (Schiller, 1975). Modern orientations toward migraine probably began with the publication of the first major treatise devoted to the subject of migraine (Liveing, 1873). Liveing believed that the analogy of migraine to epilepsy was obvious, and that the clinically apparent circulatory phenomena that occurred during the attacks were secondary to CNS discharges, or "nerve storms." These views were shared by John Hughlings Jackson and William Richard Gowers, two of the founders of modern neurology, and eminent physicans of their time. Gowers' *Manual* (1888) was the most influential textbook of neurology at the turn of the century, and remained so for a number of years.

Attention was focused on the vascular mechanism of migraine in 1925 when the Swiss chemist Rothlin recommended treating it with parenteral ergotamine tartrate, which was subsequently found to be remarkably successful (Rothlin, 1955). Although it was originally believed to be effective because of its sympathetic blocking action, Graham and Wolff (1938) showed that the adminstration of this drug reduced the amplitude of the pulsations of the temporal artery in patients with headache, and that this effect was associated with a decrease in head pain. For several years thereafter it was widely held that the mode of action of ergotamine tartrate was through a direct constricting effect upon extracerebral arteries; however, the clinical observation that this drug, used in a preventive mode, could prevent not only the headache, or vasodilatory component of a migraine attack, but also the symptoms caused by intracerebral vasoconstriction (Trautman, 1928; Tzanck, 1928; Barrie et al., 1968), cast doubt on simple peripheral vasoconstriction as the sole mode of action of ergotamine tartrate. During the past 20 years, several additional drugs have been shown to be effective in preventing migraine attacks, some of which have few, if any, peripheral vasoconstrictive effects (Fozard, 1975). Many of these drugs, including the ergot alkaloids, exert prominent effects upon the CNS, and the hypothesis that migraine is a primary disorder of the central vasoregulatory mechanism remains viable.

Migraine may be tentatively regarded as a hereditary, paroxysmal vasoregulative instability, and comprises episodes during which there is a phase of intracerebral arterial constriction and a phase of extracerebral arterial dilatation; its precise cause at present is unknown. There are lines of evidence that support the hypothesis that the modulation of synaptic serotonin — centrally as well as peripherally — is an important pathogenetic mechanism of the disorder.

NOMENCLATURE OF MIGRAINE

Because our understanding of migraine is far from complete, its definition and classification are descriptive by necessity and only partly based on mechanisms. The designation *classic migraine* denotes the syndrome of headache associated with characteristic premonitory sensory, motor or visual symptoms; *common migraine* denotes one in which there is no focal neurologic disturbance preceding the occurrence of headache (Friedman et al., 1962). However, the latter is by far the more frequent clinical problem, and it has become clear that focal neurologic disturbances are more common during headache attacks than as prodromal symptoms (Selby and Lance, 1960).

If the designation of migraine is circumscribed as a disorder consisting of two phases, intracerebral vasoconstriction accompanied or followed by extracerebral vasodilatation, there are many patients who have attacks produced by either phase, singly or in combination. Focal neurologic disturbances without headache or vomiting have come to be known as *migraine equivalents*, and appear to occur more commonly, but by no means exclusively, in older patients (Whitty and Hockaday, 1968; Airing, 1972). It is not at all unusual for the pattern of attacks to become altered over the years, many patients reporting "classic" attacks with vomiting in earlier years that eventually conform to the "common" pattern without vomiting.

These variations in pattern among different patients and in the same patient at different times are compatible with a malfunction at a high level of cerebral organization. There is at present no compelling evidence that supports the separation of classic and common migraine into biologically distinct categories, although recently Lord and Duckworth (1978) have shown that complement activation occurs at the onset of headache attacks in patients without prodromal symptoms, but not in those with focal neurologic symptoms preceding the headache.

The varied phenomenology of migraine attacks has also spawned a classification scheme, so that *ophthalmoplegic, basilar, hemiplegic, retinal* and *facial* (lower half headache, carotidynia) migraine describe distinctive clinical syndromes that generally denote the location of less commonly involved arteries, but otherwise are not different from the more common migraine syndromes. The term *complicated migraine* is somewhat ambiguous in that it has generally been used to describe migraine with dramatic focal neurologic features, and thus overlaps with classic migraine (Bruyn, 1968); it also has sometimes been used to connote a persisting neurologic deficit that is a residuum of a migraine attack.

The intriguing visual symptoms of migraine have likewise resulted in several descriptive terms that sometimes have been employed ambiguously. *Teichopsia* ("walled vision") has been used to describe both hemianopic defects and the "positive" symptoms that may occur, such as wavy lines, colors, flashes of light and zig-zag patterns. *Photòpsia* refers to the specific sensation of unformed flashes of light before the eyes. *Scotomata* are the major "negative" symptoms and are often surrounded by shiny, sparkling prismatic figures that, taken together, constitute *scintillating scotomata.* These shiny figures are very often in the shape of angles that 200 years ago were compared to the shape of fortifications seen from above (Schiller, 1975). The term *fortification spectrum* usually refers to a slowly enlarging scotoma, surrounded by luminous angles, which slowly changes shape and/or appears to move across the visual fields. This latter phenomenon is so highly characteristic of migraine that it is probably pathognomonic, never having been described in a vascular headache syndrome resulting from an intracranial anatomic lesion. The positive symptoms that occur during migraine attacks almost always persist when the eyes are closed, consistent with evidence that cerebral, and not retinal, dysfunction is the usual source of the symptoms.

PREVALENCE

Migraine occurs commonly and is the most extensively studied headache syndrome. Despite its recognition for over 2,000 years, one of the major difficulties in establishing its prevalence has been its definition. The fallacy intrinsic to most of the traditional definitions is that they are acceptable descriptions of typical attacks but do not include those patients with more nondescript forms of migraine. The validity of arriving at a diagnosis in any individual by fulfilling certain clinical criteria has never been established. For example, over the years various combinations of the following variables have been alleged to establish the diagnosis of migraine: severe, intermittent pain; unilateral pain; nausea and/or vomiting with attacks; focal neurologic symptoms preceding attacks, most commonly visual; positive family history; responsiveness to ergotamine tartrate; and tenderness of the scalp (Ziegler, 1978). It is clear that severe attacks are more likely to be described as throbbing and associated with vomiting and scalp tenderness (Olesen, 1978); however, mild headache may or may not be associated with characteristic "migrainous" features (Ziegler et al, 1977), and it is unclear whether periodic headache without such features is migrainous in mechanism.

The best presently available estimates of the annual prevalence of migraine is 20 to 25 per cent (Waters, 1973; Waters and O'Connor, 1975; Waters, 1978). This probably underestimates the true prevalence of the disorder. In surveys of large populations of people in the United States (Ziegler et al, 1977) and in Europe (Nikiforow and Hokkanen, 1978), about 40 per cent of surveyed individuals have reported severe headaches at some point in their lives; in about one-half of these subjects, the headache attacks could be recognized as migrainous in mechanism because of their reporting warning symptoms, vomiting and/or unilateral localization of headache. However, for the remainder, there were no data that supported some other mechanism of headache, and because of the lack of objective parameters it remains uncertain just how commonly migraine occurs. It is certainly possible that migraine is in fact the "ordinary" headache that almost all of us experience at highly variable intervals, at varying levels of intensity; there are no data that militate against this possibility.

The prevalence of migraine does not appreciably differ according to intelligence, social class, or educational or racial background (Waters, 1971; Markush et al, 1975). It is far commoner in women, who comprise about 75 per cent of large series of patients (Lance and Anthony, 1966; Olesen, 1978).

INHERITANCE

A parental history of migrainous headaches is obtained in 50 to 60 per cent of patients with migraine and in 10 to 20 per cent of headache-free subjects (Ely, 1930; Selby and Lance, 1960; Lance and Anthony, 1966). When extraordinary efforts were made to obtain as comprehensive reports as possible in 100 women with migraine, 90 per cent had a family history of migraine (Dalsgaard-Nielsen, 1965); the incidence of parental migraine was 73 per cent, 57 per cent maternal and 16 per cent paternal. Migraine occurred in siblings in 27 per cent and in the patients' children in 15 per cent. Waters (1971), using a questionnaire survey (probably the least rigorous method for obtaining this kind of information), found that migraine in an immediate relative was more common than in the control subjects, but the difference was not statistically significant. Goodell et al (1954) studied the occurrence of migraine in the children of families in which one or more members had migraine. Of 265 children neither of whose parents had migraine, 76 (29 per cent) had migraine; of 502 children one of whose parents had migraine, 222 (44 per cent) had migraine; and of 65 children both of whose parents were affected, 45 (69 per cent) had migrainous headaches. Thus, evidence favoring a hereditary factor in migraine is substantial; however, the mode of inheritance is not clear, largely because of the sparsity of twin studies.

In a large unselected series of 1,900 pairs of twins, Harvald and Hauge (1956) identified 84 individuals with migraine. Of these 84, 24 were members of monozygotic twin pairs that included six concordant pairs and 12 individuals who were members of discordant pairs — a concordance ratio of 33 per cent. Of 57 dizygotic twin pairs, three pairs were found to be concordant and 54 discordant. In a smaller study, Ziegler and his colleagues (1975) studied 106 twin pairs, of whom 65 were dizygotic and 41 monozygotic. Of the 212 subjects, 31 reported severe or disabling headaches; concordance was no greater among the monozygotic pairs than among the dizygotic pairs. A few other studies of small populations of twins have produced similarly conflicting results (Refsum, 1968; Ziegler, 1977).

The evidence is persuasive that a predisposition to migraine is transmitted from parent to offspring. The distribution of the disorder within families renders recessive inheritance unlikely; it may be tentatively concluded that the mode of transmission of migraine is via autosomal dominant heredity with incomplete penetrance. In the special instance of hemiplegic migraine in which affected family members sustain virtually identical stereotyped attacks, the family pedigrees point to the high likelihood of autosomal dominant inheritance (Whitty, 1953; Bradshaw and Parsons, 1965; Glista et al, 1975; Parrish and Stevens, 1977).

A major question confronting those who seek to clarify the genetic factors relevant to migraine is which aspect of the "predisposition to headache" should be measured. There are at present no biologic markers capable of identifying the potential for vasoregulatory instability that appears to underlie this predisposition; severe headache attacks, *per se*, may not necessarily be the commonest expression of the putative genetic influence upon migraine. Few of us have never experienced headache in our lives; we may all have the potential to suffer a migraine headache in the setting of an adequate stimulus. This notion is supported by the low barometric pressure experiments and other evidence cited in the previous chapter. If migraine is a lowered biologic threshold to a variety of internal as well as external stimuli, an approximation of that threshold may be the measurement that is necessary to find out what is inherited before moving on to the mode of inheritance.

DEMOGRAPHY

Over 90 per cent of patients with migraine report that their first attack occurred before the age of 40 years (Table 2–1). Migraine is encountered not uncommonly in 2- and 3-year-old children (Barlow, 1978), but quantitative epidemiologic data below the age of 7 years is not yet available. In studies of children with migraine headaches,

TABLE 2-1. AGE OF ONSET OF
MIGRAINE IN 496 PATIENTS*

AGE AT FIRST ATTACK (YEARS)	PERCENTAGE OF PATIENTS
0–10	21
10–20	25
20–30	27
30–40	19
40–50	6
50–60	2

*Selby and Lance, 1960.

between 20 and 35 per cent were under the age of 5 years when the symptoms began (Prensky, 1976). By the age of 7 years, 40 per cent of children report having experienced headache, usually infrequently, but by strict criteria less than 2 per cent of them have recognizable migraine; most of the remainder have traditionally been classified as "nonmigrainous" (Bille, 1967). Under the age of 10 years the sex ratio for migraine is reversed; whereas in adults, women comprise 75 per cent of the migraine population, among children, boys account for 60 per cent (Prensky, 1976). By the age of 10 years, 15 per cent of boys and 22 per cent of girls can be identified as having migraine headaches. In young women the appearance of menarche is not significantly related to the presence, severity or frequency of headache (Deubner, 1977).

Based on the statistics regarding the age-relatedness of migraine, the warning is often made to be wary of the diagnosis of migraine in a patient whose headache disorder commenced after the age of 50. Of course it is good advice to be careful with all patients for whose health one is responsible; but among the various causes for headache in patients in the 50- to 70-year age range, migraine ranks very high, although cerebrovascular disease and giant cell arteritis loom as important differential diagnostic possibilities.

NATURAL HISTORY

Although there is a commonly held view that migraine attacks tend to cease·with the passage of time, particularly after the menopause in women, there are surprisingly few data regarding this aspect. Whitty and Hockaday (1968) studied 92 patients, 53 of whom were women, who were followed for periods of 15 to 20 years and who at the time of the investigators' assessment had been subject to migraine attacks for 16 to 69 years. In 63 patients attacks were still occurring (Table 2–2), but were less severe in 44 of these. One-half of 18 patients over the age of 64 continued to have attacks, and only a slight tendency for the cessation of attacks with advancing years was evident. Of 40 patients in whom menopause had occurred before the follow-up study, 18 noted no change in their headaches; six were worse; two were improved; in two the attacks had ceased; and in 12 there were insufficient data to form a judgment.

Neither the age of onset nor the total duration of the disorder bore a clear relation to the persistence or cessation of attacks. Of the patients whose attacks continued, 22 noted a change in their migrainous symptoms. The most common alteration was loss or reduction of vomiting in eight patients; five noted loss of their aura, with headaches alone persisting. In four patients, the opposite was seen — headaches ceased and only auras occurred. One noted a dissociation of aura and headache, each happening separately. In one patient, episodic headaches were replaced with episodic facial pain.

The symptomatic period occupied by migrainous symptoms in the lifespan of patients is extremely variable. Some report a complete cessation of attacks in early adult life, only to experience a recurrence in the sixth or seventh decade; in some, headaches beginning in infancy persist until the eighth or ninth decade (Graham, 1968). Not uncommonly, a clear-cut migrainous pattern eventually merges into what has been described as the tension headache pattern.

ACUTE HEADACHE ATTACKS: AN OVERVIEW OF MIGRAINE

In this section, the features of acute migraine attacks will be briefly described and statistics regarding their frequency will be cited. In subsequent sections, there will be a more detailed discussion of those features of special interest.

TABLE 2-2. FOLLOW-UP STUDY OF 90 PATIENTS WITH MIGRAINE 15 TO 20 YEARS AFTER INITIAL ASSESSMENT*

| AGE (YEARS) | PERSISTING ATTACKS | | | | ATTACKS STOPPED |
	No.	Improved	No Change	Worse	No.
<25	2	1	1	0	0
25–44	21	15	4	2	8
45–64	31	22	7	2	10
>64	9	6	3	0	9
Total	63	44	15	4	27

*Modified from Whitty and Hockaday, 1968.

Headaches commonly begin upon wakening in the morning, but may occur at any time of day or night. Nocturnal headache, wakening the patient from sleep, is not uncommon in migraine; however, in an individual with recent onset of nocturnal headaches, brain tumor and glaucoma should be carefully excluded. Cluster headaches also characteristically occur nocturnally.

In a population of patients with headache disorders of sufficient seriousness to warrant attendance at a neurologic clinic, over 50 per cent reported headaches occurring between one and four times per month, and the remainder were roughly equally represented in the frequency categories of less than one, five to ten, and more than ten attacks per month (Selby and Lance, 1960). About 50 per cent of those with acute migraine attacks also have frequent mild-to-moderate headaches interictally, which often are not characteristic enough in their associated features to be identified with certainty as migrainous in mechanism (Olesen, 1978). Because these interictal headaches are relatively nondescript, it has often been assumed that their mechanism is different from those that characterize more severe attacks. However, the responsiveness of these nondescript headaches to vasoactive drugs such as methysergide, ergonovine and ergotamine appears to be at least as great as that of the severe attacks (Barrie et al, 1968), which is consistent with the variable expression of migraine in individual patients.

During severe attacks, headache is lateralized in just over one-half of the patients (Table 2–3); the entire head was painful in 22 per cent of Olesen's (1978) patients, and in 38 per cent of Selby and Lance's (1960) population. In one-half of those who report lateralized headaches, either side may be involved and this may vary from episode to episode, although the most severe attacks usually occur on a preferred side. In the other half, headache invariably affects the same side of the head (Selby and Lance, 1960). The occiput and vertex are less common sites of pain; however, the locus of pain is an insensitive criterion for the diagnosis of migraine. Pain sites on

TABLE 2–3. LOCATION OF HEADACHE IN
678 PATIENTS WITH MIGRAINE*

LOCATION	PERCENTAGE OF PATIENTS
Hemicranial	44
Holocephalic	22
Bifrontal	14
Frontal, lateralized	13
Bioccipital	4
Occipital, lateralized	2
Vertex	1

*Data from Olesen, 1978.

the face and neck have also been recorded in migraine (Bille, 1967; Raskin and Prusiner, 1977), and, much less commonly, chest and abdominal pain (Graham, 1968); abdominal pain is fairly common in childhood migraine (Prensky, 1976).

The headache is usually gradual in onset, over several minutes to an hour or two, reaches a crescendo that persists for several hours to days, and then gradually subsides over several hours. About two-thirds of the patients report that their headaches persist for less than one day; for 27 per cent, the headache duration is less than four hours; for 40 per cent, it is four to 24 hours; for 11 per cent, one to two days; and for 22 per cent, longer than two days (Selby and Lance, 1960).

The quality of headache is often dull, deep and steady at mild-to-moderate levels of intensity, and it becomes pulsatile when more severe. Many patients have observed that a dull nonthrobbing headache becomes pulsatile when they bend forward or upon rapid change in the position of their head, which may be the symptomatic expression of the dysautoregulation of cerebral arteries that occurs during migraine attacks (Sakai and Meyer, 1978). Of 750 patients attending an acute headache clinic, about one-half reported that their headaches were pulsatile or pounding in quality (Olesen, 1978). Superimposed on the dull or pulsatile pain in over 30 per cent of patients is a jabbing, sharp pain that is often compared to an icepick, nail or needle. Such icepick-like pain most often arises around the orbit or temple, and often also occurs independent of the migraine attack *per se* (Raskin and Schwartz, 1979). Superimposed icepick-like pain also arises in the cluster headache syndrome and in giant cell arteritis.

Headache may be ameliorated to a degree by pressure on an artery overlying the site of headache, or on the ipsilateral carotid artery, or at times on the eyeball ipsilateral to the pain. When such pressure is released there is a delay of three to five seconds before the previous intensity of pain is resumed. As is true of vascular headaches of all types, rapid head motion, coughing, and the vibrations produced when riding in an automobile on a rough road often aggravate migraine headaches. The pain is minimized by lying still, and may be aborted completely by a brief period of sleep.

ACCOMPANYING SYMPTOMS

Nausea is the complaint of the vast majority of patients (Table 2–4); *vomiting* in addition to nausea occurs in just over one-half of the patients. About 16 per cent experience *diarrhea* as well as nausea and vomiting (Lance and Anthony, 1966), and occasionally diarrhea alone accompanies a headache attack. These gastrointestinal

TABLE 2-4. SYMPTOMS ACCOMPANYING MIGRAINE
ATTACKS IN 500 PATIENTS°

SYMPTOM		PERCENTAGE AFFECTED
Nausea		87
Vomiting		56
Diarrhea		16
Photophobia		82
Visual disturbances		36
fortification spectra	10	
photopsia	26	
Paresthesias		33
Scalp tenderness		65
Lightheadedness		72
Vertigo		33
Alteration of consciousness		18
seizure	4	
syncope	10	
confusional state	4	

°Modified from Selby and Lance, 1960; Lance and Anthony, 1966.

disturbances usually start some time after the onset of pain, but occasionally precede headache or, as is true of all of the other symptoms of migraine, may occur without head pain at all, as migraine
equivalents. Vomiting may be central in origin, but diarrhea is not
likely to be explicable on a central basis. Studies have not been
made of gastrointestinal blood flow during migrainous attacks.

A line of evidence linking serotonin to the diarrhea that accompanies the carcinoid syndrome may be relevant to the gastrointestinal symptoms that accompany migrainous attacks. The predominant
factor in the development of diarrhea in patients with the carcinoid
syndrome is the excessive production of serotonin by the carcinoid
tumor (Feldman, 1978). Diarrhea may be aggravated by drugs that
can release serotonin from the intestinal mucosa (Melmon et al,
1965), and drugs that block the synthesis of, or the intestinal receptors for, serotonin (such as methysergide) frequently control the diarrhea (Sjoerdsma et al, 1970). There is also a line of evidence that
implicates serotonin as a neurotransmitter in the myenteric plexus,
which may account for its role in the regulation of gastrointestinal
motility (Gershon, 1968). Although the precise relationship of serotonin to the diarrhea of the carcinoid syndrome remains unclear
(Donowitz and Binder, 1975), drugs capable of suppressing migrainous attacks are capable of suppressing the diarrhea of this disorder.
The participation of serotonin in the vagal regulation of gastric contractions (Cooper et al, 1978) provides a possible mechanism for the
nausea and vomiting that accompany migrainous attacks. The tan-
talizing hypothesis arises that migraine may be a disorder in which
the neurotransmitter functions of serotonin − centrally and pe-

ripherally — are poorly modulated. Further data supporitive of this hypothesis will be reviewed in Chapter 4.

  Blurred vision is almost always reported by patients and cannot be explained by concurrent lacrimation, nor are the mechanisms known of the heightened sensitivity to light, sounds and odors that so often accompanies attacks. *Lightheadedness* is also common and is usually accentuated by stooping or bending. It generally is not appreciated that *syncope* is not uncommon during migraine attacks, occurring in about 10 per cent of patients (Weil, 1962; Barolin, 1966). Syncope occasionally may be the presenting complaint, and careful inquiry regarding the presence of other migrainous symptoms immediately preceding or succeeding the faint is often necessary to establish a diagnosis that is both benign and preventable.

  The coincidence of epilepsy with migraine is significantly greater than in the general population (Basser, 1969). Occasionally, *convulsive movements* occur in association with severe headache. It is clear that convulsions may result from cerebral ischemia (Duvoisin, 1962), but whether the mechanism of seizures that may occur in migraine are ischemic or "epileptic" and triggered by the migraine attack has not been resolved. The term *migraine-epilepsy* has sometimes been used to denote this syndrome (Ely, 1930; Critchley and Ferguson, 1933).

  Over-all, *focal neurologic symptoms* other than visual disturbances either precede or occur during migraine attacks in about 30 per cent of patients; brain stem dysfunction, probably due to constriction of the vertebrobasilar arterial system, appears to be the cause of most of these symptoms, which include vertigo, dysarthria, ataxia and diplopia. These are the *only* neurologic symptoms of an attack in 25 per cent of patients (Lance and Anthony, 1966). Therefore, *basilar migraine*, broadly defined, is a common clinical syndrome. Since the posterior cerebral arteries, branches of the basilar artery, produce the visual disturbances of migraine, it can be argued that basilar migraine is the commonest clinical form of the syndrome; however, this term has usually been reserved for a dramatic symptom complex that will be described below. Aphasia and hemihypesthesia also are not infrequently reported in association with migrainous attacks.

  Scalp tenderness occurs during or after headache in about two-thirds of the patients. This may be described as an unpleasant sensation noted when combing or brushing the hair; it may be severe enough to discourage the patient from lying on the affected side. Such tenderness may involve any portion of the head and neck, and traditionally has been attributed to widespread distention of extra-cranial arteries and/or contraction of the scalp and neck musculature. However, since muscle pain and soreness may occur as prodromal symptoms of the migraine attack (Pearce, 1977), it is possible that intramuscular vasoconstriction underlies this symptom (see Chapter 5). Distention of arterial walls clearly accounts for some portion of this tenderness; at times superficial temporal artery tenderness may be quite dramatic, prompting a mistaken diagnosis of giant cell arteritis. The superficial veins also are often distended over the forehead and temple. Occasionally the face becomes flushed, but much more commonly, facial pallor is prominent during attacks. The skin temperature is cooler by about 1° C on the affected side (Lance and Anthony, 1971). Thus, distention of veins as well as arteries, pallor and cooler skin temperature, in the presence of extracranial vasodilatation, supports the suggestion (Heyck, 1969) that the opening of cranial arteriovenous anastomoses characterizes migraine attacks; further support for this hypothesis comes from evidence that ergotamine tartrate, among its other actions, reduces the shunting of blood through these arteriovenous anastomotic channels (Johnston and Saxena, 1978).

Rarely, extracranial vasodilatation appears to be profound, resulting in the extravasation of blood, so that *subconjunctival hemorrhage, epistaxis* or *orbital ecchymoses* may appear in association with migraine attacks, usually at their termination (Sacks, 1970).

Fluid retention occurs in the vast majority of patients hours to days before a migraine attack, and about one-half become symptomatic, with, for example, tightness of rings, shoes or clothes, or the presence of frank pitting pedal edema (Ostfeld et al, 1955). For over 95 per cent of patients, the weight gain is in the order of 2 to 5 pounds, and on occasion it may be as high as 17 pounds. Polyuria occurs either immediately after the onset of headache or during the period of dwindling headache intensity. Occasionally, fluid retention persists until a series of headaches have taken place. The serum sodium concentration increases during the fluid retention phase, whereas there is evidence that between attacks the urinary output of sodium is greater than in control subjects (Campbell et al, 1951). These alterations are probably epiphenomena and not causally related to migraine, since the prevention of fluid retention by the administration of diuretic agents does not usually prevent migraine attacks, and conversely the induction of overhydration with vasopressin tannate or desoxycorticosterone acetate does not provoke headaches (Ostfeld et al, 1955). There is no consistent or predictable pattern in the excretion of sodium, potassium or corticosteroids during headache attacks. Plasma aldosterone levels drop at the onset of a migraine headache attack, whereas levels of renin, cortisol, sodium and potassium remain normal (Nattero et al, 1977).

Between 10 and 20 per cent of patients report *nasal stuffiness* during the course of a migraine attack; in some of these a profuse nasal secretion occurs as the attack terminates. These phenomena are also characteristic of the cluster headache syndrome, and these overlapping clinical features, among other similarities, have led to the contention that the two disorders are related etiologically (Medina and Diamond, 1977). Such nasal symptoms sometimes lead to a mistaken diagnosis of rhinitis or sinusitis. It should be noted in this context that sinusitis is an uncommon cause of recurring headache. Further overlapping with the cluster headache syndrome is evident in the occasional occurrence of Horner's syndrome (Vijayan and Watson, 1978) or of unilateral pupillary dilatation (Kunkle and Anderson, 1961; Edelson and Levy, 1974) in association with migraine attacks.

Mood alterations occur in most patients, sometimes before but most often during attacks; the alterations that occur range from lethargy, fatigue and anxious irritability to exhilaration. The intensity of these phenomena appears to correlate generally with the severity of headache attacks; the exceptions to this generalization are striking and render it unlikely that these changes are simply secondary to acute head pain.

Fever has occasionally arisen during attacks (Wolf and Wolff, 1942), especially in children, and may be as high as 40° C (Sacks, 1970). *Tachycardia* accompanies migraine attacks in about 3 per cent of patients (Dalsgaard-Neilsen, 1948; Briggs and Belloms, 1952), and *paroxysmal atrial tachycardia* was noted in association with migrainous attacks by Thomas and Post (1925) over 50 years ago. The frequency of classic migraine among patients with documented paroxysmal atrial tachycardia is about 40 per cent (Perera, 1971). Recent evidence implicates neural mechanisms in the genesis of cardiac arrhythmias (Levitt et al, 1976), and the pharmacologic management of some arrhythmias includes propranolol and phenytoin, which are also useful in the treatment of migraine. Thus, paroxysmal atrial tachycardia and migraine may share a common pathogenetic mechanism.

Migraine equivalents refers to the appearance of any of the accompanying symptoms of migraine attacks described above in the clinical setting in which headache may be absent or, more commonly, present but mild, and presumed to be inconsequential by the patient. Many of these patients have backgrounds in which unequivocal migraine attacks have occurred, and some do not. For example, the syndrome of episodic nausea in association with scintillating scotomata is one that we have frequently encountered, and presents little diagnostic difficulty. Periodic syncope, vertigo and vomiting comprise the commonest migraine equivalent syndromes, and the correctness of the diagnosis at present must rest on the demonstration of responsiveness to drugs such as propranolol and methysergide. Episodic tachycardia, amblyopia, mood change, diarrhea, extreme fatigue, fever, edema and somatic pain are less common, but appear to be bona-fide syndromes (Catino, 1965; Sacks,

1970). A clue that often leads to the correct diagnosis is that equivalents occur with a periodicity and duration similar to migrainous headache attacks, and are *likely to be precipitated by the same kinds of factors* (see below).

PRECIPITATING FACTORS

The wide diversity of factors capable of triggering migraine attacks suggests that there are either subgroups of patients with migraine who have different biologic abnormalities, or that there is a common single mechanism that can be triggered by a wide range of identifiable factors. Although much progress has been made during the past ten years toward understanding the biologic substrate of migraine, we are still at a relatively primitive level of comprehension. There are no compelling data that favor the unitary over the multiple mechanism hypotheses; however, there is evidence, reviewed in the preceding chapter, that supports the concept that migraine is the manifestation of a lowered biologic threshold to a variety of external and internal stimuli. Whereas the nature of the threshold may ultimately prove to be more complex than a single molecular abnormality, the latter concept is operationally useful at our current level of understanding.

The reproducible provocation of headache by stereotyped stimuli is probably the most useful way of approaching the clinical diagnosis of migraine. For example, headache occurring monthly the day before or the first day of menstrual flow, and usually at other times also (Epstein et al, 1975), is so highly characteristic of migraine as to be virtually pathognomonic, regardless of the clinical features of the headache *per se* and whether or not nausea or other migrainous symptoms are reported. Headache commencing within an hour of the ingestion of an alcoholic beverage almost always signifies a predisposition to migraine or the cluster headache syndrome. Similarly, headache occurring (1) after exposure to glare or hot, dry winds; (2) after missing a meal; or (3) on a Saturday morning after a stressful week (Table 2–5) characterizes migraine at least as well as the descriptive features of the headache attack, the latter depending a good deal on the articulateness and perceptiveness of both patient and physician.

Several aspects of these precipitants of migrainous attacks are often misunderstood by patients and physicians alike. The first of these, and one of the more puzzling, is that sometimes the sensitivity to a stimulus develops long after a spontaneous periodic headache pattern is established; it is not at all uncommon for patients to note headache after drinking a cocktail at the age of 40, having sustained recurring headaches for the preceding 20 years without hav-

TABLE 2-5. FACTORS PRECIPITATING MIGRAINE ATTACKS*

COMMON FACTORS	LESS COMMON FACTORS
Stress and worry	High humidity
Menstruation	Excessive sleep
Oral contraceptives	High altitude exposure
Glare, dazzle	Excessive vitamin A
Physical exertion, fatigue	Drugs: nitroglycerine, histamine,
Lack of sleep	reserpine, hydralazine, estrogen,
Hunger	corticosteroid withdrawal
Head trauma	Cold foods
Foods and beverages containing	Reading, refractive errors
nitrite, glutamate, salt, tyramine,	Pungent odors: perfumes, organic
and other as yet unidentified chemicals	solvents, smoke
Weather or ambient temperature change	Fluorescent lighting
	Allergic reactions

*Data from Selby and Lance, 1960; Pearce, 1971.

ing ever experienced this phenomenon previously. The same can be said of all the other stimuli, and this has relevance to the practical aspects of management. A worsening headache problem should alert the patient and physician to search for a removable environmental factor such as a dietary component (Table 2-6) or a drug that has been used for several years, *despite the fact that these factors had been tested as provocative stimuli in the past* with negative results. Furthermore, some patients lose their susceptibilities to one or more of these stimuli as the years pass and unprovoked headaches continue.

Another aspect of the precipitant phenomenology is that these stimuli only rarely are 100 per cent reproducible; unfortunately, this facet of the disorder has frustrated all attempts to achieve an objective diagnostic test for migraine. The vast majority of migraineurs report that alcohol, for example, triggers a headache after 60 to 80 per cent of exposures; this is approximately the range of reproducibility achieved with contrived diagnostic tests for migraine such as the administration of reserpine (Curzon et al, 1969), histamine (von Reis et al, 1957) nitroglycerine (Schnitker and Schnitker, 1947) or tyramine (see Chapter 3). Whereas headache occurs significantly more often after these provocational agents than by chance, the false-negative and false-positive response rate is too high (Dalsgaard-Nielsen, 1955) for any of the above agents to be useful as a diagnostic test. Similarly, the false-negative response rate of migrainous headache to ergotamine tartrate is too high to be useful diagnostically (Lennox, 1938); Curran and Lance (1964) found that 65 per cent of their patients with migraine were responsive to ergotamine.

Precipitants usually account for but a small proportion of a pa-

TABLE 2-6. FOODS CONSIDERED BY 772 FOOD-SENSITIVE
PATIENTS TO BE PRECIPITANTS OF MIGRAINE ATTACKS*

COMMON FOODS – %		LESS COMMON FOODS – %	
Chocolate	50	Beer	15
Wine and alcoholic		Fried, fatty foods	10
spirits	40	Pork	10
Dairy products	30	Onions	9
Citrus fruits	30	Tea, coffee	7
		Seafood	5

*Data from Smith et al, 1970; Moffett et al, 1974.

tient's recurring headaches (Gomersall and Stuart, 1973), and their
removal often affords only modest benefits. However, the exceptions to this generalization are well worth exploring, in view of the
many women who cease having headaches completely after stopping oral contraception or the few who benefit from revision of
their diets. For the vast majority of patients, trigger factors aggravate an underlying predisposition to headache and serve as important biologic markers of a lowered threshold to ordinary stimuli that
usually do not result in headache in nonmigraineurs.

Factors that often greatly concern patients, but which only rarely are implicated in the genesis of migrainous attacks, include ciga-
rette smoking (Volans and Castleden, 1976), refractive errors (Cameron, 1976), sinusitis (Birt, 1978) and disorders of the cervical
spine (Dutton and Riley, 1969; Edmeads, 1978).

Head trauma as a precipitant of migraine attacks will be dealt
with in Chapter 7; hunger, alcohol and food as migraine precipitants are discussed in the preceding and succeeding chapters. Regarding foods, it is often incorrectly assumed that because the common dietary precipitants of migraine have been eliminated and the
headache disorder has been unaffected, exogenous chemicals have
been ruled out as provocateurs. The varieties of foods and chemicals capable of inducing headache (Table 2–6) have only begun to
be tabulated. The authors have encountered patients who have
clearly identified such unusual factors as folic acid, the yellow dye
present in certain pharmaceutical tablets, and certain sources of tap
water.

STRESS AND ANXIETY

Emotional stress is the commonest precipitant of migrainous attacks, and in 50 per cent of a random sample of patients migraine
began for the first time ever during an emotionally-charged period
(Henryk-Gutt and Rees, 1973). However, there is no evidence that

patients with migraine are under greater stresses as compared to control subjects. Controlled psychologic studies suggest that those with migraine are disposed by biologic and not situational factors to experience a greater-than-average reaction to a given quantity of stress (Merskey, 1975). Earlier suggestions that migraineurs are especially obsessional or ambitious (Wolff, 1937) have not been confirmed in controlled studies (Henryk-Gutt and Rees, 1973).

There is a remarkable tendency to develop migraine not at the peak of stress, but during the "let-down" period of relaxation. Weekends, the beginning of a holiday, the end of June for school teachers and the 16th of April for tax accountants are common clinical settings for migrainous attacks. Children facing social, personal and learning difficulties at school may be disposed to a siege of recurring headaches. Moreover, chronic recurrent pain in itself may result in an emotional disturbance (Merskey and Boyd, 1978); mistaking the sequence of events in these instances may be harmful to some patients.

As a corollary to the above observations, many patients during periods of exhilaration — falling in love is by far the commonest circumstance — may experience a dramatic remission in their headache disorder (Raskin and Appenzeller, unpublished observations). Unfortunately, this is usually a temporary remission and the former periodicity of the attacks generally resumes within variable periods of time. Thus, there is little doubt that the personal environment of the individual may influence the course of migraine.

THE FEMALE REPRODUCTIVE CYCLE

The menstrual periodicity of migraine attacks, their amelioration during pregnancy, and their aggravation during exposure to oral contraceptive agents have led to a careful examination of gonadal hormone cycles in women with migraine attacks. Regional alterations in brain serotonin also parallel these cyclical changes (Quay and Meyer, 1978).

Menstruation. About 60 per cent of women who suffer from migrainous headaches report that at least some of their attacks are linked to their menstrual cycles (Lance and Anthony, 1966). In these women, headaches usually occur just before or during menstruation. Strictly menstrual migraine, i.e., headaches that occur *only* perimenstrually and at no other time, is much less common, occurring in only 14 per cent of female migraineurs. These latter patients are more likely to have had the onset of their migraine attacks at menarche, to have associated fluid retention as part of a periodic syndrome, and to show improvement during pregnancy (Epstein et al, 1975); there is no predictable change in the pattern of headache attacks at the menopause.

Somerville (1972a) has shown that women with menstrual migraine have estrogen–progesterone cycles that are no different from control subjects. Likewise, plasma levels obtained throughout the menstrual cycle of follicle-stimulating hormone, luteinizing hormone, prolactin and testosterone are normal (Epstein et al, 1975). The normal decline of plasma estradiol, rather than that of progesterone, appears to be the important trigger factor, since headache attacks are not affected by maintaining artificially elevated levels of progesterone, but are regularly postponed by maintenance of artificially elevated plasma estradiol levels (Somerville, 1972a). The oral administration of estrogen replacements to women during the premenstrual portions of their cycle is generally ineffectual in preventing menstrual migraine (Somerville, 1975); it appears that once the migraine mechanism is activated by falling estrogen levels, subsequent manipulation of tissue levels of estrogen does not effectively influence the appearance of an attack. There are no data that bear on the question of whether these hormonal alterations provoke migraine attacks through a direct effect upon cranial arteries or upon a central mechanism, or whether serotonergic hypothalamic regulation of gonadotropin-releasing hormone is the primary mechanism (Krieger, 1978).

Pregnancy. The alterations in the tissue levels of estradiol and progesterone, among other changes during pregnancy, are dramatic. The plasma estradiol level may be elevated one hundredfold in late pregnancy, so that the observation that pregnancy influences the course of migraine might be anticipated. In a survey of 200 women between their 36th and 40th weeks of gestation, Somerville (1972b) found 38 who reported recent migraine attacks. Of these, 31 had experienced headaches before pregnancy, and seven developed migraine for the first time during their pregnancy; in this latter group, headaches began during the first trimester in five women, and during the second and third trimesters respectively in the other two. Of the 31 women with pre-existing migraine, 24 reported improvement during pregnancy (usually during the second and third trimesters), seven of these becoming completely headache-free; the remaining seven reported either no change or a worsening of their headache disorder. Callaghan (1968) similarly found that, when migraine develops for the first time during pregnancy, it usually appears during the first trimester. The mean plasma progesterone levels in those women who experienced relief from their headache disorders did not differ significantly from the levels of those who either reported no change or who were pregnant, headache-free control subjects (Somerville, 1972b). Whether the relief from migrainous attacks during pregnancy that occurs in most female migraineurs is due to the replacement of the cyclized rises and falls in estrogen levels by rising levels of estrogenic hormones, or by one or another of the multitude of biochemical alterations that attend pregnancy, is conjectural. There are also preliminary data that suggest that, among the population of women who do not experience relief from migraine during pregnancy, there is a higher incidence of preeclampsia (Rotton et al, 1959), the latter perhaps acting as a trigger mechanism.

Oral contraception. There is an increased incidence of vascular headaches among women who use oral contraception (Carey, 1971). This is a more serious matter than simply exchanging discomfort for the convenience of this method of contraception, because there is evidence that it is this population of women that is at increased risk of cerebral infarction (Shafey and Scheinberg, 1966; Gardner et al, 1968; Collaborative Group, 1973). Intimal hyperplasia of the cerebral arterial vasculature has been found in women who had been using oral contraception and who died as a consequence of cerebral infarction (Irey et al, 1978). Hyperplasia of the arterial intima has also been reported in the pulmonic, portal, coronary and uterine circulations in women using oral contraception (Irey et al, 1970; Irey and Norris, 1973; Osterholzer et al, 1977), suggesting that this oral contraceptive-induced proliferative alteration may be important to the mechanism of thrombosis.

Headache frequency appears to correlate with the estrogen content of oral contraceptive preparations (Greene, 1975), so that many women formerly troubled by headache may successfully use a low estrogen preparation. Of those women who develop headache problems concurrent with oral contraceptive use, approximately one-half report pre-existing migrainous attacks; the other half develop migrainous attacks *de novo* (Kudrow, 1975). Upon stopping oral contraception, there may be a lag period of several months before improvement in the headache disorder occurs; the duration of this period may depend on the duration of exposure to these agents, but this point has not been studied carefully. The lag period between the commencement of oral contraception and the development or worsening of a recurring headache disorder is quite variable, and is on the order of months to years. The large majority of women who experience ill effects from oral contraception develop headache within the first months of its use (Ryan, 1978); however, the authors have occasionally encountered women who had used these agents for as long as five years before headache occurred, and then ceased suffering headache after the drug was stopped. Of women who develop headache after using hormonal agents for contraception, about 30 to 40 per cent improve after stopping their use (Dennerstein et al, 1978). For the remainder, it is not clear whether oral contraception sets in motion a mechanism that is to be unstable for years or whether migraine has coincidentally developed during the practice of oral contraception. The latter appears to be the more common explanation; however, recent evidence suggesting that oral contraceptive use may result in the clinical expression of otherwise silent pituitary adenomas (Sherman et al, 1978; Reichlin, 1979) may be analogous to the unmasking of migraine that may not stop when the stimulus is removed. The other clinical precedents for the precipitation of migraine careers of long duration are head trauma or an extraordinary emotional stress.

It generally is not appreciated that a small percentage of women report *improvement* in their headache disorders while using oral contraception (Ryan, 1978); however, there are no reliable clinical indices that might approximate the probability of headache worsening or improvement during oral contraception exposure. Although endometrial monoamine oxidase (MAO) levels are altered by these agents (Essman and Tagliente, 1978), and this enzyme has been implicated in the mechanism of migraine (see Chapter 3), there is no evidence that MAO is involved in the genesis of headache that occurs during the use of oral contraceptives.

Menopause. There is no clear pattern of migraine at or after the menopause (Epstein et al, 1975). Whereas migrainous headaches sometimes cease, headache is a common symptom among women whose menstrual cycle has recently stopped (Dennerstein et al, 1978). There are also paradoxical effects of hormone replacement therapy upon women with pre-existent migraine that persists or occurs *de novo* during the menopause. Estrogen and testosterone administration have been reported to relieve menopausal migraine in some patients (Greenblatt and Bruneteau, 1974; Shoemaker et al, 1977); several controlled studies have amplified this observation in showing that headache frequency generally correlates inversely with the estrogen dosage used for replacement therapy (Dennerstein et al, 1978). On the other hand, migraine has been shown to be improved substantially by decreasing the dosage of estrogen for women whose headaches worsened or began after estrogen replacement was commenced (Kudrow, 1975). The type as well as the dosage of estrogen replacement may be important factors to consider. The authors have seen many women whose headache disorders were remarkably improved by substituting a chemically pure synthetic estrogen, ethinyl estradiol, for an organic, equine-derived, conjugated estrogen preparation; occasionally the reverse appears to be true. There is no evidence to indicate that hysterectomy is of benefit in the treatment of migraine (Utian, 1974; Greene, 1975).

SLEEP

The fact that excessive sleep may trigger migraine attacks was recognized by Gans (1951), who reported improvement in his patients' migrainous attacks when he reduced their sleeping time and lightened the depth of their sleep by having them repeatedly touched during the night. This curious experiment has not been replicated. Some attacks of nocturnal migraine occur during dreams into the content of which the premonitory symptoms of an attack may be incorporated (Dexter and Weitzman, 1970). For some patients, too little sleep may be a stimulus for a migrainous attack. For the great majority a brief period of sleep has positive therapeutic value in aborting a migrainous attack, although there are no controlled data that bear on this common observation. These clinical observations may be more interpretable when placed into the context of the physiology of sleep, about which a great deal has been learned during the past 15 years.

Sleep comprises discrete, recurring cycles that appear to be regulated by neural mechanisms. One cycle is characterized by the appearance of rapid eye movements (REM) and a low-voltage, fast-frequency electroencephalographic pattern; this period is called REM sleep and is associated with dreaming, as well as an increase in heart rate, respiration and cerebral blood flow (Reivich et al, 1968; Sakai et al, 1979). REM cycles alternate with non-REM periods which are characterized by a high-voltage, slow-wave EEG pattern. Each REM/non-REM cycle lasts about 90 minutes, but their duration is variable throughout the night; slow-wave sleep predominates during the early sleeping hours and REM sleep occurs more frequently during the morning hours (Mendelson et al, 1977). Nocturnal migrainous headaches have been found to occur in temporal relationship to REM sleep (Dexter and Weitzman, 1970; Dexter and Riley, 1975). There is substantial evidence that serotonin is involved in the regulation of sleep cycles (Morgane and Stern, 1978). Serotonergic neurons within the lower midbrain and pons appear to regulate certain electrical events that occur within the CNS during REM cycles (Gillin et al, 1978); disruption of these neurons results in insomnia, whereas their stimulation produces slow-wave sleep (Jouvet, 1967). Inferences drawn from these findings have been applied to the syndrome of narcolepsy, one important component of which is periodic excessive sleepiness, which may be caused by dysfunction of brain stem serotonergic neurons (Broughton, 1971). Methysergide, a drug that simulates the effects of serotonin centrally (Haigler and Aghajanian, 1974) and of proved effectiveness in the prevention of migrainous attacks, was used successfully in the treatment of five patients with narcolepsy (Wyler et al, 1975).

REM sleep, as noted above, is associated with a large increase in CBF that is probably related to an increase in cerebral metabolism (Townsend et al, 1973); whether cerebral autoregulation is altered during REM sleep is unknown. REM sleep cycles are also associated with a decrease in platelet serotonin (Dexter, 1974).

That migraine headaches may be connected with a stage of sleep characterized by alterations of the cerebral vasculature and a drop in circulating serotonin, taken together with the data imputing serotonergic neurons with a role in sleep regulation, suggests the possibility that there are mechanisms common to the regulation of sleep and migraine. Furthermore, the curious predilection of migrainous attacks to the early morning hours, their precipitation by exposure to bright light, and their amelioration by exposure to darkness and/or sleep generally parallels the circadian rhythms of brain serotonin, in which peaks occur in laboratory animals during the daily light phase and the lowest levels usually occur in the dark (Quay and Meyer, 1978).

WEATHER CHANGES

Many patients report thunderstorms as a precipitant of their migraine attacks. Wilson (1972), in his diary of Scott's expedition to the Antarctic, described how he almost invariably developed such an attack 10 to 12 hours before a storm.

Weather change is reported by about 50 per cent of patients as an influence upon their migraine visitations; however, as is true of precipitants in general, only 2 per cent of all attacks are precipitated by weather. Bright dazzling sunshine, cold, thunder, wind and heat are the commonly reported weather conditions bearing on headache attacks. In an ingenious study, these conditions were shown to affect the severity rather than the frequency of attacks (Gomersall and Stuart, 1973). The various sources of dazzle in the enviroment may be neutralized to varying degrees through the use of polarized lenses. No seasonal variation in the pattern of headache has been established, although an occasional patient experiences attacks regularly during the same months each year.

Scattered throughout the world there exist weather fronts that are accompanied by hot dry winds of ill repute. These include the Sharav of Israel, the Foehn of Switzerland, Germany and Austria, the Mistral of France, the Santa Ana of southern California, the Chinook of Canada, the Sirocco of the Mediterranean, the Xlokk of Malta, the Chamsin of the Arab countries, the Zonda of Argentina and the Arizona desert winds. It has been observed for centuries that the day before the winds begin a variety of symptoms occur in a substantial proportion of the exposed population, including depression, insomnia, irritability, dyspnea and migrainous headaches (Robinson and Dirnfeld, 1963). Concurrent with the onset of symptoms, it has been shown that there is an increase both in the total number of small air ions and in the ratio of positive to negative ions (Krueger, 1972; Krueger and Reed, 1976). Moreover, Danon and Sulman (1969) have demonstrated that, parallel to these electrical alterations, urinary serotonin metabolites increase and catecholamine excretion decreases. It has been suggested, but not established, that weather-sensitive people are benefited by the administration of drugs that are peripheral serotonin-antagonists or MAO-inhibitors, agents also effective in migraine. In addition, there are reports of improvement after exposure to a negative ion environment (Sulman et al, 1971, 1974). However, it remains unclear whether either the alterations in air ions or the urinary metabolites are important to the mechanism of symptoms that occur after exposure to these hot dry winds. In an open study utilizing 20 patients with migraine who observed that weather change influenced their headaches, only one reported benefit from the daily use of a negative ion generator placed within 3 feet of the head for one month during sleep (Raskin, unpublished observations). The alterations of brain serotonin turnover that parallel changes in ambient temperature may bear on the mechanism of migraine precipitated by weather change (Myers and Waller, 1978).

PHYSICAL EXERTION

Exercise in short intense bursts, after a prolonged low-level effort in an unconditioned individual, or occasionally at any level of activity, may result in a migraine attack in susceptible persons (Dalessio, 1974). Many examples of "acute effort" migraine were encountered in highly trained participants during the Olympic games in Mexico City; the altitude of 7,000 feet probably contributed to the unusually high incidence of the syndrome. Focal neurologic symptoms usually appear immediately following exertion, followed in several minutes by nausea and what may be a severe, lateralized pulsatile headache that may last for one or more hours. Acute effort migraine may occur repeatedly, and may be prevented by ergotamine tartrate or methysergide taken before the intended exercise (Curran and Lance, 1964; Lance, 1978).

Effort migraine after prolonged noncompetitive exercise usually occurs in recent converts to physical fitness programs. Focal neurologic symptoms and vomiting arise only rarely in this syndrome (Seelinger et al, 1975), which is not apt to recur as endurance improves; however, a few individuals are prone to effort migraine at varying levels of activity. Prophylactic salicylates or ergotamine tartrate have been useful for many, but not all of these patients.

ALLERGIC REACTIONS

The fact that migraine attacks may occur in association with asthma, hay fever or angioneurotic edema upon exposure to a specific allergen was recognized over 100 years ago, and several instances of these reactions were critically recorded by Kallós and Kallós-Deffner (1955). However, over the years, patients with dietary migraine, now known to be a non-immunologic disorder, were entered into the "allergic migraine" literature because of their improvement with elimination diets; for many years allergy was erroneously believed to be causally linked to migraine (Pinnas and Vanselow, 1978).

There is no difference in the incidence of allergy nor of immunoglobulin E levels between patients with migraine and control subjects (Medina and Diamond, 1976); when allergic reactions precipitate migraine attacks, the symptoms of rhinitis, asthma and/or urticaria almost always accompany the attacks. Rarely, migraine alone is the manifestation of allergy, and one of the 500 patients of Selby and Lance (1960) was an example of this rare exception to the rule.

The provocation of migrainous attacks by (Type I) hypersensitivity reactions is understandable since histamine, prostaglandins, kinins, serotonin and platelet-activating factors are released after an antigen combines with a specific immunoglobulin E antibody, which is contained within tissue mast cells and basophilic leukocytes (Pinnas and Vanselow, 1978). Of these vasoactive mediators of allergic reactions, there is evidence that histamine and prostaglandin E may precipitate migrainous attacks (see Chapter 3).

Ergotamine tartrate is effective in preventing the migrainous features of these reactions, but antihistaminic and sympathomimetic drugs are necessary to prevent the allergic symptoms (Kallós and Kallós-Deffner, 1955). These are sparse data regarding the effectiveness of desensitization in these circumstances (Miller, 1977).

NECK DISORDERS

Headache is an uncommon feature of cervical spondylosis and herniated discs (Brain, 1963). Some afferent fibers of the upper two, and possibly the third and fourth, cervical roots converge upon the same dorsal horn cells that receive afferent innervation from the descending trigeminal spinal tract (Kerr, 1961a), which probably explains the observation that stimulation of the first cervical dorsal root results in orbital and frontal pain (Kerr, 1961b). There is some evidence that stimulation of the second, third and fourth cervical nerve roots may produce headache, but no evidence that lesions below C4 may do so (Edmeads, 1978). The vertebral artery, a pain-sensitive structure, may be compressed by cervical osteophytes and result in episodic vertebral insufficiency, a syndrome that includes a lateralized pulsatile headache in 20 per cent of such patients, and which may be confused with migraine (Dutton and Riley, 1969). Attacks of headache and neurologic symptoms are almost always associated with certain positions of the head and neck, such as hyperextension of the neck, turning the head to one side, or neck flexion; this is a rare syndrome.

The term *migraine cervicale* was originally applied to the syndrome that may follow head and neck trauma (Bärtschi-Rochaix, 1968) and which now appears to be more appropriately included in the post-traumatic group of disorders (see Chapter 7).

Patients with cervical spondylosis that involves the upper cervical spine often report neck and shoulder pain and occasionally suboccipital headache in conjunction with other symptoms of cervical nerve root compression. When headache is severe, it may radiate to the forehead, eye or temple; it often occurs in the morning and appears intermittently throughout the day. Occasionally, headache is ' pulsatile in quality and is aggravated by neck movements and by coughing and straining. Thus, headache resulting from upper cervical spine disorders may occasionally be confused with migraine. Edmeads (1978) has proposed that certain features of a headache syndrome may suggest its origin from the cervical spine. They are: (1) persistent, unilateral suboccipital pain; (2) reproduction or alteration of headache with neck motion; (3) abnormal postural attitudes of the head and neck; (4) aggravation or reproduction of headache by deep suboccipital pressure; (5) painful limitation of neck movements; and, most importantly, (6) signs and symptoms referable to cervical nerve roots.

Whether headache results from lesions of the lower cervical spine is controversial; patients with pre-existing migraine may experience a worsening of their headache disorder concurrent with the development of a low cervical disc, but *de novo* headache disorders resulting from lesions of the lower cervical spine have not been well documented.

To summarize, neck disorders are an uncommon cause of headache. Occasionally, patients with disorders that involve the upper cervical spine report recurring headache that may resemble migraine, but there is almost always a prominent suboccipital component and clinical evidence of nerve root compression; patients with pre-existing migraine may undergo an exacerbation of their headache problem. It may be concluded that cervical spine disorders only rarely mimic migraine.

ASSOCIATED DISORDERS

A variety of disorders have been linked with migraine, some for as yet inexplicable reasons. In addition, several conditions have been described which rarely give rise to *de novo* migraine or more frequently aggravate pre-existing migraine. Essential hypertension was discussed in Chapter 1.

Motion Sickness

About 60 per cent of migraineurs report severe motion sickness during early childhood (Selby and Lance, 1960). The kinds of motion most likely to result in nausea are very similar to those that induce or aggravate migraine attacks. Moreover, there are other factors common to both motion sickness and migraine: (1) females are more susceptible than males; (2) odors may trigger attacks; (3) there is increased susceptibility during menses; and (4) vomiting, vertigo and headache are common to both syndromes (Money, 1970). However, less is known about the mechanism of motion sickness than that of migraine, so that speculation about the nature of the relationship of these disorders is difficult.

Mitral Valve Prolapse

There is a remarkably high incidence of migraine among patients with mitral valve prolapse (Litman and Friedman, 1978), a disorder predominantly of young women. The symptoms of paroxysmal tachycardia, syncope and vertigo are common to both conditions, and propranolol is effective in the treatment of both. (Naggar, 1979).

Transient ischemic attacks and cerebral infarction also occur in patients with the mitral valve prolapse syndrome for reasons that are not yet clear (Barnett et al, 1976). Platelet adherence and aggregation may occur at the altered margins of prolapsed valves and this may result in the formation of a platelet fibrin embolus, but supportive evidence for this mechanism has not been obtained. Whether the cerebral ischemic events in these patients are embolic in mechanism or caused by the vasomotor dysregulation that characterizes migraine is not clear. A possibly related problem is the high (33 per cent) incidence of transient monocular visual obscurations in patients with rheumatic heart disease (Swash and Earl, 1970).

Prosthetic Cardiac Valve

Five patients have been described who, several months after the insertion of a prosthetic heart valve, developed transient focal neurologic symptoms with or without headache that were highly characteristic of migraine (Caplan et al, 1976). No valvular dysfunction could be demonstrated and the administration of anticoagulant drugs was of no benefit. The syndrome was self-limited to a period of several months and remains unexplained; it appears to be analogous to the mitral valve prolapse syndrome.

PAGET'S DISEASE

Whereas the skull is a frequent site of involvement of Paget's disease, headache is an uncommon complaint in such cases. Two patients have been described: one developed migraine *de novo*, and the second reported a marked worsening of lifelong migraine, concurrent with the appearance of Paget's disease of the skull (Hamilton and Quesada, 1973). Ergotamine tartrate and methysergide were ineffective, but in both patients headache attacks were impressively improved after partial control of the Paget's disease with calcitonin or mithramycin, and not after placebo injections.

Paget's disease is associated with increased blood flow to involved osseous structures; this was clinically evident in both of the aforementioned patients by cranial bruits, bounding scalp artery pulses, and by angiographically dilated meningeal and extracranial arteries. Both individuals were genetically disposed to migraine, and Paget's disease may have unmasked this predisposition.

ADRENAL DYSFUNCTION

One patient with lifelong migraine reported a worsening of her headache attacks concurrent with the development of Conn's syndrome. Following subtotal adrenalectomy the migraine attacks ceased (Stanford and Greene, 1970). Similarly, Cushing's syndrome and the hypoadrenal state following steroid withdrawal may be the source of *de novo* migraine headaches (Graham, 1976). The adrenal regulation of tryptophan hydroxylase activity, the rate-limiting catalyst of serotonin synthesis in brain (Costa and Meek, 1974), may contribute to the mechanism of headache in these circumstances.

HEMODIALYSIS

Headache occurs with varying degrees of severity during dialysis in about 70 per cent of dialyzed patients. The commonest form of "dialysis headache" is the precipitation of migraine headaches in those with pre-existing migraine. Other patients without previous headache disorders experience headache only in association with dialysis, usually during the third or fourth hour. It is usually reported as bilateral and throbbing, without focal neurologic symptoms (Bana et al, 1972). Headaches may disappear after nephrectomy or after a successful transplant; if the latter is subsequently rejected, headache may reappear as a symptom of rejection and may continue until nephrectomy is carried out (Graham, 1976). There is some evidence that arterial renin and 18-hydroxy-11-deoxycorticosterone levels, obtained during hemodialysis, are lower in patients who are subject to headache (Graham, 1976; Bana and Graham, 1976, 1978). However, the preponderance of evidence points to shifts of water into the brain as the major cause of "dysequilibrium," the term denoting a conglomeration of symptoms, including headache, that occur during or after dialysis (Arieff et al, 1978).

The mechanism of these symptoms was originally believed to be based on the lag in the reduction of brain urea compared to the rate of reduction of blood urea because of the influence of the blood-brain barrier. This effect was thought to produce an osmotic gradient between blood and brain, resulting in movement of water into brain leading to cerebral edema, increased intracranial pressure and symptoms of encephalopathy. This hypothesis became known as the reverse urea effect, and the unequal effects of dialysis upon tissue and blood solutes, resulting in an osmotic gradient, underlies the naming of this disorder "the dysequilibrium syndrome." Experimental models of dysequilibrium support the hypothesis that osmotically active substances ("idiogenic osmoles") are present in brain in the dialyzed uremic animal (and not in the dialyzed non-uremic animal), creating an osmotic gradient between brain and blood that results in shifts of water into brain (Raskin and Fishman, 1976). The nature of the idiogenic osmoles is not clear, although there is some evidence that this moiety comprises middle-to-large-sized molecules. It is now clear that the amount of urea transiently retained in brain is not sufficient to account for cerebral edema, nor are alterations in brain or plasma sodium likely to underlie dysequilibrium. The marked lowering of CSF pH that occurs in dialyzed uremic animals may reflect the cerebral accumulation of organic acids, and such osmotically active solutes may also be important to the genesis of the neurologic disturbances that take place in relation to hemodialysis.

HYPERLIPIDEMIA

Migraine probably occurs with a higher-than-chance frequency among patients with hyperlipidemias. Restoration of serum lipids to normal levels with clofibrate dramatically improved the headache problem in a well-studied patient (Leviton and Camenga, 1969). Whether the alteration in serum viscosity that accompanies hyperlipidemia is important to the trigger mechanism of headache is not clear.

HYPERAMMONEMIA

Russell (1973) administered ammonium loads to 15 children with migraine and cyclical vomiting; in eight there was an abnormally high rise in blood ammonium levels, and in six migraine attacks were provoked. Seven of the children with abnormal ammonium tolerance tests were studied further and were found to have lower-than-normal activities of ornithine transcarbamylase (OTC) in jejunal mucosal biopsy specimens, which was believed to be an indication that they were heterozygotes of OTC deficiency. Liver biopsies were not obtained and it is not entirely clear how or whether urea cycle enzyme defects bear on the problem of migraine. Ammonia intoxication in monkeys results in cerebral vasomotor paralysis, i.e., a loss of autoregulation (Altenau, 1977), and this phenomenon may explain the precipitation of migraine in these children.

MIGRAINOUS SYNDROMES

Transient disturbance of cerebral function occurs in over 60 per cent of migraine attacks. Visual disturbances are the commonest of these symptoms, occurring in almost 40 per cent of patients (Hachinski et al, 1973), but the frequency and nature of the other neurologic symptoms that may accompany headache attacks is not generally appreciated.

VISUAL PHENOMENA

The moving shapes often experienced upon closing the eyes, the light sensation upon opening them, and the fine moving particles sometimes seen against a uniform background are normal physiologic phenomena that almost always are very brief in duration (Priestly and Foree, 1955; Nebel, 1957). The visual displays that arise during migraine can take several forms but are likely to be stereotyped for the same individual. In over 75 per cent of patients visual hallucinations appear in both visual fields, and are of unformed objects or shapes (stars, spots, circles, angles), suggesting a disturbance of the occipital lobe which is within the distribution of supply of the posterior cerebral artery. In 15 per cent there are illusions of altered size, shape or position of structured objects (metamorphopsia) and/or frank hallucinations of structured objects, characteristic of a disturbance of function of the posterior temporal lobe (optic radiation) which is within the distribution of the middle cerebral artery. In approximately 5 per cent the visual symptoms are monocular, suggesting a prechiasmal disturbance in the distribution of the ophthalmic artery (Hachinski et al, 1973).

PHOTOPSIA AND TEICHOPSIA

Flashes of color, wavy lines, heat waves, spots or stars, very often appearing in the central portion of the visual fields, but sometimes occurring temporally or dispersed throughout the entire visual field, are the commonest visual hallucinations, accounting for over 75 per cent of the visual symptoms reported by migraineurs (Lance and Anthony, 1966). Many patients report that the most accurate simile for their symptoms is that of the visual experience that follows the ignition of a flash bulb. These last for varying time intervals — seconds to several minutes — and are more likely to occur concurrent with the most severe headaches than as premonitory symptoms. The figures are sometimes described as pulsatile, but more commonly they flicker, shine, sparkle or shimmer; the margins most often are well defined. Rapid postural change, whether a migraine attack is in progress or not, such as in reaching for the soap on the shower floor and standing up quickly, may reproduce a migraineur's teichopsia (Raskin and Knittle, 1976). The teichopic figures very often move within the visual field, but on occasion are stationary. As noted above, they almost invariably persist when the eyes are closed, consistent with their cerebral, and not retinal, origin.

OBSCURATION

Total blindness is not uncommon, occurring more frequently than homonymous hemianopia, but precise statistics are lacking. In many patients visual loss begins bitemporally and progresses to involve the binasal fields in a slow march. Others report a central scotoma that slowly enlarges until the entire field of vision is obscured; the blind area is often surrounded by or contains sparkling zigzag figures, a "scintillating scotoma." Still others report sudden total blindness. Occasionally the visual field is only partially obscured as a "grayout" or as if a thick black film were being held before the eyes, so that shapes may continue to be perceived. Infrequently, patients have reported that within the blind visual field several "holes" of clear vision are preserved, so that they attempt to see during these interludes by scanning their environment. Very often, within the darkened visual field, hallucinated bright figures are present, sometimes transiently and recurrently. Some patients experience this kind of visual disturbance as a "whiteout" in which their vision is obscured by a dazzling, bright white light; such whiteouts are highly characteristic of migraine and take place much less commonly in vertebrobasilar insufficiency. Altitudinal and quadrantic visual field defects also occur, but are much less common.

Monocular amblyopia, or amaurosis fugax, also arises in migraine and must be distinguished from embolic transient ischemic attacks, temporal arteritis and occlusion of the central retinal artery. An embolic ischemic attack in the carotid distribution producing monocular amblyopia is often described as a black curtain slowly descending or ascending until vision is obscured (Marshall and Meadows, 1968); retinal artery occlusion is usually an acute, single event, and the visual symptoms are sometimes reported as a pattern of horizontal "venetian blinds" crossing the visual field of one eye. These two latter visual syndromes fortunately are rare in migraine. A monocular visual whiteout is very likely to be migrainous in mechanism.

DISTORTIONS AND HALLUCINATIONS

The illusion that people or objects are smaller (micropsia) or larger (macropsia) than normal without change in their proportions is the commonest metamorphoptic symptom. Occasionally, patients experience an alteration of their own body size, feeling unusually large or small; many describe leaving their bodies and viewing themselves from above (Klee, 1975). Some report that a scene turns upside down or that an hallucinated person walks by tilted or upside down, or that the entire environment tilts. Rarely, there are elaborate hallucinations (Fig. 2–1), such as seeing oneself lying on a railroad track with a train about to roll by. Other symptoms referable to temporal lobe dysfunction, not necessarily visual in nature, are worth noting here. *Déjà vu* and *jamais vu*, the overwhelming sensations that the present circumstances or scene have already occurred or have never occurred, respectively, arise on occasion as migrainous symptoms.

FORTIFICATION SPECTRA

Probably the visual disturbance most characteristic and easily recognized by most physicians, the typical spectral march of fortification figures, occurs in only 10 per cent of migraine patients (Lance and Anthony, 1966). Several detailed and precise accounts of this symptom complex, all remarkable for their similarity, have been written by migraineurs (Lashley, 1941; Hare, 1966; Richards, 1971; Airing, 1972). In about 50 per cent of patients who report fortification spectra, the syndrome begins with an ill-defined alteration of visual acuity shortly followed by hallucinated unformed figures throughout the visual fields, usually with a preponderance for one-half of the visual field (Baumgartner, 1977). Seconds to minutes following these symptoms, a small, indefinitely circumscribed paracentral scotoma appears and slowly expands into a "C" or horseshoe shape. Luminous 45°

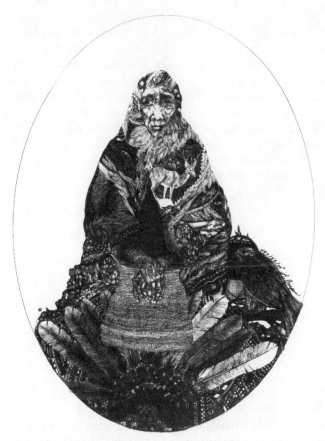

Figure 2-1. Reproduction of the visual hallucination of an artist-migraineur. The complex intricate detail of the hallucination suggests temporal lobe malfunction. (*From* Atkinson, R. A. and Appenzeller, O. 1978: Headache *17*:229–232. Reproduced by permission of the editor of Headache.)

angles appear at the enlarging outer edge, becoming more distinct, larger, and colored or prismatic as the scintillating scotoma drifts slowly toward the periphery of the involved half visual field at the rate of 3 mm per minute (Fig. 2–2). Some patients describe several C-shaped arcs of serrated fortification figures within the advancing scotoma. The bright zigzags usually oscillate in brightness at a fast rate, 10 cycles per second, early in the attack, and then become constant at about 5 cycles per second; their angles increase to about 70° as they reach the periphery of the visual field. The scintillating scotoma appears to expand with increasing speed as if growing larger, until it eventually disappears over the horizon of peripheral vision, the entire process usually consuming 20 to 25 minutes; its termination may be followed by a headache that is usually contralateral to the involved visual field. The putative neuronal mechanism underlying fortification spectra is discussed in Chapter 3. Although these spectra often occur without an ensuing headache, this phenomenon has never been reported to take place *during* the headache phase of a migraine attack; this temporal sequence is also the rule for other neurologic symptoms that are complex and highly organized, such as structured hallucinations and metamorphopsia.

Inquiries of patients regarding the presence or absence of visual symptoms should be made fairly directly, somewhat contrary to the general principles of eliciting a medical history. General nondirective questions, such as whether the patient experiences any visual abnormalities in association with headache attacks, are often met with false-negative responses for several reasons:

(1) Patients have often had visual hallucinations from an early age, have been assured of their benignity and, not unreasonably, do not regard such phenomena as abnormalities;

(2) Many patients experience visual symptoms only infrequently and briefly, in association with their most severe headaches or dissociated temporally from their headache attacks, so that they may not have connected these symptoms with their headache disorder;

(3) Everyone in the patient's family experiences these symptoms so that they long ago assumed them to be universal and irrelevant.

In view of these influences, it is the authors' practice to inquire directly as to the occurrence, *with* or *without headache*, of "sparkles,"

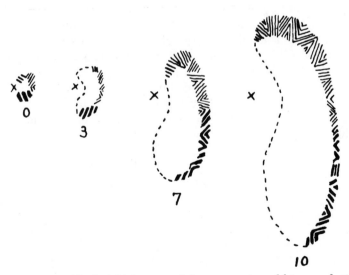

Figure 2-2. Lashley's (1941) maps of the progression of his own fortification spectra at varying time intervals after the onset of a migrainous attack. The "X" in each instance indicates the visual fixation point. The numbers represent minutes. (*From* Lashley, K.S., 1941: Arch. Neurol. Psychiatry 46:331–339. Copyright 1941, American Medical Association: reproduced with permission.)

heat waves, visual fuzziness or clouds, grayouts, whiteouts, zigzags or spots; asking whether such symptoms have ever occurred after rapid postural change may further jog a patient's memory for what he has regarded as an inconsequential phenomenon. If there is any doubt about a false-positive response, further inquiries as to the portion of the visual field involved, size, shape, color, quantity and duration of hallucinated figures, the effects of eye closure, and the temporal relationship to headache usually leave no doubt as to the validity of the symptom. The false-positive response frequency is remarkably low.

PARESTHESIA

Unilateral paresthesia in association with headache is reported by one-third of patients with migraine attacks (Table 2–4); it is described most commonly as tingling or numbness in the hand or forearm, but numbness of both hands, all four limbs, half the face and the perioral area, and hemihypesthesia, are also reported (Heyck, 1973). These symptoms are usually transient, persisting for several seconds to 20 minutes, but occasionally they last several hours and (rarely) days; they bear the same significance in establishing the diagnosis of migraine as do the more characteristic visual symptoms.

The distribution of paresthesias shows a peculiar preference for the face and hand (Bruyn, 1968). The ulnar digits are more often involved than the other fingers, and numbness may slowly progress proximally to the elbow, skip the rest of the upper limb and neck, and appear around the mouth, involving half the tongue, lips and buccal mucosa, and occasionally the cheek and nose. This distribution of numbness has differential diagnostic value; in carotid TIAs that result in hemihypesthesia, numbness of half the inside of the mouth, including the tongue, is quite rare. The slow spread of sensory symptoms is comparable to the march of fortification spectra, and usually requires 10 to 20 minutes for its full expression. This is considerably slower than the sensory march that may be an expression of focal epilepsy.

HEMIPLEGIC MIGRAINE

Attacks of frank paralysis of the limbs of one side in association with headache is uncommon, but those cases described appear to fall into two groups. In one, hemiparesis is one of the features of the prodromal phase, with recovery in 20 to 30 minutes, like the visual symptoms, as the headache begins; the affected side may vary from attack to attack. In the other group, hemiparesis usually affects the same side consistently; it persists for hours or days, long after headache subsides, and is associated with a strong family history of highly comparable attacks (Whitty, 1953; Parrish and Stevens, 1977). The term *familial hemiplegic migraine* has been used to denote this latter group, in which the pattern of affected family members suggests autosomal dominant inheritance (Glista et al., 1975).

In both groups headache usually follows the onset of hemiparesis and is ipsilateral in about one-third of the patients. Dysarthria and/or aphasia occurs in over 50 per cent of patients in association with hemiparesis, and the sensorium is impaired in one-third (Heyck, 1973). Hemihypesthesia accompanies hemiparesis in virtually every case (Bradshaw and Parsons, 1965). Of 17 lumbar punctures performed during hemiparetic episodes, three CSF specimens contained excessive leukocytes, 185, 10 and 124 cells/mm^3 (Bradshaw and Parsons, 1965). Cerebral angiography performed during hemiparetic attacks has revealed no abnormalities. Computerized axial tomography performed during and between attacks has been normal in most patients (Masland et al, 1978) but Mathew (1978) has found one or more low-density areas in several of those with complicated migraine. Presumably because of prolonged neuronal ischemia, persisting hemiparesis occasionally occurs, and probably represents cerebral infarction.

In general, hemiplegic migrainous attacks take place infrequently and irregularly, so that management with daily preventive vasoactive drugs usually is not elected; systematic studies of the effectiveness of these drugs in complicated migraine have not been done. There is preliminary uncontrolled evidence that propranolol (Glista et al, 1975) and papaverine (Vijayan, 1977) are effective in preventing attacks of complicated migraine. Although migraine therapy will be dealt with separately, this special circumstance, when it occurs, often poses a dilemma to the physician who is concerned about using ergotamine tartrate, a drug that constricts arteries, for a circumstance in which the effects of cerebral ischemia are dramatic. Edmeads (1977) and Hachinski et al (1978) have summarized the literature regarding CBF studies performed on patients during migrainous attacks, and the effects of ergotamine; the intracerebral carotid circulation appears to be unaffected by therapeutically effective parenteral doses of ergotamine tartrate. Moreover, Sakai and Meyer (1978) have confirmed these findings, and have also found that ergotamine reduces cerebral hyperperfusion in the basilar artery distribution to normal but not subnormal levels. Heyck (1973) noted that, in one patient who had had hemiplegic attacks that lasted for up to three hours, the duration of the attacks was shortened to 30 minutes or less on 50 occasions by the intravenous administration of dihydroergotamine. Simard and Paulson (1973) showed that 1 mg of intravenous ergotamine had no effect on regional CBF during a prolonged migrainous aura, nor three months later, when the patient was asymptomatic. However, in one of the patients of Bradshaw and Parsons

(1965) a severe hemiplegic attack may have been triggered that did not completely resolve after the parenteral administration of a large (0.75-mg) dose of ergotamine. More data are necessary to completely resolve this important therapeutic issue. At the moment, the evidence points to the relative safety of ergotamine in the presence of cerebral vasoconstriction, if used in judicious dosage.

OPHTHALMOPLEGIC MIGRAINE

There are occasional patients who report infrequent attacks of orbital or periorbital pain that usually radiates to the hemicranium, is often accompanied by vomiting, and lasts one to four days. Concurrent with this pain, or more often as it subsides, ipsilateral ptosis appears, and within the next several hours a complete third nerve palsy becomes evident, usually including pupillary dilatation. Occasionally, the sixth nerve or the ophthalmic division of the fifth nerve also may be involved (Pearce, 1975). After the headache ceases, the ophthalmoplegia usually persists for several days, with a range of 45 minutes to two months (Cruciger and Mazow, 1978). The ophthalmoplegia usually resolves completely, but after many attacks some extraocular muscle paresis may persist. Occasionally, attacks on alternating sides occur. The age-relatedness of this disorder is similar to the more common forms of migraine, many patients experiencing their first attack below the age of 12 years (Friedman et al, 1962; Bickerstaff, 1964). Several infants with this disorder have been reported (Robertson and Schnitzler, 1978); however, adults in the fourth and fifth decade also may develop their first attack (Pearce, 1968). Ophthalmoplegic migraine is usually, but not always, preceded by a history of more common forms of migraine.

The fact that this syndrome may involve the oculomotor nerves and the ophthalmic division of the fifth nerve suggests that the anatomic localization of the lesion is close to the cavernous sinus. Angiographic evidence of constriction of the internal carotid artery in the region of the cavernous sinus has been demonstrated in a few patients during attacks of ophthalmoplegic migraine (Walsh and O'Doherty, 1960; Bickerstaff, 1964). It seems reasonable to suppose that edema of the internal carotid artery wall could account for the angiographic findings and result in compression of neighboring cranial nerves. The shortening of ophthalmoplegic attacks in two patients with intravenous norepinephrine (Ostfeld and Wolff, 1957), a vasoconstrictor, supports the possibility that dilated arteries produce the neural compression that may result in ophthalmoplegia.

Ophthalmoplegic migraine is rare, and more common causes of recurring painful ophthalmoplegia include internal carotid aneurysm; the Tolosa-Hunt syndrome; diabetic ophthalmoplegia; sphenoid sinus infection or tumor; and meningeal inflammation due to syphilis, tuberculosis, fungi and carcinoma.

BASILAR MIGRAINE

Symptoms referable to a disturbance of brain stem function are common during migrainous attacks, occurring as the only neurologic symptoms of the attack in about 25 per cent of patients (Lance and Anthony, 1966). However, a stereotyped sequence of dramatic neurologic events, often involving total blindness and an alteration of consciousness, followed by headache, arises more often than is reflected by the literature on the subject, and is deserving of attention.

Although the syndrome of basilar migraine was recognized by Aretaeus, Bickerstaff (1961a,b, 1962) called attention to it when he culled 34 patients with this disorder out of a consecutive series of 300 patients with migraine, giving an incidence of over 10 per cent. Twenty-six of his patients were adolescent girls and all were under the age of 35 years; he noted that these attacks often occurred in relationship to menstruation. The episodes usually began with blindness, or with the appearance of a vivid visual hallucination of unformed images or photopsia involving the whole of the visual fields, so as completely to obscure vision; this was accompanied or followed by varying admixtures of vertigo, ataxia, dysarthria, tinnitus, and distal and perioral paresthesias. In eight patients the appearance of neurologic symptoms heralded a gradual loss of consciousness which was sometimes preceded by a curious dreamlike, confusional state. The degree of obtundation was not profound, and developed despite the patients' lying flat; they generally were rousable with vigorous stimulation. The neurologic segment of the attack usually persisted for 10 to 30 minutes (the range was two to 45 minutes), and upon its cessation a severe throbbing headache, usually occipital, appeared, often accompanied by vomiting, and lasted for hours or until the patient went to sleep. For most of these patients these dramatic attacks occurred only infrequently, and more common forms of migraine had taken place before and between the attacks. The basilar attacks tended to cease with time and appeared to be replaced by common migraine.

Several additional examples of this syndrome have been recorded (Watson and Steele, 1974; Golden and French, 1975; Lapkin et al, 1977) and in one instance an attack was captured electroencephalographically. Whereas the EEG before the attack was normal, high rates (20 per second) of photic stimulation induced a basilar attack accompanied by unconsciousness, during which a discharge of regular repetitive spikes at four per second developed in both occipital regions, persisting for 40 seconds after flash stimulation had ceased (Swanson and Vick, 1978). Paroxysmal responses such as this are consistent with cerebral hyperexcitability and most often are found in, but not restricted to, patients with epilepsy. Ziegler and Wong (1967) found that as many as 33 per cent of migrainous children develop paroxysmal EEG responses after photic activation. However, this response may also be found in individuals who have never had a seizure.

The generation of cortical excitability by the attack may explain why seizures occur during some attacks of basilar migraine (Lee and Lance, 1977; Emery, 1977; Camfield et al, 1978) sometimes, but not always, in patients with co-existing epilepsy. The fact that cerebral ischemia may serve as a precipitant of an epileptic attack in a patient with a lowered seizure threshold (epilepsy) has been amply documented (Basser, 1969). For many patients this is the only circumstance in which convulsions occur and, although rigorous data have not been collected on this point, the authors have seen six individuals whose headache-associated convulsive attacks ceased concurrent with prophylactic therapy with propranolol or ergonovine maleate, and who had failed to respond to phenytoin, phenobarbital or primidone. It is possible that these patients are predisposed to cortical electrical discharges by their genetic constitution, especially in view of data revealing an increased incidence of epilepsy in the migrainous patient population. Until these data become clearer, the potentially important therapeutic inference noted above should not be overlooked.

The basilar migraine syndrome, it is now clear, is not confined to adolescent girls; children (Lapkin and Golden, 1978) as well as patients as old as 56 years have been reported, and the accompanying headache is often hemicranial in location. The sensorial alterations that occur during an attack, although usually brief, may last for as long as five days; they may take the form of confusional states that appear to be psychotic reactions during which agitated, aggressive and hysterical behavior may be seen (Gascon and Barlow, 1970; Emery, 1977; Lee and Lance, 1977; Ehyai and Fenichel, 1978). Three out of seven of the patients of Lee and Lance (1977) manifested unilaterally dilated pupils during their attacks. In children, minor head trauma may produce a syndrome indistinguishable from basilar migraine that develops minutes to hours following the traumatic event (Haas et al, 1975).

Substantial evidence favors brain stem ischemia as the mechanism of this syndrome. The midbrain appears to be at least one ischemic site, since it contains both the third nerve nuclei (pupillary dilatation) and the reticular activating system (alteration in consciousness). Hauge (1954), in a study of the symptoms that accompany selective angiography of the vertebral artery, virtually reproduced the spectrum of symptoms and signs that have been recorded as features of basilar migraine, including occipital headache, visual hallucinations, stupor and alterations in pupillary size. The inhalation of 5-per-cent carbon dioxide, a potent cerebral vasodilator, has improved a patient's stuporous state, with subsequent deterioration when the inhalation ceased (Lee and Lance, 1977). Moreover, although this syndrome is usually benign, at least one fatality has occurred; pathologic examination of this case revealed brain stem infarction (Guest and Woolf, 1964). Visualization of the posterior circulation with angiography interictally has been unrevealing, even in the presence of a fixed neurologic deficit (Connor, 1962; Pearce and Foster, 1965).

It should be noted that loss of consciousness and confusional states are not restricted to patients who report symptoms referable to the basilar artery territory; these symptoms also occur often in association with symptoms referable to the perfusion area of the internal carotid artery (Lance and Anthony, 1966). It appears likely that migraine is not a disorder of only one major artery and its branches, but rather that it commonly affects multiple loci of the cerebral circulation, with focal symptoms resulting from ischemia of the brain most prominently involved during an attack. Sakai and Meyer (1978) have provided evidence that supports this clinical inference; in at least one patient studied during the prodromal phase of a migraine attack, regional blood flow was diffusely reduced, but the maximal reduction occurred focally in the area of brain corresponding to the neurologic symptoms. Focal impairment of cerebral autoregulation has also been found (Marshall, 1978).

Alterations of the posterior circulation during migraine, not evident by earlier methods of measurement of CBF, may have importance in regard to the mechanism of the headache phase during migraine attacks. Therapeutically effective doses of ergotamine tartrate do not decrease cerebral hemispheric flow, but markedly decrease the hyperfusion present in the basilar artery territory (Sakai and Meyer, 1978). Since the mode of action of ergotamine in migraine remains unclear, further studies will be necessary to clarify the meaning of these data; it is possible that the drug exerts a selective effect upon certain dilated cerebral arteries and/or upon brain stem serotonergic neurons that may regulate arterial tone.

CAROTIDYNIA

The term "carotidynia" (lower half headache, facial migraine) was first used by Fay (1932) 50 years ago to denote a syndrome comprising facial pain and other symptoms that he judged to be atypical facial neuralgia. This latter disorder remains poorly understood today and its vagaries have resulted, until recently, in some uncertainty about its nature. Carotidynia is more prominent in an older population of patients, with peak incidence in the fourth through sixth decades, and is much more common in women.

Pain is usually reported to be located at the jaw or neck, although sometimes periorbital or maxillary pain occurs; it is deep, dull and aching, and becomes throbbing or pounding episodically. Occasionally, there are also sharp, icepick-like jabs. Attacks take place from one to several times per week, each one lasting minutes to hours. Tenderness and prominent pulsations of the cervical carotid artery, and soft tissue swelling overlying the carotid, are usually present ipsilateral to the pain, and many patients also report throbbing ipsilateral headache concurrent with carotidynia attacks as well as interictally (Lovshin, 1977; Raskin and Prusiner, 1977). Dental trauma appears to be a common precipitant of this syndrome.

Head and neck pain may result from electric stimulation of the carotid artery wall at its bifurcation (Fig. 2–3); there may be pain in the teeth and gums, eye, nose, scalp, cheek and jaw, depending on the precise area of the carotid artery that is stimulated (Fay, 1932). Thus, carotid artery wall lesions may result in pain about the face, head and neck, and this phenomenon probably explains the symptoms of carotidynia. The episodic pain associated with tenderness and dilatation

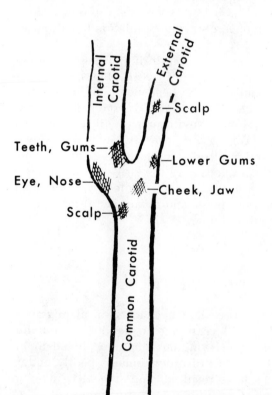

Figure 2-3. Effect of electric stimulation of the carotid artery at its bifurcation. Hatched areas show specific sites of pain referral, as determined by the patient during stimulation. (*From* Raskin, N.H. and Prusiner, S., 1977: Neurology 27:43–46. Reproduced by permission of the editor of Neurology.)

of the carotid artery in this syndrome appears to be analogous to the episodic hemicranial pain more easily recognized as migraine, which is often associated with tenderness and pulsation of the superficial temporal artery. Further support for the relatedness of carotidynia to migraine stems from the therapeutic responsiveness of the former to vasoactive drugs such as ergotamine tartrate (Lovshin, 1960), methysergide, and nortriptyline (Raskin and Prusiner, 1977).

As a corollary to these observations, over 50 per cent of patients with frequent migraine headaches have been found to have tenderness of the carotid artery at several points ipsilateral to the cranial side preponderantly involved during their attacks. In 100 consecutively examined patients with neurologic problems other than headache, carotid tenderness was not found (Raskin and Prusiner, 1977). The differential diagnosis of recurring carotid artery pain includes dissecting cervical carotid aneurysm (Fisher et al, 1978), thrombosis of the internal carotid artery, giant cell arteritis, and post-traumatic neck pain (Vijayan and Dreyfus, 1975); however, carotidynia is probably the commonest cause of this syndrome.

CHILDHOOD MIGRAINE

Migraine is probably the commonest cause of recurring headache in children. Krupp and Friedman (1953) found that, of 100 children with recurring headache, migraine was apparent in 75 and tension headache in 17. Millichap (1978) noted migraine to be the cause of chronic recurring headache in 42 of 100 children and tension headache in 18. Migraine has been relatively neglected in the pediatric literature, however, largely because of a disproportionate concern with emotional sources of headache, and failure to consider anxiety as a precipitating factor rather than an etiologic factor in children with chronic headache disorders. Although rigorous psychologic data have not been obtained, psychogenic headaches appear to be uncommon before adolescence (Barlow, 1978).

Acute migrainous attacks in children are quite similar phenomenologically to those that occur later in life; however, some of the differences are notable (Table 2–7). About 60 per cent of children with migraine are male. The attacks tend to be shorter in duration, lasting for fractions of an hour to several hours, and rarely more than 12 hours; vomiting is usually more prominent. Lateralization of headache and visual symptoms occur with lower frequencies, and the incidence of convulsions between headache episodes is considerably higher (Prensky, 1976). Visible pulsation of the temporal arteries during attacks is rare. Vertigo, motion-sickness and lightheadedness, both in association with headache and interictally, are common (Fenichel, 1967), and there appears to be a greater-than-chance coincidence of

TABLE 2-7. FEATURES DISTINCTIVE
OF CHILDHOOD MIGRAINE

Male preponderance
Shorter attacks, prominent vomiting
Interictal seizure incidence of 10 per cent
Common equivalents: abdominal pain, cyclic vomiting, vertigo
Sleep disturbances
Minor head trauma a common trigger
Favorable prognosis

sleep disturbances that include bedwetting, night terrors and sleep-walking (Bille, 1962). Cycles of frequent and severe headaches usually last less than 6 months (Prensky and Sommer, 1979).

The commonest precipitants of migraine attacks in children are school stress and changes in lighting, the latter including exposure to glare, television and motion pictures (Bille, 1967). Some children have found that attacks may be prevented by sitting farther away from the motion-picture screen or by increasing the illumination in the television room. Children who are light-sensitive commonly report headache developing upon leaving the motion-picture theater and encountering the glare of broad daylight, suggesting that the dark–light transition under conditions of dark adaptation is an important trigger factor. In addition, physical exertion, hunger, noise, traveling, and cold weather (Congdon and Forsythe, 1979) are among the more common precipitants, whereas food and allergies are very uncommon trigger factors. The first appearance of migraine after minor head injury appears to be more common in children than in adults (Haas et al, 1975).

Two common periodic syndromes of childhood (Cullen and Mac-Donald, 1963), cyclic vomiting and periodic abdominal pain, are probably migraine equivalents. Cyclic vomiting episodes, sometimes associated with abdominal pain, headache and fever, and lasting hours to days, occur predominantly in school-age children. Approximately 75 per cent of children with cyclic vomiting develop unequivocal migraine in later years (Hammond, 1974). Periodic abdominal pain may occur in association with vomiting and fever, so that the boundaries between these two syndromes are indistinct. The episodes are generally briefer, lasting for several minutes, and convulsions take place frequently among these children either in association with abdominal pain or between attacks. Paroxysmal electroencephalograms are seen in over 20 per cent of these children, which is significantly higher than in their migrainous peers (Prensky, 1976).

The distinction between abdominal pain as a migraine equivalent and as an epileptic equivalent may not be obvious, and responsiveness to anticonvulsants is not a useful way of discerning between the two mechanisms, since children with migraine derive substantial benefit from these drugs (Millichap, 1978). Migraine appears to be far more common than epilepsy as a cause of recurring abdominal pain in children (Barlow, 1978). In those children who do not develop convulsions in association with attacks of pain, the occurrence of seizure disorders later in life is rare, and their symptoms improve greatly or subside when they reach adolescence; they have a greater chance of developing typical migraine attacks than do control subjects (Apley and Hale, 1973). The evidence supports the conclusion that migraine constitutes an important mechanism of periodic abdominal pain in children; there probably is also a less frequent epileptic mechanism (Chao et al, 1964). A very brief episode without migrainous symptoms, associated with depression of the sensorium and a substrate of familial epilepsy, favors epilepsy, but the distinction can be difficult. It is possible that central neuronal excitability is a mechanism common to both migraine and epilepsy (see Chapter 4).

The natural history of childhood migraine appears to be more favorable than the adult-onset disorder. Bille (1962) reported on 67 patients who were 13 to 21 years of age, six years after the initial evaluation. Headache attacks had ceased in 51 per cent, 34 per cent had improved and 15 per cent were unimproved or worse. Hinrichs and Keith (1965) described 58 patients whose mean age was 21 years, nine to 14 years after the initial diagnosis was made. Cessation of headache had occurred in one-third, and 47 per cent had improved; substantially more males than females had improved. Hockaday's (1978) figures were not quite as hopeful; she reviewed 99 patients whose migrainous attacks began before the age of 20 years, eight to 25 years after the diagnosis was made. In 28 patients attacks had ceased, significantly more often in males than in females, and 52 others reported improvement. Only seven reported worsening and 12 no change. The preponderance of women in adult migraine may be due, at least in part, to the more favorable prognosis for cessation of migraine in boys.

The same general principles of therapy in migraine apply to children. Acute attacks are most easily controlled with simple analgesics taken early during an attack; the rectal suppository form of aspirin or acetaminophen is especially useful when nausea or vomiting preclude oral medication. For frequent severe headache, prophylaxis with vasoactive drugs seems to be as effective in children as in adults (Ludvigsson, 1974; Bille et al, 1977; Sillanpää and Koponen, 1978). Anticonvulsant drugs appear to be especially effective in this age group, and phenytoin or phenobarbital control over 70 per cent of childhood headache attacks; this effect is not related to the presence or absence of electroencephalographic abnormalities (Millichap, 1978; Barlow, 1978). After three to six months of control, medication should be slowly tapered, and reinstituted if headaches recur. There are no long-term outcome studies in children or adults regarding the effectiveness of prophylactic medication versus placebo.

PHYSICAL FINDINGS IN MIGRAINE

A tender cervical carotid artery, ipsilateral to the more severely affected hemicranium, is found between attacks in over 50 per cent of patients with frequent migrainous headaches (Raskin and Prusiner, 1977). Of those with point tenderness, approximately 10 per cent report that their head pain is transiently reproduced after carotid examination. This procedure is optimally carried out with the examiner standing behind the seated patient, with the latter's neck slightly flexed. There are no other physical signs of migraine interictally. A coincidental orbital bruit may be heard in about 2 per cent of patients (Selby and Lance, 1960). During an attack, there usually is prominence of the scalp arteries and veins, and facial pallor is evident, although some patients manifest facial suffusion. Although compression of a pulsating and dilated temporal artery often relieves the pain temporarily (Graham and Wolff, 1938), no systematic study of the effectiveness of this maneuver has been done; it is sometimes erroneously concluded that a headache is not vascular in mechanism because of a lack of response to this maneuver. Some patients develop distention of the scalp arteries to the point that they are tender, and in these instances manipulation is often met with worsening of the discomfort. These patients aside, it is the authors' experience that carotid or temporal artery compression is a diagnostic maneuver of low sensitivity, with positive responses of diminished pain in only 50 to 70 per cent of those examined during headache attacks. The maneuver itself can be controlled by compressing nonarterial structures, and it is useful to inquire, after compression is begun, whether the pain is worse. After digital compression is released there is invariably a lag period of several seconds after which pain resumes its former intensity; the presence of this lag is a further control of the validity of the response.

Occasionally, neck stiffness and Kernig's sign are present, and in a setting of vomiting, prostration and pallor may be confused with the features of meningitis or subarachnoid hemorrhage (Pearce and Foster, 1965). A lumbar puncture is almost always necessary in such patients. Complete recovery is the rule for such patients with "meningeal migraine," and the syndrome is not likely to recur (Pearce, 1975).

Slowed cerebration, irritability and somnolence accompany migraine attacks in many patients, and appear to be out of proportion to their level of pain or lack of attentiveness (Pearce, 1975). These symptoms are not readily explained by our current level of understanding of the vascular alterations that accompany migrainous attacks, and may eventually prove to be related to alterations of central neurotransmitter turnover.

LABORATORY INVESTIGATIONS

Whereas there are no objective studies of value in the clinical diagnosis of migraine, high frequencies of abnormalities are found in the electroencephalograms and visual-evoked potentials of patients subject to migraine attacks, which may have bearing on the pathogenesis of the disorder. Furthermore, the role of cerebral angiography and its hazards in the migrainous population is an issue that is often raised and will be considered here.

ELECTROENCEPHALOGRAPHY

The incidence of interictal EEG abnormalities in patients with migraine is about three times higher than the incidence of abnormalities in control subjects (Parsonage, 1975). However, there are no specific abnormalities peculiar to migraine, and the patterns range from normality to focal or generalized slow waves, spike-wave discharges, local spike or sharp waves, and abnormal responses to hyperventilation or to photic flash stimulation. Focal EEG abnormalities occur with highest frequency in patients with focal hemispheric symptoms accompanying their attacks, and is usually lateralized to the appropriate hemisphere (Hockaday and Whitty, 1969). Although focal slow waves have been recorded during the prodromal phase of migraine attacks, their occurrence is rare (Goldensohn, 1976). The incidence of EEG abnormality does not correlate with the duration or frequency of migraine attacks, data that neither support nor exclude the hypothesis that the EEG alterations are secondary to migraine attacks. However, the hypothesis that migraine is accompanied by a hyperexcitable nervous system is supported by the high incidence of dysrhythmic abnormalities and the exaggerated EEG responsiveness to high-frequency photic stimulation (Goldensohn, 1976).

VISUAL-EVOKED POTENTIALS

Among patients who sustain migrainous attacks accompanied or preceded by focal visual symptoms, visual-evoked potential latencies, obtained with pattern reversal stimuli, are prolonged compared to control subjects (Kennard et al, 1978) during headache-free periods. Repeated episodic ischemia to portions of the visual pathways may slow conduction velocity or depress synaptic transmission within the visual system, to explain these findings; alternatively, synaptic delay caused by alterations in neurotransmitter regulation that may underlie the mechanism of migraine may be important (MacLean et al, 1975).

However, the frequency of these abnormalities is not high enough to be useful diagnostically. The visual-evoked potential measurement is often used to assess patients for the possibility of multiple sclerosis, and the abnormalities noted above underline the nonspecificity of the test.

CEREBRAL ANGIOGRAPHY

The tenuous association of intracranial aneurysms or arteriovenous malformations and migraine is reviewed in Chapter 8. There are no compelling data that support an etiologic role for these vascular lesions in migraine, so that there is little reason to perform angiography in a patient who has experienced neither a subarachnoid hemorrhage nor epileptic attacks, and manifests a normal neurologic examination and a normal CAT scan. Furthermore, at a pragmatic level, the detection of an unruptured coincidental vascular anomaly in a patient whose sole problem is headache may convert a difficult management problem into a psychologic disaster! The ominous possibilities of subarachnoid hemorrhage, epilepsy and death present themselves in a situation in which surgical extirpation carries a high risk and uncertain benefit toward the original problem, headache.

For the patient whose diagnosis is not certain, and in whom the question of aneurysm arises because of the occurrence of ophthalmoplegia, for example, there is no doubt that angiography must be carried out. Early angiographic experiences when direct carotid puncture was employed in patients with migraine revealed a high morbidity (Patterson et al, 1964); direct carotid puncture now is rarely employed, and the risks may not be any greater than for age-matched control subjects.

SEQUELAE OF MIGRAINOUS ATTACKS

Transient low-density areas have been found in the CAT scans of several patients with migraine, especially those whose attacks were preceded by hemiplegia. The lesions were maximally visualized three to four days after the migrainous attack and persisted for at least two weeks (Mathew, 1978). These findings are consistent with cerebral edema or infarction, but the frequency of such abnormalities is not clear; reports of cortical atrophy or ventricular enlargement in patients with longstanding migraine have not been confirmed (Masland et al, 1978). Cerebral atrophy as seen on the CAT scan has yet to be correlated with postmortem atrophy, so that some caution should be exercised in interpreting the appearance of ventricular size by this relatively new diagnostic procedure.

Many individual cases of persisting hemiplegic, aphasic, hemianopic and retinal sequelae of migraine attacks have been described (Connor, 1962; Pearce and Foster, 1965; Pearce, 1975; Dorfman et al, 1979). Pathologic verification has been rare (Guest and Woolf, 1964; Buckle et al, 1964), revealing ischemic necrosis of neural tissue without vascular occlusion or thrombosis. It seems reasonable that focal ischemia on occasion may become prolonged and result in edema and infarction, but this occurs in patients whose previous migrainous attacks are unremarkable and in whom there is no demonstrable arterial disease (Pearce, 1968); the factors that determine the prolonged nature of the ischemic episode leading to infarction are unknown.

On the whole, fortunately, permanent sequelae from migraine are decidely rare even in those patients with hemiplegic migraine. When fixed deficits occur, they are usually, but not always, persisting focal neurologic syndromes that had arisen transiently many times over a period of years. However, there are many examples of patients whose permanent neurologic deficit was the first neurologic symptom experienced in association with an attack of migraine, or was in a vascular distribution that was different from preceding attacks (O'Connor, 1973). A curious clinical point has been made by Graveson (1949) and Symonds (1951): many patients who sustain fixed deficits continue to experience their prodromal symptoms, but these are never again followed by headache. This is analogous to patients who sustain atherosclerotic cerebral infarction (see Chapter 1) or giant cell arteritis (Russell, 1959), in whom headache ceases as the infarction becomes maximal. A clue to the mechanism of headache in migraine is undoubtedly buried within these observations, but it is presently obscure.

REFERENCES

Airing, C. D. (1972): The migrainous scintillating scotoma. J.A.M.A. 220:519–522.

Altenau, L. L. and Kindt, G. W. (1977): Cerebral vasomotor paralysis produced by ammonia intoxication. Acta Neurol. Scand. (suppl.) 64:19.2–19.3.

Apley, J. and Hale, B. (1973): Children with recurrent abdominal pain: how do they grow up? Br. Med. J. 3:7–9.

Arieff, A. I., Lazarowitz, V. C. and Guisado, R. (1978): Experimental dialysis dysequilibrium syndrome prevention with glycerol. Kidney Int. 14:270–278.

Atkinson, R. A. and Appenzeller, O. (1978): Deer woman. Headache 17:229–232.

Bana, D. S. and Graham, J. R. (1976): Renin response during hemodialysis headache. Headache 16:168–172.

Bana, D. S. and Graham, J. R. (1978): Plasma 18-hydroxy-11-deoxycorticosterone in dialysis patients with headache. Headache 18:23–25.

Bana, D. S., Yap, A. U. and Graham, J. R. (1972): Headache during hemodialysis. Headache 12:1–14.

Barlow, C. F. (1978): Migraine in childhood. Res. Clin. Stud. Headache 5:34–46.

Barnett, H. J. M., Jones, M. W., Boughner, D. R. and Kostuk, W. J. (1976): Cerebral ischemic events associated with prolapsing mitral valve. Arch. Neurol. 33:777–782.

Barolin, G. (1966): Migraines and epilepsies — a relationship? Epilepsia 7:53–66.
Barrie, M. A., Fox, W. R., Weatherall, M. and Wilkinson, M. I. P. (1968): Analysis of symptoms of patients with headaches and their response to treatment with ergot derivatives. Q. J. Med. 37:319–336.
Bärtschi-Rochaix, W. (1968): Headaches of cervical origin. In Handbook of Clinical Neurology, Vol. 5, eds. P. J. Vinken and G. W. Bruyn. John Wiley and Sons, New York, pp. 192–203.
Basser, L. S. (1969): The relation of migraine and epilepsy. Brain 92:285–300.
Baumgartner, G. (1977): Neuronal mechanisms of the migrainous visual aura. In Physiological Aspects of Clinical Neurology, ed. F. C. Rose. Blackwell, London, pp. 111–121.
Bickerstaff, E. R. (1961a): Basilar artery migraine. Lancet 1:15–17.
Bickerstaff, E. R. (1961b): Impairment of consciousness in migraine. Lancet 2:1057–1059.
Bickerstaff, E. R. (1962): The basilar artery and the migraine–epilepsy syndrome. R. Soc. Med. Proc. 55:167–169.
Bickerstaff, E. R. (1964): Ophthalmoplegic migraine. Rev. Neurol. 110:582–588.
Bille, B. (1962): Migraine in school children. Acta Paediatr. (suppl. 136) 51:14–151.
Bille, B. (1967): Juvenile headache; the natural history of headaches in children. In Headaches in Children, eds. A. P. Friedman and E. Harms. Charles C Thomas, Springfield, Ill., pp. 10–28.
Bille, B., Ludvigsson, J. and Sanner, G. (1977): Prophylaxis of migraine in children. Headache 17:61–63.
Birt, D. (1978): Headaches and head pains associated with diseases of the ear, nose, and throat. Med. Clin. North Am. 62:523–531.
Bradshaw, P. and Parsons, M. (1965): Hemiplegic migraine, a clinical study. Q. J. Med. 34:65–85.
Brain, W. R. (1963): Some unsolved problems of cervical spondylosis. Br. Med. J. 1:771–777.
Briggs, J. F. and Belloms, J. (1952): Precordial migraine. Dis. Chest. 21:635–640.
Broughton, R. (1971): Neurology and sleep research. Can. Psychiatr. Assoc. J. 16:283–293.
Bruyn, G. W. (1968): Complicated migraine. In Handbook of Clinical Neurology, Vol. 5, eds. P. J. Vinken and G. W. Bruyn. John Wiley and Sons, New York, pp. 59–95.
Buckle, R. M., duBoulay, G. and Smith, B. (1964): Death due to cerebral vasospasm. J. Neurol. Neurosurg. Psychiatry 27:440–444.
Callaghan, N. (1968): The migraine syndrome in pregnancy. Neurology 18:197–199.
Cameron, M. E. (1976): Headaches in relation to the eyes. Med. J. Aust. 1:292–294.
Camfield, P. R., Metrakos, K. and Andermann, F. (1978): Basilar migraine, seizures, and severe epileptiform EEG abnormalities. Neurology 28:584–588.
Campbell, D. A., Hay, K. M. and Tonks, E. M. (1951): An investigation of the salt and water balance in migraine. Br. Med. J. 2:1424–1429.
Caplan, L.-R., Weiner, H., Weintraub, R. M. and Austen, W. G. (1976): "Migrainous" neurologic dysfunction in patients with prosthetic cardiac valves. Headache 16:218–221.
Carey, H. M. (1971): Principles of oral contraception. 2. Side effects of oral contraceptives. Med. J. Aust. 2:1242–1250.
Catino, D. (1965): Ten migraine equivalents. Headache 5:1–11.
Chao, D., Sexton, J. A. and Davis, S. D. (1964): Convulsive equivalent syndrome of childhood. J. Pediatr. 64:499–508.
Collaborative Group for the Study of Stroke in Young Women (1973): Oral contraception and increased risk of cerebral ischemia or thrombosis. N. Engl. J. Med. 288:871–878.
Congdon, P. J. and Forsythe, W. I. (1979): Migraine in childhood: A study of 300 children. Develop. Med. Child. Neurol. 21:209–216.
Connor, R. C. R. (1962): Complicated migraine. A study of permanent neurological and visual defects caused by migraine. Lancet 2:1072–1075.
Cooper, J. R., Bloom, F. E. and Roth, R. H. (1978): Serotonin (5-hydroxytryptamine). In The Biochemical Basis of Neuropharmacology, 3rd ed. Oxford University Press, New York, pp. 196–222.

Costa, E. and Meek, J. (1974): Regulation of the biosynthesis of catecholamines and serotonin in the CNS. Annu. Rev. Pharmacol. 14:491–511.

Critchley, M. (1967): Migraine: from Cappadocia to Queen Square. In Background to Migraine. First Migraine Symposium, ed. R. Smith. Springler-Verlag, New York, pp. 28–38.

Critchley, M. and Ferguson, F. R. (1933): Migraine. Lancet 1:123–126.

Cruciger, M. P. and Mazow, M. L. (1978): An unusual case of ophthalmoplegic migraine. Am. J. Ophthalmol. 86:414–417.

Cullen, K. J. and MacDonald, W. B. (1963): The periodic syndrome: its nature and prevalence. Med. J. Aust. 2:167–173.

Curran, D. A. and Lance, J. W. (1964): Clinical trial of methysergide and other preparations in the management of migraine. J. Neurol. Neurosurg. Psychiatry 27:463–469.

Curzon, G., Barrie, M. and Wilkinson, M. I. P. (1969): Relationships between headache and amine changes after administration of reserpine to migrainous patients. J. Neurol. Neurosurg. Psychiatry 32:555–561.

Dalessio, D. J. (1974): Effort migraine. Headache 14:53.

Dalsgaard-Nielsen, T. (1948): Migraine and paroxysmal tachycardia. Nord. Med. 37:28.

Dalsgaard-Nielsen, T. (1955): Migraine diagnostics with special reference to pharmacological tests. Int. Arch. Allergy Appl. Immunol. 7:312–322.

Dalsgaard-Nielsen, T. (1965): Migraine and heredity. Acta Neurol. Scand. 41:287–300.

Danon, A. and Sulman, F. G. (1969): Ionizing effect of winds of ill repute on serotonin metabolism. Int. J. Biometeorol. (suppl.) 13:135–136.

Dennerstein, L., Laby, B., Burrows, G. D. and Hyman, G. J. (1978): Headache and sex hormone therapy. Headache 18:146–153.

Deubner, D. C. (1977): An epidemiologic study of migraine and headache in 10–20 year olds. Headache 17:173–180.

Dexter, J. D. (1974): Studies in nocturnal migraine. Arch. Neurobiol. (Madr.) 37:281–300.

Dexter, J. D. and Riley, T. L. (1975): Studies in nocturnal migraine. Headache 15:51–62.

Dexter, J. D. and Weitzman, E. D. (1970): The relationship of nocturnal headaches to sleep stage patterns. Neurology 20:513–518.

Donowitz, M. and Binder, H. J. (1975): Jejunal fluid and electrolyte secretion in carcinoid syndrome. Am. J. Dig. Dis. 20:1115–1122.

Dorfman, L. J., Marshall, W. H. and Enzmann, D. R. (1979): Cerebral infarction and migraine: clinical and radiologic correlations. Neurology 29:317–322.

Dutton, C. B. and Riley, L. H. (1969): Cervical migraine. Am. J. Med. 47:141–148.

Duvoisin, R. C. (1962): Convulsive syncope induced by the Weber maneuver. Arch. Neurol 7:219–226.

Edelson, R. N. and Levy, D. E. (1974): Transient benign unilateral pupillary dilation in young adults. Arch. Neurol. 31:12–14.

Edmeads, J. (1977): Cerebral blood flow in migraine. Headache 17:148–152.

Edmeads, J. (1978): Headaches and head pains associated with diseases of the cervical spine. Med. Clin. North Am. 62:533–544.

Ehyai, A. and Fenichel, G. M. (1978): The natural history of acute confusional migraine. Arch. Neurol. 35:368–369.

Ely, F. A. (1930): The migraine–epilepsy syndrome. Arch. Neurol. Psychiatry 24:943–949.

Emery, E. S. (1977): Acute confusional state in children with migraine. Pediatrics 60:110–114.

Epstein, M. T., Hockaday, J. M. and Hockaday, T. D. R. (1975): Migraine and reproductive hormones throughout the menstrual cycle. Lancet 1:543–548.

Essman, W. B. and Tagliente, T. (1978): Monoamine oxidase and serotonin regulation. In Serotonin in Health and Disease, Vol. 1, ed. W. B. Essman. Spectrum, New York, pp. 301–362.

Fay, T. (1932): Atypical facial neuralgia, a syndrome of vascular pain. Ann. Otol. Rhinol. Laryngol. 41:1030–1062.

Feldman, J. M. (1978): Serotonin metabolism in patients with carcinoid tumors: incidence of 5-hydroxytryptophan-secreting tumors. Gastroenterology 75:1109–1114.

Fenichel, G. M. (1967): Migraine as a cause of benign paroxysmal vertigo of childhood. J. Pediatr. 71:114–115.

Fisher, C. M., Ojemann, R. G. and Roberson, G. H. (1978): Spontaneous dissection of cervico-cerebral arteries. Can. J. Neurol. Sci. 5:9–19.

Fozard, J. R. (1975): The animal pharmacology of drugs used in the treatment of migraine. J. Pharm. Pharmacol. 27:297–321.

Friedman, A. P., Finley, K. H., Graham, J. R. et al (1962): Classification of headache. The Ad Hoc Committee on the Classification of Headache. Arch. Neurol. 6:173–176.

Friedman, A. P., Harter, D. H. and Merritt, H. H. (1962): Ophthalmoplegic migraine. Arch. Neurol. 7:320–327.

Gans, M. (1951): Part II. Treating migraine by "sleep-rationing." J. Nerv. Ment. Dis. 113:405–429.

Gardner, J. H., Horenstein, S. and Van den Noort, S. (1968): The clinical characteristics of headache during impending cerebral infarction in women taking oral contraceptives. Headache 8:108–111.

Gascon, G. and Barlow, C. (1970): Juvenile migraine presenting as an acute confusional state. Pediatrics 45:628–635.

Gershon, M. D. (1968): Serotonin and the motility of the gastrointestinal tract. Gastroenterology 54:453–456.

Gillin, J. C., Mendelson, W. B., Sitaram, N. and Wyatt, R. J. (1978): The neuropharmacology of sleep and wakefulness. Annu. Rev. Pharmacol. Toxicol. 18:563–579.

Glista, G. G., Mellinger, J. F. and Rooke, E. D. (1975): Familial hemiplegic migraine. Mayo Clin. Proc. 50:307–311.

Golden, G. S. and French, J. H. (1975): Basilar artery migraine in young children. Pediatrics 56:722–726.

Goldensohn, E. S. (1976): Paroxysmal and other features of the electroencephalogram in migraine. Res. Clin. Stud. Headache 4:118–128.

Gomersall, J. D. and Stuart, A. (1973): Variations in migraine attacks with changes in weather conditions. Int. J. Biometeorol. 17:285–299.

Goodell, H., Lewontin, R. and Wolff, H. G. (1954): Familial occurrence of migraine headache. A study of heredity. Arch. Neurol. Psychiatry 72:325–334.

Gowers, W. R. (1888): A Manual of Diseases of the Nervous System. Churchill, London, 789 pp.

Graham, J. R. (1968): Migraine. Clinical aspects. In Handbook of Clinical Neurology, Vol. 5, eds. P. J. Vinken and G. W. Bruyn. John Wiley and Sons, New York, pp. 45–58.

Graham, J. R. (1976): Headache related to a variety of medical disorders. In Pathogenesis and Treatment of Headache, ed. O. Appenzeller. Spectrum, New York, pp. 49–67.

Graham, J. R. and Wolff, H. G. (1938): Mechanism of migraine headache and action of ergotamine tartrate. Arch. Neurol. Psychiatry 39:737–763.

Graveson, G. S. (1949): Retinal occlusion in migraine. Br. Med. J. 2:838–840.

Greenblatt, R. B. and Bruneteau, D. W. (1974): Menopausal headache — psychogenic or metabolic? J. Am. Geriatr. Soc. 22:186–190.

Greene, R. (1975): The endocrinology of headache. In Modern Topics in Migraine, ed. J. Pearce. Wm. Heinemann, London, pp. 64–71.

Guest, I. A. and Woolf, A. L. (1964): Fatal infarction of brain in migraine. Br. Med. J. 1:225–226.

Haas, D. C., Pineda, G. and Lourie, H. (1975): Juvenile head trauma syndromes and their relationship to migraine. Arch. Neurol. 32:730–737.

Hachinski, V., Norris, J. W., Edmeads, J. and Cooper, P. W. (1978): Ergotamine and cerebral blood flow. Stroke 9:594–596.

Hachinski, V. C., Porchawka, J. and Steele, J. C. (1973): Visual symptoms in the migraine syndrome. Neurology 23:570–579.

Haigler, H. J. and Aghajanian, G. K. (1974): Peripheral serotonin antagonists: failure to antagonize serotonin in brain areas receiving a prominent serotonergic input. J. Neural Trans. 35:257–273.

Hamilton, C. R. and Quesada, O. (1973): Paget's disease of the skull and migraine headache. Johns Hopkins Med. J. 132:179–185.

Hammond, J. (1974): The late sequelae of recurrent vomiting of childhood. Dev. Med. Child. Neurol. 16:15–22.

Hare, E. H. (1966): Personal observations on the spectral march of migraine. J. Neurol. Sci. 3:259–264.

Harvald, B. and Hauge, M. (1956): A catamnestic investigation of Danish twins. A preliminary report. Dan. Med. Bull. 3:150–158.

Hauge, T. (1954): Catheter vertebral angiography. Acta Radiol. (suppl.) 109:28–118.

Henryk-Gutt, R. and Rees, W. L. (1973): Psychological aspects of migraine. J. Psychosom. Res. 17:141–153.

Heyck, H. (1969): Pathogenesis of migraine. Res. Clin. Stud. Headache 2:1–28.

Heyck, H. (1973): Varieties of hemiplegic migraine. Headache 12:135–142.

Hinrichs, W. L. and Keith, H. M. (1965): Migraine in childhood: a follow-up report. Mayo Clin. Proc. 40:593–596.

Hockaday, J. M. (1978): Late outcome of childhood onset migraine and factors affecting outcome, with particular reference to early and late EEG findings. In Current Concepts in Migraine Research, ed. R. Greene. Raven Press, New York, pp. 41–48.

Hockaday, J. M. and Whitty, C. W. M. (1969): Factors determining the electroencephalogram in migraine. A study of 560 patients according to clinical type of migraine. Brain 92:769–788.

Irey, N. S., Manion, W. C. and Taylor, H. B. (1970): Vascular lesions in women taking oral contraceptives. Arch. Pathol. 89:1–8.

Irey, N. S., McAllister, H. A. and Henry, J. M. (1978): Oral contraceptives and stroke in young women: a clinicopathologic correlation. Neurology 28:1216–1219.

Irey, N. S. and Norris, H. J. (1973): Intimal vascular lesions associated with female reproductive steroids. Arch. Pathol. 96:227–234.

Johnston, B. M. and Saxena, P. R. (1978): The effect of ergotamine on tissue blood flow and the arteriovenous shunting of radioactive microspheres in the head. Br. J. Pharmacol. 63:541–549.

Jouvet, M. (1967): Neurophysiology of the states of sleep. Physiol. Rev. 47:117–177.

Kallós, P. and Kallós-Deffner, L. (1955): Allergy and migraine. Int. Arch. Allergy Appl. Immunol. 7:367–372.

Kennard, C., Gawel, M., Rudolph, N. de M. and Rose, F. C. (1978): Visual evoked potentials in migraine subjects. Res. Clin. Stud. Headache 6:73–80.

Kerr, F. W. L. (1961a): Trigeminal and cervical volleys. Arch. Neurol. 5:171–178.

Kerr, F. W. L. (1961b): A mechanism to account for frontal headache in cases of posterior fossa tumors. J. Neurosurg. 18:605–609.

Klee, A. (1975): Perceptual disorders in migraine. In Modern Topics in Migraine, ed. J. Pearce. Wm. Heinemann, London, pp. 45–51.

Krieger, D. (1978): Endocrine processes and serotonin. In Serotonin in Health and Disease, Vol. 3, ed. W. B. Essman. Spectrum, New York, pp. 51–67.

Krueger, A. P. (1972): Are air ions biologically significant? A review of a controversial subject. Int. J. Biometeorol. 16:313–322.

Krueger, A. P. and Reed, E. J. (1976): Biological impact of small air ions. Science 193:1209–1213.

Krupp, G. R. and Friedman, A. P. (1953): Recurrent headache in children; a study of 100 clinic cases. N.Y. State J. Med. 53:43–45

Kudrow, L. (1975): The relationship of headache frequency to hormone use in migraine. Headache 15:36–40.

Kunkle, E. C. and Anderson, W. B. (1961): Significance of minor eye signs in headache of migraine type. Arch. Ophthalmol. 65:504–507.

Lance, J. W. (1978): Mechanism and Managment of Headache, 3rd ed. Butterworths, Boston, pp. 77–78.

Lance, J. W. and Anthony, M. (1966): Some clinical aspects of migraine. A prospective survey of 500 patients. Arch. Neurol. 15:356–361.

Lance, J. W. and Anthony, M. (1971): Thermographic studies in vascular headache. Med. J. Aust. 1:240–243.

Lapkin, M. L., French, J. H., Golden, G. S. and Rowan, A. J. (1977): The electroencephalogram in childhood basilar artery migraine. Neurology 27:580–583.

Lapkin, M. L. and Golden, G. S. (1978): Basilar artery migraine. Am. J. Dis. Child. 132:278–281.

Lashley, K. S. (1941): Patterns of cerebral integration indicated by scotomas of migraine. Arch. Neurol. Psychiatry 46:331–339.

Lee, C. H. and Lance, J. W. (1977): Migraine stupor. Headache 17:32–38.

Lennox, W. G. (1938): Ergonovine vs. ergotamine as a terminator of migraine headaches. Am. J. Med. Sci. 195:458–468.

Leviton, A. and Camenga, D. (1969): Migraine associated with hyper-pre-beta-lipoproteinemia. Neurology 19:963–966.

Levitt, B., Cagin, N., Kleid, J., Somberg, J. and Gillis, R. (1976): Role of the nervous system in the genesis of cardiac rhythm disorders. Am. J. Cardiol. 37:111–113.

Litman, G. I. and Friedman, H. M. (1978): Migraine and the mitral valve prolapse syndrome. Am. Heart J. 96:610–614.

Liveing, E. (1873): On Megrim, Sick-headache, and some Allied Disorders: A Contribution to the Pathology of Nerve-Storms. Churchill, London, 512 pp.

Lord, G. D. A. and Duckworth, J. W. (1978): Complement and immune complex studies in migraine. Headache 18:255–260.

Lovshin, L. L. (1960): Vascular neck pain — a common syndrome seldom recognized. Cleveland Clin. Quart. 27:5–13.

Lovshin, L. L. (1977): Carotidynia. Headache 17:192–195.

Ludvigsson, J. (1974): Propranolol used in prophylaxis of migraine in children. Acta Neurol. Scand. 50:109–115.

MacLean, C., Appenzeller, O., Cordaro, J. T. and Rhodes, J. (1975): Flash-evoked potentials in migraine. Headache 14:193–198.

Markush, R. E., Karp, H. R., Heyman, A. and O'Fallon, W. M. (1975): Epidemiologic study of migraine symptoms in young women. Neurology 25:430–435.

Marshall, J. (1978): Cerebral blood flow in migraine without headache. Res. Clin. Stud. Headache 6:1–5.

Marshall, J. and Meadows, S. (1968): The natural history of amaurosis fugax. Brain 91:419–433.

Masland, W. S., Friedman, A. P. and Buchsbaum, H. W. (1978): Computerized axial tomography of migraine. Res. Clin. Stud. Headache 6:136–140.

Mathew, N. T. (1978): Computerized axial tomography in migraine. In Current Concepts in Migraine Research, ed. R. Green. Raven Press, New York, pp. 63–71.

Medina, J. L. and Diamond, S. (1976): Migraine and atopy. Headache 15:271–274.

Medina, J. L. and Diamond, S. (1977): The clinical link between migraine and cluster headaches. Arch. Neurol. 34:470–472.

Melmon, K. L., Sjoerdsma, A., Oates, J. A. and Laster, L. (1965): Treatment of malabsorption and diarrhea of the carcinoid syndrome with methysergide. Gastroenterology 48:18–24.

Mendelson, W. B., Gillin, J. C. and Wyatt, R. J. (1977): Human Sleep and its Disorders. Plenum Press, New York, pp. 1–20.

Merskey, H. (1975): Psychiatric aspects of migraine. In Modern Topics in Migraine, ed. J. Pearce. Wm. Heinemann, London, pp. 52–63.

Merskey, H. and Boyd, D. (1978): Emotional adjustment and chronic pain. Pain 5:173–178.

Miller, J. B. (1977): A double-blind study of food extract injection therapy: a preliminary report. Ann. Allergy 38:185–191.

Millichap, J. G. (1978): Recurrent headaches in 100 children. Child's Brain 4:95–105.

Moffett, A. M., Swash, M. and Scott, D. F. (1974): Effect of chocolate in migraine: a double-blind study. J. Neurol. Neurosurg. Psychiatry 37:445–448.

Money, K. E. (1970): Motion sickness. Physiol. Rev. 50:1–39.

Morgane, P. J. and Stern, W. C. (1978): Serotonin in the regulation of sleep. In Serotonin in Health and Disease, Vol. 2, ed. W. B. Essman. Spectrum, New York, pp. 205–245.

Myers, R. D. and Waller, M. B. (1978): Thermoregulation and serotonin. In Serotonin in Health and Disease, Vol. 2, ed. W. B. Essman. Spectrum, New York, pp. 1–67.

Naggar, C. Z. (1979): The mitral valve prolapse syndrome: spectrum and therapy. Med. Clin. North Am. 63:337–353.

Nattero, G., Bisbocci, D., Bottini, A. et al (1977): Humoral and hormonal changes in menstrual migraine. Headache 17:23–24.

Nebel, B. R. (1957): The phosphene of quick eye motion. Arch. Ophthalmol. 58:235–243.

Nikiforow, R. and Hokkanen, E. (1978): An epidemiological study of headache in an urban and a rural population in northern Finland. Headache 18:137–145.

O'Connor, P. J. (1973): Strokes in migraine. In Background to Migraine, 5th Migraine Symposium, ed. J. N. Cumings. Springer-Verlag, New York, pp. 40–44.

Olesen, J. (1978): Some clinical features of the acute migraine attack. An analysis of 750 patients. Headache 18:268–271.

Osterholzer, H. O., Grillo, D., Kruger, P. S. et al (1977): The effect of oral contraceptive steroids on branches of the uterine artery. Obstet. Gynecol. 49:227–232.

Ostfeld, A. M., Reis, D. J., Goodell, H. and Wolff, H. G. (1955): Headache and hydration. Arch. Intern. Med. 96:142–152.

Ostfeld, A. M. and Wolff, H. G. (1957): Studies on headache: participation of ocular structures in the migraine syndrome. Bibl. Ophthalmol. 1:634–647.

Parrish, R. M. and Stevens, H. (1977): Familial hemiplegic migraine. Minn. Med. 60:709–715.

Parsonage, M. (1975): Electroencephalographic studies in migraine. In Modern Topics in Migraine, ed. J. Pearce. Wm. Heinemann, London, pp. 72–84.

Patterson, R. H., Jr., Goodell, H. and Dunning, H. S. (1964): Complications of carotid arteriography. Arch. Neurol. 10:513–520.

Pearce, J. (1968): The ophthalmological complications of migraine. J. Neurol. Sci. 6:73–81.

Pearce, J. (1971): Some aetiological factors in migraine. In Background to Migraine, 4th Migraine Symposium, ed. J. N. Cumings. Springer-Verlag, New York, pp. 1–7.

Pearce, J. (1975): Complicated migraine. In Modern Topics in Migraine, ed. J. Pearce. Wm. Heinemann, London, pp. 30–44.

Pearce, J. (1977): Migraine: a psychosomatic disorder. Headache 17:125–128.

Pearce, J. M. S. and Foster, J. B. (1965): An investigation of complicated migraine. Neurology 15:333–340.

Perera, G. A. (1971): Paroxysmal arrhythmias and migraine. J.A.M.A. 215:488.

Pinnas, J. L. and Vanselow, N. A. (1978): Relationship of allergy to headache. Res. Clin. Stud. Headache 4:85–95.

Prensky, A. L. (1976): Migraine and migrainous variants in pediatric patients. Pediatr. Clin. North Am. 23:461–471.

Prensky, A. L. and Sommer, D. (1979): Diagnosis and treatment of migraine in children. Neurology 29:506–510.

Priestley, B. S. and Foree, K. (1955): Clinical significance of some entoptic phenomena. Arch. Ophthalmol. 53:390–397.

Quay, W. B. and Meyer, D. C. (1978): Rhythmicity and periodic functions of the central nervous system and serotonin. In Serotonin in Health and Disease, Vol. 2, ed. W. B. Essman. Spectrum, New York, pp. 159–204.

Raskin, N. H. and Fishman, R. A. (1976): Neurologic disorders in renal failure. N. Engl. J. Med. 294:204–210.

Raskin, N. H. and Knittle, S. C. (1976): Ice cream headache and orthostatic symptoms in patients with migraine. Headache 16:222–225.

Raskin, N. H. and Prusiner, S. (1977): Carotidynia. Neurology 27:43–46.

Raskin, N. H. and Schwartz, R. K. (1979): Icepick-like pain. Neurology 29:550.

Refsum, S. (1968): Genetic aspects of migraine. In Handbook of Clinical Neurology, Vol. 5, eds. P. J. Vinken and G. W. Bruyn. John Wiley and Sons, New York, pp. 258–269.

Reichlin, S. (1979): The prolactinoma problem. N. Engl. J. Med. 300:313–315.

Reivich, M., Isaacs, G., Evarts, E. and Kety, S. (1968): The effect of slow wave sleep and REM sleep on regional cerebral blood flow in cats. J. Neurochem. 15:301–306.

Richards, W. (1971): The fortification illusions of migraines. Sci. Am. 224:89–96 (May).

Robertson, W. C. and Schnitzler, E. R. (1978): Ophthalmoplegic migraine in infancy. Pediatrics 61:886–888.

Robinson, N. and Dirnfeld, F. S. (1963): The ionization state of the atmosphere as a function of the meteorological elements and various sources of ions. Int. J. Biometeorol. 4:101–110.

Rothlin, E. (1955): Historical development of the ergot therapy of migraine. Int. Arch. Allergy 7:205–209.

Rotton, W. N., Sachtleben, M. R. and Friedman, E. A. (1959): Migraine and eclampsia. Obstet. Gynecol. 14:322–330.

Russell, A. (1973): The implications of hyperammonemia in rare and common disorders, including migraine. Mt. Sinai J. Med. 40:723–735.

Russell, R. W. R. (1959): Giant-cell arteritis; a review of 35 cases. Q. J. Med. 28:471–489.

Ryan, R. E., Sr. (1978): A controlled study of the effect of oral contraceptives on migraine. Headache 17:250–252.

Sacks, O. W. (1970): Migraine: The Evolution of a Common Disorder. University of California Press, Berkeley, pp. 35–53.

Sakai, F. and Meyer, J. S. (1978): Regional cerebral hemodynamics during migraine and cluster headaches measured by the 133Xe inhalation method. Headache 18:122–132.

Sakai, F., Meyer, J. S., Karacan, I., Yamaguchi, F. and Yamamoto, M. (1979): Narcolepsy: regional cerebral blood flow during sleep and wakefulness. Neurology 29:61–67.

Schiller, F. (1975): The migraine tradition. Bull. Hist. Med. 49:1–19.

Schnitker, M. T. and Schnitker, M. A. (1947): A clinical test for migraine. J.A.M.A. 135:89.

Seelinger, D. F., Coin, G. C. and Carlow, T. J. (1975): Effort headache with cerebral infarction. Headache 15:142–145.

Selby, G. and Lance, J. W. (1960): Observations on 500 cases of migraine and allied vascular headache. J. Neurol. Neurosurg. Psychiatry 23:23–32.

Shafey, G. and Scheinberg, P. (1966): Neurological syndrome occurring in patients receiving steroids (oral contraceptives). Neurology 16:205–211.

Sherman, B. M., Harris, C. E., Schlecte, J. et al (1978): Pathogenesis of prolactin-secreting pituitary adenomas. Lancet 2:1019–1021.

Shoemaker, E. S., Forney, J. P. and MacDonald, P. C. (1977): Estrogen treatment of postmenopausal women. J.A.M.A. 238:1524–1530.

Sillanpää, M. and Koponen, M. (1978): Papaverine in the prophylaxis of migraine and other vascular headache in children. Acta Paediatr. Scand. 67:209–212.

Simard, D. and Paulson, O. B. (1973): Cerebral vasomotor paralysis during migraine attack. Arch. Neurol. 29:207–209.

Sjoerdsma, A., Lovenberg, W., Engleman, K., Carpenter, W. T., Wyatt, R. J. and Gessa, G. L. (1970): Serotonin now: clinical implications of inhibiting its synthesis with para-chlorophenylalanine. Ann. Intern. Med. 73:607–629.

Smith, I., Kellow, A. H. and Hanington, E. (1970): A clinical and biochemical correlation between tyramine and migraine headache. Headache 10:43–52.

Somerville, B. W. (1972a): The role of estradiol withdrawal in the etiology of menstrual migraine. Neurology 22:355–365.

Somerville, B. W. (1972b): A study of migraine in pregnancy. Neurology 22:824–828.

Somerville, B. W. (1975): Estrogen withdrawal migraine. I and II. Neurology 25:239–244, 245–250.

Stanford, E. and Greene, R. (1970): A case of migraine cured by treatment of Conn's syndrome. In Background to Migraine, 3rd Migraine Symposium, ed. A. L. Cochrane. Springer-Verlag, New York, pp. 53–57.

Sulman, F. G., Danon, A., Pfeifer, Y. et al (1971): The exhaustion syndrome in climatic heat stress and its treatment. Int. J. Biometeorol. 15:93.

Sulman, F. G., Levy, D., Levy, A. et al (1974): Air-ionometry of hot, dry desert winds (Sharav) and treatment with air ions of weather-sensitive subjects. Int. J. Biometeorol. 18:313–318.

Swanson, J. W. and Vick, N. A. (1978): Basilar artery migraine. Neurology 28:782–786.

Swash, M. and Earl, C. J. (1970): Transient visual obscurations in chronic rheumatic heart disease. Lancet 2:323–326.

Symonds, C. (1951): Migrainous variants. Trans. Med. Soc. Lond. 67:237–250.

Thomas, W. A. and Post, W. E. (1925): Paroxysmal tachycardia in migraine. J.A.M.A. 84:569–570.

Townsend, R. E., Prinz, P. N. and Obrist, W. D. (1973): Human cerebral blood flow during sleep and waking. J. Appl. Physiol. 35:620–625.

Trautman, E. (1928): Die Beeinflussung migräneartiger Zustände durch ein sympathi-kushemmendes Mittel (Gynergen). Münch. Med. Wochenschr. 75:513.
Tzanck, A. (1928): Le traitement des migraines par le tartrate d'ergotamine. Bull. Soc. Med. Paris 44:1057.
Utian, W. H. (1974): Oestrogen, headache, and oral contraceptives. S. Afr. Med. J. 48:2105–2108.
Vijayan, N. (1977): Brief therapeutic report: papaverine prophylaxis of complicated migraine. Headache 17:159–162.
Vijayan, N. and Dreyfus, P. (1975): Posttraumatic dysautonomic cephalalgia. Arch. Neurol. 32:649–652.
Vijayan, N. and Watson, C. (1978): Pericarotid syndrome. Headache 18:244–254.
Volans, G. N. and Castleden, C. M. (1976): The relationship between smoking and migraine. Postgrad. Med. J. 52:80–82.
von Reis, G., Lund, F. and Sahlgren, E. (1957): Experimental histamine headache. Acta Med. Scand. 157:451–460.
Walsh, J. P. and O'Doherty, D. S. (1960): A possible explanation of the mechanism of ophthalmoplegic migraine. Neurology 10:1079–1084.
Waters, W. E. (1971): Migraine: intelligence, social class and familial prevalence. Br. Med. J. 2:77–81.
Waters, W. E. (1973): The epidemiological enigma of migraine. Int. J. Epidemiol. 2:189–194.
Waters, W. E. (1978): The prevalence of migraine. Headache 18:53–54.
Waters, W. E. and O'Connor, P. J. (1975): Prevalence of migraine. J. Neurol. Neurosurg. Psychiatry 38:613–616.
Watson, P. and Steele, J. C. (1974): Paroxysmal dysequilibrium in the migraine syn-drome of childhood. Arch. Otolaryngol. 99:177–179.
Weil, A. A. (1962): Observations on "dysrhythmic" migraine. J. Nerv. Ment. Dis. 134:277–281.
Whitty, C. W. M. (1953): Familial hemiplegic migraine. J. Neurol. Neurosurg. Psychia-try 16:172–177.
Whitty, C. W. M. and Hockaday, J. M. (1968): Migraine: a follow-up study of 92 patients. Br. Med. J. 1:735–736.
Wilson, E. (1972): Diary of the 'Terra Nova' Expedition to the Antarctic, 1910–1912, ed. H. G. R. King. Blandford Press, London, pp. 129–134.
Wolf, S. and Wolff, H. G. (1942): Intermittent fever of unknown origin. Arch. Intern. Med. 70:293–302.
Wolff, H. G. (1937): Personality features and reactions of subjects with migraine. Arch. Neurol. Psychiatry 37:895–921.
Wyler, A. R., Wilkus, R. J. and Troupin, A. S. (1975): Methysergide in the treatment of narcolepsy. Arch. Neurol. 32:265–268.
Ziegler, D. K. (1977): Genetics of migraine. Headache 16:330–331.
Ziegler, D. K. (1978): The epidemiology and genetics of migraine. Res. Clin. Stud. Headache 5:21–33.
Ziegler, D. K., Hassanein, R. S. and Couch, J. R. (1977): Characteristics of life headache histories in a nonclinic population. Neurology 27:265–269.
Ziegler, D. K., Hassanein, R. S., Harris, D. and Stewart, R. (1975): Headache in a non-clinic twin population. Headache 14:213–218.
Ziegler, D. K. and Wong, G., Jr. (1967): Migraine in children: clinical and electroen-cephalographic study of families. The possible relation to epilepsy. Epilepsia 8:171–187.

CHAPTER 3

MIGRAINE: PATHOGENESIS

The available evidence supports the contention that migraine is an hereditary disorder characterized by paroxysmal vascular instability, episodes during which there is often a phase of intracranial arterial constriction and/or a phase of extracranial (and probably intracranial) arterial dilatation. The two phases often occur sequentially, but also commonly appear concurrently. Although substantial data have been generated describing the vascular changes that characterize migraine attacks, the mechanisms by which these alterations take place remain enigmatic. In reviews of the subject, there is often an implicit supposition that a single disordered mechanism must be found to account for migrainous phenomena. Although the multivariate features of migraine do not necessarily require different mechanisms for their explanation, the diversity of precipitating factors raises the possibility that several disordered mechanisms underlie what is usually assumed to be one disorder.

There is hardly a single study concerning the biologic aspects of migraine that has not been challenged. In this section, an effort has been made to draw attention to those data that have been obtained by rigorous application of the scientific method. The biologic phenomena that characterize a migrainous headache attack are listed in Table 3–1. Whether any of these alterations are only epiphenomena of the migraine attack is uncertain at present.

The two major hypotheses currently being tested regarding causation are that migraine is the manifestation of: (1) a central nervous system disorder of vasomotor regulation; and (2) a systemic metabolic disorder. The lack of an animal model of migraine thus far has precluded much testing of the former hypothesis, so that much of the accumulated data bear on possible circulating biochemical factors. Psychologic factors are of great importance in the production of

84

TABLE 3-1. BIOLOGIC PHENOMENA OCCURRING DURING HEADACHE ATTACKS

Intra- and extracranial vasodilatation
Opening of cephalic arteriovenous shunts
Cerebral vasomotor dysautoregulation
Release of platelet serotonin
Increased concentration of plasma free fatty acids
Platelet activation
Decreased concentration of plasma norepinephrine
Decreased platelet monoamine oxidase activity
Increased CSF concentrations of:
    γ-aminobutyrate, lactate, 3',5'-cyclic adenosine monophosphate

migrainous headaches, but they are almost certainly a trigger mechanism with the same import as bright light exposure, hunger and the menstrual cycle.

VASCULAR ALTERATIONS

The widely-held hypothesis concerning the behavior of arteries in migraine is that the phase of neurologic symptoms that occurs prior to (the "aura") or concurrent with headache is caused by constriction of intracerebral arteries resulting in focal cerebral ischemia, and that a second phase of dilatation of extracranial and probably intracranial arteries results in headache.

INTRACEREBRAL VASOCONSTRICTION

That cerebral blood flow is reduced in the region of brain appropriate to the clincal symptom complex is supported by direct measurement (Skinhøj, 1973; Hachinski et al, 1977; Sakai and Meyer, 1978). CBF may reach levels that imperil the structural integrity of brain (Simard and Paulson, 1973), thus explaining the occasional occurrence of cerebral infarction in migraine (Connor, 1962). The angiographic appearance of larger cerebral arteries is often normal (Hachinski et al, 1977) in the face of gross neurologic deficit and a reduction of regional blood flow of as much as 50 per cent, suggesting that cerebrovascular resistance is increased at the arteriolar level. Such data are consistent with the transient elevation of CSF concentrations of lactate, gamma-aminobutyrate (GABA) and 3', 5'-cyclic adenosine monophosphate (cyclic AMP) found in patients during headache attacks, and which also accompany occlusive cerebrovascular disease (Welch et al, 1978). The mechanisms whereby GABA and cyclic AMP increase in ischemic brain, however, are uncertain.

The neurologic symptoms that often accompany migrainous attacks characteristically develop and progress over 20 minutes or so. Lashley (1941) estimated that the evolution of his own visual scotomata proceeded at a rate of 3 mm per minute, and speculated that his visual cortex was suppressed electrophysiologically by a spreading inhibitory wave. A few years later, the phenomenon that has come to be known as "spreading depression" was described by Leão (1944) in the cerebral cortex of experimental animals. It is a slowly moving (2 to 3 mm per minute) potassium-liberating depression of cortical activity that can be produced by a variety of experimental stimuli, including hypoxia, electrical tetanus and the topical application of potassium. This inhibitory wave is associated with pial artery dilatation, cerebral edema and an increase in the metabolic rate of the involved cerebral cortex (Shinohara et al, 1979); some observers have found a vasoconstrictive phase preceding dilatation (Marshall, 1959). Since ischemia is an adequate stimulus for spreading depression to occur, and since the rate of progression is quite similar to the ischemic phase of migraine, it is plausible that spreading depression is mechanistically relevant to the spectral march of migraine (Basser, 1969).

Extracranial Vasodilatation

The theory that dilatation of arteries lying outside the brain, especially scalp arteries, is important to the mechanism of pain production in migraine is supported by several lines of evidence (Graham and Wolff, 1938). There is a positive correlation between the severity of headache and the pulse amplitude of scalp arteries; artificial distention of the superficial temporal artery can reproduce a migraine headache; physical compression or chemical vasoconstriction of scalp arteries often at least temporarily alleviates headache; and direct measurement confirms that extracranial blood flow is elevated (Sakai and Meyer, 1978). However, headache does not generally develop after physical exertion or a hot bath, two circumstances that also produce extracranial dilatation; perhaps in migraine different rates of dilatation between arteries, arterioles and capillaries result in overdistention of arteries.

A factor that may be important to the production of pain is the appearance during headache of a substance, "neurokinin," in the extravascular space at the site of pain (Chapman et al, 1960); this material, perhaps a polypeptide, has yet to be clearly identified, but has been shown to lower local tissue pain threshold, increase capillary permeability and increase tissue vulnerability to injury. Thus, in addition to vasodilatation, a local sterile inflammatory reaction may occur resulting in pain.

Biopsies of the superficial temporal artery, taken at the time of headache, have shown no abnormality (Adams et al, 1968). Heyck (1974) has suggested that cephalic arteriovenous anastomoses become patent during migraine attacks. This idea is supported by the observations that: (1) facial pallor occurs in the presence of external carotid dilatation; (2) there is increased prominence of *both* veins and arteries of the scalp; and (3) the oxygen saturation of external jugular and frontal venous blood approaches a level similar to that of arterial blood during a headache attack.

INTRACRANIAL VASODILATATION

It is unclear whether intracranial vasodilatation is important to the genesis of headache. The brain responds to pain with an increase in metabolic rate, and subsequent vasodilatation (Ingvar, 1976). Therefore, the increased CBF recorded during the headache phase of migraine may well be secondary to pain *per se*; evidence often cited to support this inference is the fact that ergotamine tartrate, administered parenterally in an amount sufficient to terminate a headache, has no effect on cerebral hemispheric blood flow (Hachinski et al., 1978). However, the vertebrobasilar circulation has been largely neglected in these studies; Sakai and Meyer (1978) have recently corroborated other data (Hachinski et al, 1977) in finding that the posterior circulation blood flow is substantially increased during the headache phase and is markedly affected by ergotamine tartrate administration. Since the vertebral and basilar arteries are pain-sensitive structures (Ray and Wolff, 1940), posterior circulation vasodilatation may play an important role in the mechanism of headache.

CEREBRAL DYSAUTOREGULATION

During migrainous attacks and for about two days thereafter, the responsivity of the cerebral arteries to alterations in mean arterial blood pressure or to the concentration of arterial carbon dioxide is markedly reduced (Simard and Paulson, 1973; Sakai and Meyer, 1978, 1979). Thus, increased severity of headache during physical exertion or when the head is lowered, and the appearance of vertigo or scintillating scotomata with rapid postural change (Raskin and Knittle, 1976), are probably explained by impaired autoregulation. Whether dysautoregulation occurs as a response to cerebral ischemia (Agnoli et al, 1968; Paulson et al, 1970) or whether it is a feature peculiar to the vascular alterations of migraine is not entirely clear; however, since it has been found during some migrain-

ous attacks in which neither clinical evidence of ischemia nor a reduction of CBF were seen (Sakai and Meyer, 1978), it appears
unlikely that loss of autoregulation is secondary to cerebral ischemia.

SEROTONIN

Interest in the possible role of serotonin (5-hydroxytryptamine)
in migraine was initiated by the observation that urinary levels of
5-hydroxyindoleacetic acid (5-HIAA), a serotonin metabolite, were
increased in some patients during headache attacks (Sicuteri, 1961).
Subsequently, it has become clear that during headache attacks, in
about 85 per cent of patients, platelet serotonin levels fall and urinary serotonin levels increase (Anthony and Lance, 1975), whereas
urinary 5-HIAA is increased only occasionally (Curzon et al., 1966).
To place these data (Table 3–2) into context, the physiologic role of
serotonin will be briefly reviewed.

Serotonin is widely distributed in body tissues, with 90 per
cent of it contained in the enterochromaffin cells of the gastrointestinal tract, and the remainder in platelets (8 per cent) and brain
(predominantly the pineal body); only trace amounts are found free,
unbound to platelets, in plasma. It originally was thought that serotonin was implicated only in the mechanisms of intestinal motility
and vasoconstriction, but subsequent data have imputed serotonin
with actions on a variety of smooth muscles, collagen tissue and
nerves, and there is good evidence that it is an important neurotransmitter within the CNS (Christian and Smythies, 1978; Gerschenfeld et al, 1978). This multisystem activity is compatible with
the variegated symptoms of migraine.

Serotonin originates from dietary tryptophan, and its enzymatic
synthesis occurs in neurons and in enterochromaffin cells; however,
platelets have no capacity for synthesis, and acquire serotonin by
uptake of serotonin released into the plasma by the cells of the intestine (Sneddon, 1973). Neuronal and intestinal serotonin turnover
times are fairly short (one and 17 hours, respectively), but platelet-

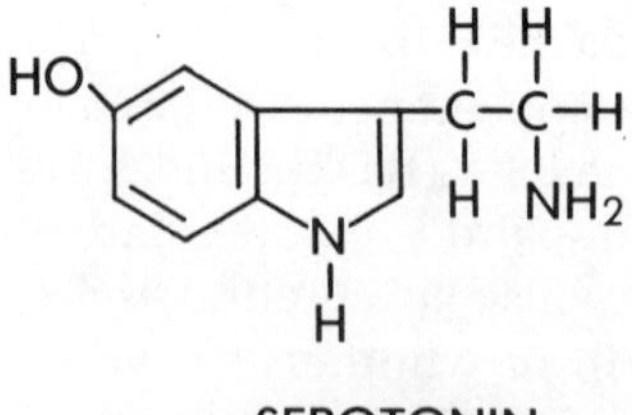

Figure 3-1.

SEROTONIN
(5-HYDROXYTRYPTAMINE)

TABLE 3–2. SEROTONIN IN MIGRAINE

Urinary 5-hydroxyindoleacetic acid and serotonin increased
Platelet-bound and free plasma serotonin decreased
Plasma serotonin releasing factor appears during headache attacks
Headache — precipitated by reserpine
      relieved by serotonin and its metabolic precursors
Migraine drugs depress central serotonergic neuronal activity

bound serotonin is released only upon the destruction of platelets, during the thrombin-induced release reaction, or by drugs such as reserpine (Douglas, 1975).

Within brain, serotonin is contained within specific nerve circuits located near the midline regions of the medulla, pons and upper brain stem (Heller, 1972). Serotonergic circuits have been implicated in such functions as sleep (see Chapter 2), mood, extrapyramidal motor activity and pain perception (Edelman et al, 1977; Fields and Basbaum, 1978). One role of serotonergic circuits may be to dampen overreaction to a variety of stimuli, extrinsic as well as intrinsic. The medullary serotonergic projection has recently been implicated in the central control of cardiovascular function (Cabot et al, 1979). Transient cerebral ischemia results in a depletion of cerebral serotonin (Welch et al, 1977).

Serotonin has a dual action upon blood vessels; vasoconstriction or vasodilatation may be produced, depending on the vascular bed, its resting tonus and the concentration of serotonin (Haddy, 1960). In general, serotonin constricts large arteries and dilates smaller arterioles and capillaries; it is the most potent vasoconstrictor amine in the cerebral circulation (Edvinsson and MacKenzie, 1976). In vivo human and primate studies clearly demonstrate that both the internal and external carotid arterial circulations are constricted by serotonin (Anthony and Lance, 1975; Spira et al, 1978). However, the concentration of serotonin required for this effect greatly exceeds free plasma concentrations of serotonin in man. In vitro studies of human pial arterioles and superficial temporal arteries have also shown pronounced vasoconstriction after application of serotonin; the effect of serotonin is greater upon pial arterioles (Hardebo et al, 1978). Small pial arterioles dilate in response to serotonin by a mechanism that may involve β-adrenergic receptors (Edvinsson et al, 1975), whereas large pial arterioles and small arteries consistently constrict, by a mechanism mediated by specific serotonin receptors (Edvinsson and Hardebo, 1976).

During headache attacks, both free and platelet-bound serotonin plasma levels decrease (Somerville, 1976). There is no difference in serotonin levels between the external jugular and forearm venous blood samples in this regard. CSF serotonin levels remain unmeasurable (Barrie and Jowett, 1967). Platelets drawn during attacks retain their ability to take up serotonin and contain normal levels of adenine nucleotides; however, plasma specimens drawn during attacks have the capacity to release serotonin from normal platelets (Anthony and Lance, 1975; Dvilansky et al, 1976). The as yet unidentified plasma-releasing factor has a molecular weight of less than 50,000. Serotonin-induced aggregation, a phenomenon seen more easily when platelet serotonin uptake sites are unoccupied (Hilton and Cumings, 1971), occurs more readily in platelets from migrainous subjects. These data suggest that, in migraine, platelets are less capable of accepting or retaining serotonin (Hilton and Cumings, 1972). These platelet abnormalities may be of no direct consequence *per se,* but may reflect a more systematic abnormality of serotonin metabolism. In other words, the platelet release of serotonin may be a model for a pathophysiologically more important but inaccessible system, such as the serotonergic neuronal circuit within the brain stem.

The intramuscular injection of reserpine (2.5 mg), an agent that releases serotonin from platelets and depletes the brain of serotonin, norepinephrine and dopamine, precipitates a headache attack within four to six hours in most migraine patients, but only occasionally and to a lesser degree in normal subjects (Anthony et al, 1967). The intravenous administration of serotonin often relieves spontaneous or reserpine-induced migraine headache; platelet serotonin decreases after reserpine admininstration in migraine patients, whether or not a headache is produced, and the prior administration of methysergide is effective in preventing reserpine-induced headache, but has no effect upon the reserpine-induced diminution of platelet serotonin (Carroll and Hilton, 1973). Early data pointed to serotonin antagonism as a likely mode of action of vasoactive drugs such as methysergide; however, serotonin receptor agonism occurs at lower dosages than antagonism (Hardebo et al, 1978). Although there is no single property of the drugs effective in migraine that can be unequivocally correlated with their clinical effectiveness (Fozard, 1975), *alterations of central serotonergic neuronal activity have been demonstrated,* for those drugs that have been examined regarding this action, in laboratory animals (see Chapter 4).

Of all the vasoactive substances thus far put forth as agents of the migraine mechanism, the data regarding alterations of serotonin levels are the most consistent and specific to migraine headache attacks. Furthermore, the curious dual effect of this substance upon cranial vessels correlates well with the biphasic vascular alterations that parallel the symptomatology of migraine. Moreover, vasoactive drugs have biphasic actions toward the effects of serotonin upon the cranial vasculature. Alterations of serotonergic circuits within the brain stem have not been studied as yet in migraine. Could the migraine attack be triggered by the release of a factor resulting in the sudden circulatory withdrawal of serotonin and an attendant biphasic vascular response? The major challenges to this hypothesis are:

(1) There are no data confirming the supposition that the plasma serotonin changes observed during migraine have an important role in the regulation of arterial tone;

(2) Serotonin levels do not fall in some patients — indeed, there is occasionally an increase in platelet-bound serotonin (Anthony et al, 1967; Somerville, 1976);

(3) Since the depletion of serotonin from platelets is not confined to the cranial circulation, why are only the cranial arteries responsive to the diminution in serotonin levels?

The responses to these objections may reside in studies of arterial fluctuations of serotonin, serotonergic circuits in brain, and/or identification of the serotonin-releasing factor. There are no compelling arguments that exclude a fundamental role for serotonin in migraine.

PROSTAGLANDINS

The prostaglandins (PG) are a group of chemically distinct, naturally occurring lipids which are synthesized by virtually all body tissues (Christ and Van Dorp, 1972). Their production increases in response to a broad variety of stimuli and their effects are equally diverse, sparing very few biologic functions. Since prostaglandins are not stored in tissue, release probably reflects *de novo* biosynthesis (Piper and Vane, 1971). Prostaglandins generally are almost undetectable in arterial blood, largely because of effective pulmonary destruction. These compounds are thus local hormones produced at their site of action (Needleman and Kaley, 1978). They are classified alphabetically (PGA, PGB, etc.) according to the constituents of their common cyclopentane rings. Brain contains many different prostaglandins, predominantly PGF, which are distributed fairly ho-

Figure 3–2.

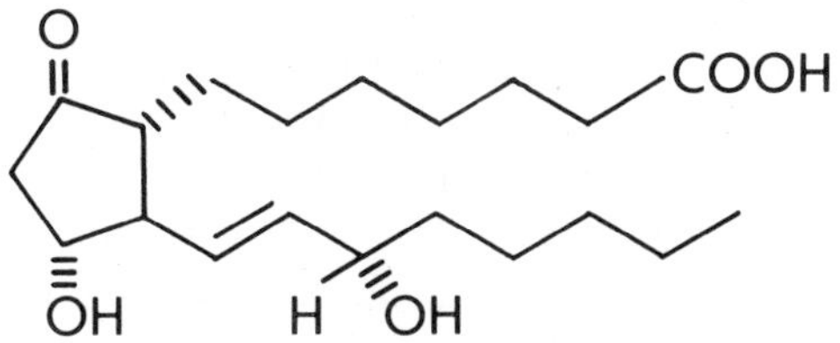

PROSTAGLANDIN E_1

mogeneously (Cooper et al, 1978). The prostaglandins inhibit or activate adenylate cyclase in many cells, thus affecting cyclic AMP levels, and they may act as local modulating agents within brain.

The possible relationship of prostaglandins to migraine (Horrobin, 1977) was first suggested by the observation that intravenous infusion of PGE_1 in nonmigrainous subjects consistently resulted in a vascular headache accompanied by nausea, sometimes preceded by characteristically migrainous visual symptoms (Carlson et al, 1968). Further studies in laboratory animals have shown that infusion of serotonin into the pulmonary artery releases prostaglandins into the pulmonary vein (Alabaster and Bakhle, 1970); this response can be blocked by methysergide and ergotamine tartrate (Bakhle and Smith, 1972; Sandler, 1975). Moreover, serotonin is one of but few compounds which, when perfused into the cerebral ventricles, results in a substantial release of PGE into the ventricular fluid (Holmes, 1970).

In most vascular beds, the prostaglandin Es are potent vasodilators. In the monkey, intracarotid PGE_1 produces substantial extracranial vasodilatation and loss of cerebral vasomotor autoregulation (Welch et al, 1974a,b), but its effects upon the internal carotid artery are more variable. At low doses a minimal dilator effect occurs, but at high doses there is a reduction of internal carotid artery flow (Spira et al, 1978) that is probably due to "steal" by the external carotid artery. A biphasic response to PGE_1 has been observed in the mesenteric vascular bed, vasoconstriction occurring at low concentrations and vasodilatation at higher ones (Manku et al, 1977). Blood vessels themselves synthesize and release vasoactive prostaglandins (Needleman et al, 1973) and can thereby regulate arterial tone (Needleman and Kaley, 1978). Cranial arteries per se have only begun to be studied (Gaudet et al, 1979), so that the contribution of prostaglandins to cranial vasomotor tone is unknown at present. At least some of the vasomotor effects of systemically administered PGE_1 are mediated by a central serotonergic mechanism (Lin, 1979).

PGE_1 levels have been measured in arterial and venous blood during migrainous attacks, and no alterations noted (Welch and Lance, 1975; Anthony, 1976); Sandler (1975) was likewise unable to find any changes in venous blood samples. However, for prostaglandins to function mechanistically in migraine does not necessitate release into arterial blood from a distant site such as lung. Rather, consistent with the general mode of action of the prostaglandins, release may occur locally at the arterial wall in response to neural or chemical stimuli.

Flufenamic acid (not available in the United States) was shown to be remarkably effective in aborting individual migraine attacks, but was ineffectual in preventing attacks when used regularly (Vardi et al, 1976). This drug is known to be an inhibitor of prostaglandin

TABLE 3-3. PROSTAGLANDINS IN MIGRAINE

Intravenous administration produces vascular headache in nonmigrainous subjects.

Inhibitors of prostaglandin synthesis alleviate migraine headache attacks.

Biphasic effects upon vascular beds; profound dilation of extracranial arterial circulation.

Infusion of serotonin into pulmonary artery releases prostaglandins into pulmonary vein; antagonized by methysergide, ergotamine tartrate.

PGE_1 impairs cerebral autoregulation

synthesis, as is aspirin; however, whether the mode of action of flufenamic acid or aspirin in aborting migraine attacks is via prostaglandin inhibition or by some other mechanism is uncertain. Indomethacin, another PG antagonist, has been shown to be no better than placebo in the treatment of migraine (Anthony and Lance, 1968).

The prostaglandins are an exciting group of compounds currently commanding widespread interest, and much more needs to be learned about them before assessing their role in migraine (Table 3-3). Since serotonin is a prostaglandin-releasing factor, hypotheses implicating either of these agents are not mutually exclusive.

HISTAMINE

Histamine was one of the first biologically vasoactive substances identified, and its possible involvement in the mechanism of migraine has been speculated on ever since Pickering (1933) showed that its parenteral administration regularly resulted in a vascular headache. The idea of using histamine to establish an experimental model of headache came to him after observing that circulation time measurements, which at the time were obtained with intravenous histamine, were regularly followed by headache. Subsequently, evidence was put forth that distinguished histamine headache from migrainous headaches. Histamine headache is: (1) primarily an intracranial and not an extracranial arterial disorder (Pickering, 1939; Schumacher and Wolff, 1941); (2) regularly blocked by the prior administration of an H_1 receptor antagonist, whereas migraine is not (Ostfeld et al, 1957); and (3) unaffected by the administration of ergotamine tartrate (Graham and Wolff, 1938).

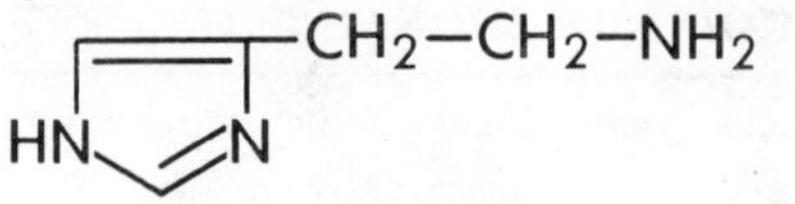

$$\text{HN} \diagdown \text{N} \diagup \text{---CH}_2\text{--CH}_2\text{--NH}_2$$

Figure 3–3.

HISTAMINE

Despite these clinical distinctions, recent data have once again implicated histamine as a putative mediator of migraine.

Histamine is stored in the granules of mast cells in tissues and within basophilic leukocytes in blood; it may be released from these stores by trauma, toxins, histamine-releasing agents such as compound 48/80 (Paton, 1951) and by IgE-antigen-mediated immune reactions. Once released, histamine is rapidly metabolized, disappearing from plasma within minutes; it is highly polar and does not cross cell membranes readily (Beaven, 1978).

Within the CNS, histamine may be a neurotransmitter. It is present in highest concentration in the hypothalamus and is rapidly turned over (Dismukes and Snyder, 1974). It is not restricted to mast cells (Edvinsson et al, 1977) and is not depleted by compound 48/80. Injected into the lateral ventricle, histamine releases serotonin from the hypothalamus (Pilc and Nowak, 1979).

Sicuteri (1963) showed that mast cells were degranulated in skin biopsy specimens taken from the involved cranial side of patients with migrane. Later, Anthony and Lance (1971), assaying whole blood, demonstrated a slight increase in histamine levels during, and 24 hours after, migraine attacks; the post-headache levels achieved statistical significance. Sicuteri (1967) showed that the release of endogenous histamine was capable of provoking pain by injecting compound 48/80 into the superficial temporal or external carotid artery, producing ipsilateral mast cell degranulation and a brief intense headache. Curiously, the injection of 48/80 into a limb artery produced erythema and edema, but no pain,

There are pitfalls in the measurement of whole blood histamine and drawing inferences about the role of this substance in clinical conditions (Sjaastad, 1975). Moreover, there are several circumstances under which histamine release occurs where headache is either a rare or uncommon symptom (Lorenz and Doenicke, 1978). Furthermore, there is now evidence that there are at least two histamine receptors, H_1 and H_2 (Black et al, 1972), and intracranial arteries contain both receptors whereas extracranial arteries contain primarily H_2 receptors (Spira et al, 1978). However, therapeutic trials of H_1 and H_2 antagonists, alone and in combination, in patients with migraine have been ineffectual (Anthony et al, 1978). On balance, it is doubtful whether histamine is mechanistically involved in migraine other than as an epiphenomenon; the degranulation of mast cells and the modest elevations of histamine levels may be secondary to the tissue injury that may result from a migraine attack.

CATECHOLAMINES

It has sometimes been suggested that migraine is an exaggerated response to stress and anxiety. Since the catecholamines, epinephrine and norepinephrine, are vasoactive components of stress, and vascular headache is an important symptom in the syndrome resulting from norepinephrine- and (less commonly) epinephrine-secreting pheochromocytomas (Lance and Hinterberger, 1976), measurement has been made of levels of, and pharmacologic responsiveness to, the catecholamines.

The conjunctival arterioles are constricted by norepinephrine, and Ostfeld et al (1955) found that the reactivity to conjunctival norepinephrine was increased during the premonitory phase of a migrainous attack and decreased during headache. Infusions of norepinephrine during migrainous attacks, at a rate sufficient to reduce extracranial arterial pulsations, usually result in a diminution of headache. After infusions during headache-free periods, headache generally does not occur, indicating that migrainous headache is not a rebound phenomenon following the constriction of cranial arteries (Ostfeld and Wolff, 1955).

Although elevations of urinary vanillylmandelic acid (VMA), a major product of norepinephrine and epinephrine metabolism, have been reported during migrainous attacks (Curran et al, 1965), Curzon et al (1966) found no consistent relationship between migrainous attacks and VMA excretion.

In patients whose headaches waken them from sleep, plasma norepinephrine is significantly elevated during the three hours before wakening (Hsu et al, 1977). Plasma levels of norepinephrine decline during headache attacks, and gradually return to normal over a period of hours as the intensity of headache diminishes (Føg-

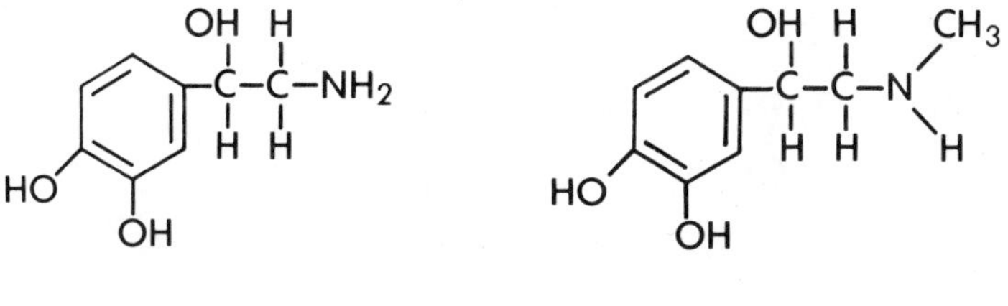

NOREPINEPHRINE   EPINEPHRINE

Figure 3–4.

Moller et al, 1978). Plasma epinephrine levels remain unaltered. In general, stressful conditions result in an increased turnover of catecholamines which is often reflected by an elevation of the plasma norepinephrine level (Taggart et al, 1973; Kopin et al, 1978). However, different types of stress may produce decreases as well as increases in peripheral catecholamine concentrations (Stone, 1975), so that the plasma alterations associated with migraine attacks may be the manifestation of this particular form of stress. The elevation of serum dopamine-beta-hydroxylase activity found interictally in migraineurs is also consistent with a stress response (Gotoh et al, 1976).

TYRAMINE, PHENYLETHYLAMINE AND MONOAMINE OXIDASE

It was Liebig (1846) who named tyrosine after the Greek word for cheese, tyrisine, from which he first isolated it. By the turn of the century the amine derivative, tyramine, had been extracted from cheese and was found to cause hypertension in man and animals (Dale and Dixon, 1909). In this early report, one of the investigators recorded a rise in his own blood pressure together with a feeling of fullness in the head after taking tyramine by mouth. Findlay (1911) showed that parenterally-administered tyramine (20 to 80 mg) elicited rises of blood pressure within ten minutes and that the largest increases were accompanied by excruciating headaches. Subsequently, it was shown that the pressor effects of tyramine were mediated by the release of norepinephrine from its binding sites (Burn and Rand, 1958).

Worldwide attention was accorded tyramine when it was implicated in a syndrome of intense throbbing headache, sometimes associated with hypertension, that occurred in some patients receiving antidepressant monoamine oxidase inhibitors (MAOI) after they had eaten certain foods rich in tyramine (Blackwell et al, 1967). Hanington and Harper (1968) observed that the foodstuffs implicated in these untoward reactions were similar to those foods most

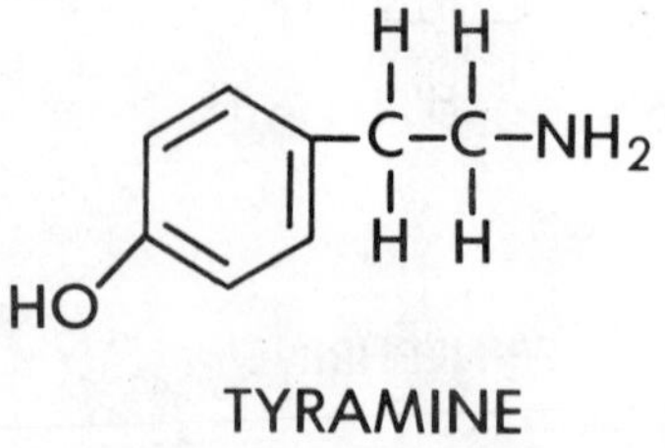

Figure 3–5.

TYRAMINE

TABLE 3-4. RESPONSE TO 125 mg OF TYRAMINE AND
LACTOSE OF 45 PATIENTS WITH DIETARY
MIGRAINE AND 104 NORMAL SUBJECTS*

| | DIETARY MIGRAINE | | NORMAL SUBJECTS | |
	No Effect	Headache	No Effect	Headache
Lactose	55	5	97	4
Tyramine	19	75**	97	5

*Smith, Kellow and Hanington, 1970; Hanington, Horn and Wilkinson, 1970.
**P<.01

often cited by migraine sufferers as precipitants of their attacks, a
condition that has come to be designated as "dietary migraine."
These authors later convincingly demonstrated that this subpopulation of migraine patients was sensitive to tyramine; a migrainous
attack was provoked within hours of the ingestion of tyramine in
over 80 per cent of instances (Table 3-4), whereas neither the non-
dietary migraine patients nor the headache-free control subjects experienced headache attacks to any significant extent (Smith et al,
1970; Hanington et al, 1970). These results were partially confirmed by Bonnet and Lepreux (1971), who identified 63 tyramine-
sensitive migraineurs among a series of 213 cases. Ghose et al
(1977), using intravenous tyramine, precipitated headache in 46 per
cent of 31 migraine sufferers and not at all in 27 control subjects.
On the other hand, Moffett et al (1972) and Shaw et al (1978), in
studies of eight and nine diet-sensitive migraineurs, were unable to
demonstrate tyramine sensitivity. Hanington (1974) has responded
to the earlier failure of confirmation, pointing out some of the methodologic pitfalls that may account for the discrepant results. On balance, the data supporting tyramine sensitivity in dietary migraine
are persuasive.

Sulfate conjugation forms an important inactivation mechanism
for ingested monoamines (Connolly et al, 1972), and two reports
have suggested that this mechanism is defective in tyramine-
sensitive migraineurs (Smith et al, 1971; Youdim et al, 1971). A
subsequent study from one of these laboratories in which methods
of greater precision were employed failed to confirm the original
observation (Smith et al, 1973).

Although endogenous tyramine is located primarily within the
CNS (Spector et al, 1963), where it may have a role as a modulator
of norepinephrine release, the mechanism by which tyramine is implicated in migraine is not clear. It appears likely that exogenous
tyramine can trigger migraine headaches, but blood pressure elevations do not occur at the doses used. Tyramine releases serotonin
from platelets in vitro (Bartholini and Pletscher, 1964), but this phenomenon has not been correlated with headache responsiveness.

Although tyramine-containing dairy products are frequently implicated as headache precipitants in patients with dietary migraine, other provocative foodstuffs such as ethyl alcohol and chocolate contain little or no tyramine (Sandler, 1975). Another vasoactive amine, phenylethylamine (PEA), has been identified in a variety of chocolates as well as in many cheeses and some red wines (Chaytor et al, 1975; Schweitzer et al, 1975); unsweetened chocolate contains the highest concentration of PEA, approximately 0.4 mg per ounce. Like tyramine, endogenous PEA has been identified in human brain, and is believed to modulate functions influenced by catecholamines (Sabelli et al, 1978); exogenous PEA crosses the blood-brain barrier and can effect large changes in CBF (McCulloch and Harper, 1979). Using 3 mg of PEA, Sandler et al (1974) showed that patients with chocolate-sensitive migraine experienced headache attacks about 50 per cent of the time after PEA ingestion, compared to a 15 per cent incidence after placebo ingestion (Table 3–5). Moffett et al (1974), using 44- to 62-gm samples of two types of chocolate of unknown PEA content, were unable to provoke headache significantly more often than after placebo ingestion.

This latter study notwithstanding, Sandler et al (1974) formulated the ingenious hypothesis that chocolate-sensitive migraineurs are sensitive to PEA because of a deficiency of an isomer of monoamine oxidase (MAO) that is substrate-specific for PEA. This was a reasonable suggestion since PEA is inactivated predominantly via oxidative deamination which is catalyzed by MAO (Edwards and Blau, 1973), and there are separable forms of MAO (A and B) that possess distinct substrate preferences (McCauley and Racker, 1973; Murphy, 1978). Type A is relatively specific for serotonin and norepinephrine, whereas type B is relatively specific for PEA. Therefore, a specific defect of MAO-B was hypothesized as the mechanism of chocolate-induced migraine. Sandler et al (1974) used platelets (which contain solely the B form) as the source of MAO and showed significantly depressed enzyme activity in the chocolate-sensitive patients; however, the activities of the non-chocolate-sensitive migraine patients were equally depressed, and in both groups the diminution in activity was apparent with all four monoamine substrates utilized: PEA, tyramine, serotonin and dopamine.

Thus, although the hypothesis was not supported, attention should be drawn to the low platelet MAO activities found in this

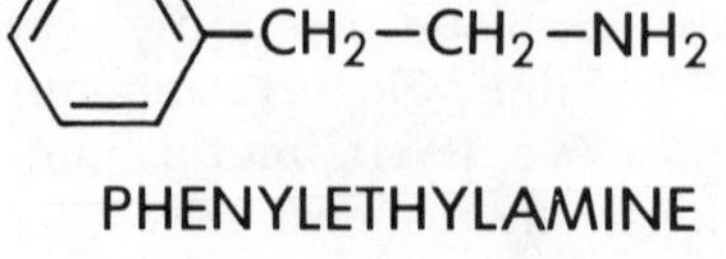

Figure 3–6.

PHENYLETHYLAMINE

TABLE 3-5. *RESPONSE TO 3 mg OF β-PHENYLETHYLAMINE AND LACTOSE OF 36 PATIENTS WITH CHOCOLATE-INDUCED MIGRAINE*[*]

	No Effect	Headache
Lactose	30	6
Phenylethylamine	18	18[**]

[*]Sandler, Youdim and Hanington, 1974.
[**]$p < .01$

study and others (Sicuteri, 1972; Glover et al, 1977); this depression of activity is more apparent when platelet samples are drawn *during* migrainous attacks (Sandler, 1977). It remains to be determined whether these alterations of platelet MAO activity are reflected in other tissues. The large concentrations of MAO in cerebral capillary endothelial cells may be relevant to this point; since enzymatic degradation by brain capillary MAO contributes to the blood-brain barrier mechanism for monoamines (Bertler et al, 1966), reduced capillary MAO activity may result in the sensitivities that appear to occur clinically. These ideas are difficult, at present, to reconcile with the observation that phenelzine, a MAO-inhibitor, is effective in migraine (Anthony and Lance, 1969), although it is certainly possible that the pharmacologic activity of this drug is unrelated to its capacity to inhibit MAO.

CARBOHYDRATE AND FATTY ACID METABOLISM

The precipitation of migrainous attacks by hunger and fasting (Blau and Cumings, 1966) in certain migrainous subjects has led to several studies of carbohydrate metabolism in search of a metabolic explanation for this phenomenon. Although headache is a common symptom of insulin-induced hypoglycemia (Hockaday, 1975), it clearly is not hypoglycemia *per se* that is responsible for the precipitation of migrainous attacks by hunger (Pearce, 1971), since the lowest blood glucose levels recorded during fasting in subjects experiencing an attack are not different from those in subjects who do not develop headache (Hockaday et al, 1971).

During extended standard insulin hypoglycemia tests, migrainous subjects demonstrate hypoglycemia unresponsiveness (Rao and Pearce, 1971). Since the cortisol response to insulin-induced hypoglycemia and the metapyrone test is normal in migraineurs, a defect of the hypothalamic-pituitary-adrenal axis is not likely to be contributory. A diminished hyperglycemic response to glucagon (DeSilva et al, 1974) is consistent with an impairment in the hepatic mobilization of glucose. During migrainous attacks, there are decreased glucose tolerance, low plasma insulin levels, and elevations of free fatty acids, glycerol, ketone bodies, secretin (McLoughlin et al., 1978) and growth hormone (Shaw et al, 1977). These findings (Table 3–6), taken together, are consistent with a chronic stress reaction with heightened sympathetic activity (Taggart et al, 1973). Fasting results in increased turnover of brain serotonin (Curzon et al, 1972) which may be important to the mechanism of headache provoked by hunger.

PLATELET FUNCTION

Platelets aggregate in response to conditions such as stress and tissue injury, and are somehow activated to synthesize prostaglandins and thromboxane A. This results in further aggregation and the initiation of a secretory process, the release reaction, during which substances stored in the platelets (including serotonin, β-thromboglobulin, ADP and proteolytic enzymes) are extruded from the cell (Weiss, 1975). The involvement of serotonin in platelet activation has led to a series of studies (Hilton and Cumings, 1971; Couch and Hassanein, 1977) which have shown that heightened platelet aggregability is present in migrainous subjects. Since hyperaggregability is also demonstrable in patients who have sustained cerebral infarction (Kalendovsky et al, 1975), it is possible that this finding is relevant to the elevated risk of stroke in the migraine population (Collaborative Group, 1975).

Deshmukh and Meyer (1977) performed platelet function tests in 14 migraineurs during the headache-free period, and restudied three patients during their prodromal symptoms and 11 during the headache phase. They showed an increase in platelet aggregation during the aura and a decrease during the headache; platelet adhesiveness, however, increased during the headache phase. Because the biochemical basis for the attachment of platelets to surfaces (ad-

TABLE 3–6. *CARBOHYDRATE METABOLISM DURING MIGRAINE ATTACKS*°

Decreased glucose tolerance
Low plasma insulin levels
Elevated plasma free fatty acids,
glycerol, ketone bodies,
growth hormone
Plasma lactate, pyruvate unchanged

°Shaw, Johnson and Keogh, 1977.

hesion) and to each other (aggregation) is poorly understood at present, the interpretation of these findings is difficult. Whether the release of platelet serotonin that occurs during headache attacks is directly related to these alterations in platelet function is unclear. Informal therapeutic trials with antiplatelet drugs such as dipyridamole and sulfinpyrazone (Weiss, 1978) in migrainous patients have been disappointing (Hawkes, 1978). It is similarly unclear whether the benefits received from aspirin are related to its effects on platelet functions. Moreover, platelet hyperaggregability is found in many other conditions, such as diabetes mellitus, and no association of diabetes with migraine was found by Hockaday (1975).

Damasio and Beck (1978) have shown that attacks of migraine may be associated with the thrombocytopenia that occurs in idiopathic thrombocytopenic purpura (ITP), and that may arise in systemic lupus erythematosus (SLE). Six migraine patients were studied, only one of whom had migraine (to a lesser degree) before the discovery of the hematologic disorder. All six had migrainous attacks during periods in which they tended to bruise easily and had low platelet counts. Three of the six underwent splenectomy, following which their migraine improved remarkably; two patients were kept going on corticosteroids with maintenance of adequate platelet counts and little headache, but one experienced recurrence of headache despite steroid therapy during periods of thrombocytopenia. In patients with SLE and ITP, platelet serotonin is very low and the free plasma serotonin is elevated; this is also true in those with other forms of immune complex diseases such as glomerulonephritis and rheumatoid arthritis (Parbtani and Cameron, 1978). Plasma from patients with ITP contains a serotonin-releasing factor in that it releases much more serotonin from normal platelets than does plasma from normal subjects (Hirschman and Shulman, 1973). These data linking migraine to abnormalities of serotonin metabolism and of platelets in immune complex diseases, taken together with the recent demonstration of complement activation during migrainous attacks (Lord et al, 1977), suggest that further attention to immune responses in migraine may be fruitful.

CENTRAL VASOMOTOR DYSREGULATION

Before a migraine attack, many patients have noted a variety of symptoms, including increased appetite and thirst, exhilaration, specific food cravings, fatigue and nausea, that suggest a central, possibly hypothalamic disturbance (Herberg, 1975). An increased frequency of electroencephalographic abnormalities in migraineurs has been taken to support this inference (Parsonage, 1975), although it remains possible that these central alterations are secondary to the disorder itself; the responsiveness of at least some migraine patients to phenytoin (Fields and Raskin, 1976), especially children (Millichap, 1978), is likewise supportive of a central hypothesis.

An additional line of evidence that suggests the possibility of a central disorder of vasomotor regulation is provided by a series of observations regarding the vascular responses of migraineurs. Although systemic orthostatic hypotension does not occur with increased frequency in migraine patients, there is a much higher incidence of symptomatic transient cerebral ischemia that is provoked by ordinary postural change, suggesting imprecise regulation of the cranial vasculature (Raskin and Knittle, 1976). Similarly, the amplitude of the superficial temporal artery pulse is orthostatically reduced to a greater degree in migraineurs than in control subjects (Wennerholm, 1961). Vasodilatation in the hand in response to radiant heating of the trunk is mediated by a neural reflex (Kerslake and Cooper, 1950). Evidence has been advanced that this reflex is defective in migraineurs (Appenzeller et al, 1963; Appenzeller, 1969, 1978) and these results have been replicated (Downey and Frewin, 1972; Elliot et al, 1973). MacMillan and Hockaday (1967) showed that the mean responsiveness of migraine patients to thermal stimuli was less than that of normal subjects, but this difference between the means did not reach statistical significance. Another group of investigators found no differences in the reflex vasomotor responses of migraineurs (French et al, 1967). Morley (1977) has critically reviewed the evidence regarding defective vasomotor function in patients with migraine; he pointed out major methodologic problems that make it difficult to compare these studies. Although the evidence is not as yet conclusive, it appears likely that vasoregulatory mechanisms are defective in migraine patients.

Surgical procedures in migraine aimed at disconnecting the neural regulation of cranial arteries have been unsuccessful in preventing migraine attacks. Cervical sympathectomy, greater superfi-

TABLE 3-7. FEATURES CONSISTENT WITH MIGRAINE AS A
DISORDER OF CENTRAL VASOMOTOR REGULATION

"Central" symptoms precede attacks:
    exhilaration, increased thirst and appetite, nausea

Increased frequency of electroencephalographic abnormalities

Vasomotor dysregulation:
    increased frequency of postural symptoms
    decreased temporal artery pulse amplitude with postural shifts
    decreased vascular responsiveness to hot and cold stimuli

Effective drugs produce substantial alterations within the central nervous
    system

cial petrosal neurectomy, external carotid or middle meningeal artery ligation and carotid body resection are all without lasting benefit in migraine (Lance and Anthony, 1977). Resection of the sensory portion of the trigeminal nerve is generally effective at the expense of permanent facial numbness (Olevicrona, 1947); it is not a procedure to be recommended. These data have been used to refute the idea that migraine is a disturbance of central vasoregulatory mechanisms, whereas they neither confirm nor deny the hypothesis.

Thus, the data supporting the hypothesis that migraine is a disturbance of central regulatory mechanisms are not substantial (Table 3–7). On the other hand, the idea remains viable, with no compelling evidence that excludes this possibility.

PSYCHOLOGIC FACTORS

Developments during the third and fourth decades of this century included the detailed study of personality and psychodynamics, and the presentation of psychoanalytic theories relevant to migraine. Over several years some of these views were adopted and disseminated by Wolff (1937); he noted that migraine patients were apt to be rigid, ambitious and perfectionistic, and responded with headache attacks to repressed hostility and a variety of frustrations. The inability to express anger was held to be caused by guilt since the object of resentment was so often a loved one. Acceptance of these views, unsupported by data, persisted for many years.

It is clear that there is no personality type specific for migraine. Selby and Lance (1960) found that only 23 per cent of 500 patients with migraine displayed obsessive-compulsive traits; nor are there differences in social standing or intelligence (Waters, 1971). Projective tests demonstrate a somewhat higher incidence of "neuroticism" and of anxiety in patients with migraine; however, these results are also seen when patients with chronic pain of various causation are tested (Merskey, 1975). Psychologic reactions to pain certainly occur, and there are data which support the view that a significant proportion of the emotional disturbance associated with chronic pain is a secondary effect (Merskey and Boyd, 1978). Emotional reactions to migraine attacks, as with any other illness, may potentiate mechanisms that may exacerbate or perpetuate headache attacks, and some patients may derive benefit from psychotherapy (Hunter and Ross, 1960). No adequately controlled study of psychotherapy in migraine has been carried out.

A large variety of experiences can precipitate migraine attacks, many of which would be generally regarded as potentially stressful; however, the nonmigrainous population-at-large is subject to similar or greater stresses without experiencing headache. These circumstances appear to hold for exposure to glare or high altitudes, the ingestion of chocolate or cheese, or receiving an injection of reserpine. Stress, worry and anxiety appear to be important and frequent precipitants of migraine attacks, and exemplify the wide variety of stimuli toward which migraineurs are sensitive. However, it appears to be quite uncommon for stress to be the *sole* circumstance in which headache attacks arise. The view that migraine is primarily a psychosomatic disorder is not supportable by the evidence at hand; furthermore, there are data that militate against it (Rees, 1971; Pearce, 1977)

Further data regarding the pathogenesis of migraine drawn from clinical and biochemical pharmacologic studies will be reviewed in the following chapter.

REFERENCES

Adams, C. W. M., Orton, C. C. and Zilkha, K. J. (1968): Arterial catecholamine and enzyme histochemistry in migraine. J. Neurol. Neurosurg. Psychiatry 31:50–56.
Agnoli, A., Fieschi, C., Bozzao, L. et al (1968): Autoregulation of cerebral blood flow. Studies during drug-induced hypertension in normal subjects and in patients with cerebrovascular disease. Circulation 38:800–812.
Alabaster, V. A. and Bakhle, Y. S. (1970): The release of biologically active substances from isolated lungs by 5-hydroxytryptamine and tryptamine. Br. J. Pharmacol. 40:582–583P.
Anthony, M. (1976): Plasma free fatty acids and prostaglandin E₁ in migraine and stress. Headache 16:58–63.
Anthony, M., Hinterberger, H. and Lance, J. W. (1967): Plasma serotonin in migraine and stress. Arch. Neurol. 16:544–552.
Anthony, M., Hinterberger, H. and Lance, J. W. (1969): The possible relationship of serotonin to the migraine syndrome. Res. Clin. Stud. Headache 2:29–59.
Anthony, M. and Lance, J. W. (1968): Indomethacin in migraine. Med. J. Aust. 1:56–57.
Anthony, M. and Lance, J. W. (1969): Monoamine oxidase inhibition in the treatment of migraine. Arch. Neurol. 21:263–268.
Anthony, M. and Lance, J. W. (1971): Histamine and serotonin in cluster headache. Arch. Neurol. 25:225–231.
Anthony, M. and Lance, J. W. (1975): The role of serotonin in migraine. In Modern Topics in Migraine, ed. J. Pearce. Wm. Heinemann, London, pp. 107–123.
Anthony, M., Lord, G. D. A. and Lance, J. W. (1978): Controlled trials of cimetidine in migraine and cluster headache. Headache 18:261–264.
Appenzeller, O. (1969): Vasomotor function in migraine. Headache 9:147–155.
Appenzeller, O. (1978): Reflex vasomotor function: clinical and experimental studies in migraine. Res. Clin. Stud. Headache 6:160–166.
Appenzeller, O., Davison, K. and Marshall, J. (1963): Reflex vasomotor abnormalities in the hands of migrainous subjects. J. Neurol. Neurosurg. Psychiatry 26:447–450.
Bakhle, Y. S. and Smith, T. W. (1972): Release of spasmogenic substances by vasoactive amines from isolated lungs. Br. J. Pharmacol. 46:543–544P.
Barrie, M. and Jowett, A. (1967): A pharmacological investigation of cerebrospinal fluid from patients with migraine. Brain 90:785–794.
Bartholini, G. and Pletscher, A. (1964): Two types of 5-hydroxytryptamine release from isolated blood platelets. Experientia 20:376–378.
Basser, L. S. (1969): The relation of migraine and epilepsy. Brain 92:285–300.
Beaven, M. A. (1978): Histamine: its role in physiological and pathological processes. In Monographs in Allergy, Vol. 13, eds. P. Dukor, P. Kallós, Z. Trnka, B. Waksman and A. L. deWeck. S. Karger, New York, pp. 1–113.

Bertler, A., Falck, B., Owman, C. et al (1966): The localization of monoaminergic blood-brain barrier mechanisms. Pharmacol. Rev. 18:369–385.

Black, J. W., Duncan, W. A. M., Durant, C. J. et al (1972): Definition and antagonism of histamine H_2 receptors. Nature 236:385–390.

Blackwell, B., Marley, E., Price, J. and Taylor, D. (1967): Hypertensive interactions between monoamine oxidase inhibitors and foodstuffs. Br. J. Psychiatry 113:349–365.

Blau, J. N. and Cumings, J. N. (1966): Methods of precipitating and preventing some migraine attacks. Br. Med. J. 2:1242–1243.

Bonnet, G. F. and Lepreux, P. (1971): Les migraines tyraminiques. Sem. Hop. Paris 47:2441–2445.

Burn, J. H. and Rand, M. J. (1958): The action of sympathomimetic amines in animals treated with reserpine. J. Physiol. 144:314–336.

Cabot, J. B., Wild, J. M. and Cohen, D. H. (1979): Raphe inhibition of sympathetic preganglionic neurons. Science 203:184–186.

Carlson, L. A., Ekelund, L.-G. and Orö, L. (1968): Clinical and metabolic effects of different doses of prostaglandin E_1 in man. Acta Med. Scand. 183:423–430.

Carroll, J. D. and Hilton, B. P. (1973): The effects of reserpine injection on methysergide treated control and migrainous subjects. In Background to Migraine, 5th Migraine Symposium, ed. J. N. Cumings. Springer-Verlag, New York, pp. 122–133.

Chapman, L. F., Ramos, A. O., Goodell, H., Silverman, G. and Wolff, H. G. (1960): A humoral agent implicated in vascular headache of the migraine type. Arch. Neurol. 3:223–229.

Chaytor, J. P., Crathorne, B. and Saxby, M. J. (1975): The identification and significance of 2-phenylethylamine in foods. J. Sci. Food Agric. 26:593–598.

Christ, E. J. and Van Dorp, D. A. (1972): Comparative aspects of prostaglandin biosynthesis in animal tissues. In Advances in the Biosciences, ed. G. Raspe. Pergamon Press, New York, pp. 35–38.

Christian, S. T. and Smythies, J. R. (1978): Molecular interactions with serotonin. In Serotonin in Health and Disease, Vol. 1, ed. W. B. Essman. Spectrum, New York, pp. 363–374.

Collaborative Group for the Study of Stroke in Young Women (1975): Oral contraceptives and stroke in young women, associated risk factors. J.A.M.A. 231:718–722.

Connolly, M. E., Davies, D. S., Dollery, C. T., Morgan, C. D., Paterson, J. W. and Sandler, M. (1972): Metabolism of isoprenaline in dog and man. Br. J. Pharmacol. 46:458–472.

Connor, R. C. R. (1962): Complicated migraine: a study of permanent neurological and visual defects caused by migraine. Lancet 2:1072–1075.

Cooper, J. R., Bloom, F. E. and Roth, R. H. (1978): The Biochemical Basis of Neuropharmacology. Oxford University Press, New York, pp. 294–304.

Couch, J. R. and Hassanein, R. S. (1977): Platelet aggregability in migraine. Neurology 27:843–848.

Curran, D. A., Hinterberger, H. and Lance, J. W. (1965): Total plasma serotonin, 5-hydroxyindoleacetic acid and p-hydroxy-m-methoxymandelic acid excretion in normal and migrainous subjects. Brain 88:997–1010.

Curzon, G., Joseph, M. H. and Knott, P. J. (1972): Effects of immobilization and food deprivation on rat brain tryptophan metabolism. J. Neurochem. 19:1967–1974.

Curzon, G., Theaker, P. and Phillips, B. (1966): Excretion of 5-HIAA in migraine. J. Neurol. Neurosurg. Psychiatry 29:85–90.

Dale, H. H. and Dixon, W. E. (1909): Action of pressor bases produced by putrefaction. J. Physiol. 34:25–44.

Damasio, H. and Beck, D. (1978): Migraine, thrombocytopenia, and serotonin metabolism. Lancet 1:240–242.

Deshmukh, S. V. and Meyer, J. S. (1977): Cyclic changes in platelet dynamics and the pathogenesis and prophylaxis of migraine. Headache 17:101–108.

DeSilva, K. L., Ron, M. A. and Pearce, J. (1974): Blood sugar response to glucagon in migraine. J. Neurol. Neurosurg. Psychiatry 37:105–107.

Dismukes, K. and Snyder, S. H. (1974): Histamine turnover in the brain. Brain Res. 78:467–480.

Douglas, W. W. (1975): Autacoids. In The Pharmacological Basis of Therapeutics, 5th ed., eds. L. S. Goodman and A. Gilman, Macmillan, New York, pp. 589–629.

Downey, J. A. and Frewin, D. B. (1972): Vascular responses in the hands of patients suffering from migraine. J. Neurol Neurosurg. Psychiatry 35:258–263.

Dvilansky, A. Rishpon, S., Nathan, I., Zolotow, Z. and Korczyn, A. (1976): Release of platelet 5-hydroxytryptamine by plasma taken from patients during and between migraine attacks. Pain 2:315–318.

Edelman, A. M., Berger, P. A. and Reson, J. F. (1977): 5-hydroxytryptamine: basic and clinical perspectives. In Neuroregulators and Psychiatric Disorders, eds. E. Usdin, D. Hamburg and J. Barchas. Oxford University Press, New York, pp. 177–187.

Edvinsson, L., Cervos-Navarro, J., Larsson, L-I., Owman, Ch. and Rönnberg, A-L. (1977): Regional distribution of mast cells containing histamine, dopamine, or 5-hydroxytryptamine in the mammalian brain. Neurology 27:878–883.

Edvinsson, L. and Hardebo, J. E. (1976): Characterization of serotonin-receptors in intracranial and extracranial vessels. Acta Physiol. Scand. 97:523–525.

Edvinsson, L., Hardebo, J. E., MacKenzie, E. T. and Stewart, M. (1975): Dual action of serotonin on pial arterioles in situ and the effect of propranolol on the response. Blood Vessels 14:366–371.

Edvinsson, L. and MacKenzie, E. T. (1976): Amine mechanisms in the cerebral circulation. Pharmacol. Rev. 28:275–348.

Edwards, D. J. and Blau, K. (1973): Phenylethylamine in brain and liver of rats with experimentally-induced phenylketonuria-like characteristics. Biochem. J. 132:95–100.

Elliot, K., Frewin, D. B. and Downey, J. A. (1973): Reflex vasomotor responses in hands of patients suffering from migraine. Headache 13:188–196.

Fields, H. L. and Basbaum, A. O. (1978): Brainstem control of spinal pain-transmission neurons. Annu. Rev. Physiol. 40:217–248.

Fields, H. L. and Raskin, N. H. (1976): Anticonvulsants and pain. In Clinical Neuropharmacology, Vol. 1, ed. H. L. Klawans. Raven Press, New York, pp. 173–184.

Findlay, J. (1911): The systolic pressure at different points of the circulation in the child and the adult. Q. J. Med. 4:489–497.

Føg-Moller, F., Genefke, I. K. and Bryndum, B. (1978): Changes in concentration of catecholamines in blood during spontaneous migraine attacks and reserpine-induced attacks. In Current Concepts in Migraine Research, ed. R. Greene. Raven Press, New York, pp. 115–119.

Fozard, J. R. (1975): The animal pharmacology of drugs used in the treatment of migraine. J. Pharm. Pharmacol. 27:297–321.

French, E. B., Lassers, B. W. and Desai, M. G. (1967): Reflex vasomotor responses in the hands of migrainous subjects. J. Neurol. Neurosurg. Psychiatry 30:276–278.

Gaudet, R. J., Maurer, P., Levine, L. and Moskowitz, M. A. (1979): Prostaglandins: accumulation in brain after transient ischemia and in vitro synthesis by cerebral microvessels. Heachache 19:245.

Gerschenfeld, H. M., Hamon, M. and Paupardin-Tritsch, D. (1978): Release of endogenous serotonin from two identified serotonin-containing neurones and the physiological role of serotonin re-uptake. J. Physiol. 274:265–278.

Ghose, K., Coppen, A. and Carroll, D. (1977): Intravenous tyramine response in migraine before and during treatment with indoramin. Br. Med. J. 1:1191–1193.

Glover, V., Sandler, M., Grant, E., Rose, F. C., Orton, D., Wilkinson, M. and Stevens, D. (1977): Transitory decrease in platelet monoamine-oxidase activity during migraine attacks. Lancet 1:391–393.

Gotoh, F., Kanda, T., Sakai, F. et al (1976): Serum dopamine-beta-hydroxylase activity in migraine. Arch. Neurol. 33:656–657.

Graham, J. R. and Wolff, H. G. (1938): Mechanism of migraine headache and action of ergotamine tartrate. Arch. Neurol. Psychiatry 39:737–763.

Hachinski, V., Norris, J. W., Edmeads, J. and Cooper, D. W. (1978): Ergotamine and cerebral blood flow. Stroke 9:594–596.

Hachinski, V. C., Olesen, J., Norris, J. W., Larsen, B., Enevoldsen, F. and Lassen, N. A. (1977): Cerebral hemodynamics in migraine. Can. J. Neurol. Sci. 4:245–249.

Haddy, F. J. (1960): Serotonin and the vascular system. Angiology 11:21–24.

Hanington, E. (1974): Monoamine oxidase and migraine. Lancet 2:1148–1149.

Hanington, E. and Harper, A. M. (1968): The role of tyramine in the etiology of migraine, and related studies on the cerebral and extracerebral circulations. Headache 8:84–97.

Hanington, E., Horn, M. and Wilkinson, M. (1970): Further observations on the effect of tyramine. In Background to Migraine, 3rd Migraine Symposium, ed. J. N. Cumings. Springer-Verlag, New York, pp. 113–119.

Hardebo, J. E., Edvinsson, L., Owman, C. and Svendgaard, N.-Aa. (1978): Potentiation and antagonism of serotonin effects on intracranial and extracranial vessels. Neurology 28:64–70.

Hawkes, C. H. (1978): Dipyridamole in migraine. Lancet 2:153.

Heller, A. (1972): Neuronal control of brain serotonin. Fed. Proc. 31:81–90.

Herberg, L. J. (1975): The hypothalamus and aminergic pathways in migraine. In Modern Topics in Migraine, ed. J. Pearce. Wm. Heinemann, London, pp. 85–95.

Heyck, J. R. S. (1974): Pathogenesis of migraine. Res. Clin. Stud. Headache. 2:1–28.

Hilton, B. P. and Cumings, J. N. (1971): An assessment of platelet aggregation induced by 5-hydroxytryptamine. J. Clin. Pathol. 24:250:258.

Hilton, B. P. and Cumings, J. N. (1972): 5-hydroxytryptamine levels and platelet aggregation responses in subjects with acute migraine headache. J. Neurol Neurosurg. Psychiatry 35:505–509.

Hirschman, R. J. and Shulman, N. R. (1973): The use of platelet serotonin release as a sensitive method for detecting antiplatelet antibodies. Br. J. Haematol. 24:793–802.

Hockaday, J. M. (1975): Anomalies of carbohydrate metabolism. In Modern Topics in Migraine, ed. J. Pearce. Wm. Heinemann, London, pp. 124–137.

Hockaday, J. M., Williamson, D. H. and Whitty, C. W. M. (1971): Blood glucose levels and fatty acid metabolism in migraine related to fasting. Lancet 1:1153–1156.

Holmes, S. W. (1970): The spontaneous release of prostaglandins into the cerebral ventricles of the dog and the effect of external factors on this release. Br. J. Pharmacol. 38:653–658.

Horrobin, D. F. (1977): Prostaglandins and migraine. Headache 17:113–117.

Hsu, L. K. G., Crisp, A. H., Kalucy, R. S., Koval, J. and Chen, C. N. (1977): Early morning migraine. Nocturnal plasma levels of catecholamines, tryptophan, glucose, and free fatty acids and sleep encephalographs. Lancet 2:447–451.

Hunter, R. A. and Ross, I. P. (1960): Psychotherapy in migraine. Br. Med. J. 1:1084–1088.

Ingvar, D. H. (1976): Pain in the brain — and migraine. Hemicrania 7:2–5.

Kalendovsky, Z., Austin, J. and Steele, P. (1975): Increased platelet aggregability in young patients with stroke. Arch. Neurol. 32:13–20.

Kerslake, D. McK. and Cooper, K. E. (1950): Vasodilatation in the hand in response to heating the skin elsewhere. Clin. Sci. 9:31–47.

Kopin, I. J., Lake, R. C. and Ziegler, M. (1978): Plasma levels of norepinephrine. Ann. Intern. Med. 88:671–680.

Lance, J. W. and Anthony, M. (1977): The cephalgias, with special reference to vascular and muscle-contraction headaches. In Scientific Approaches to Clinical Neurology, eds. E. Goldensohn and S. H. Appel. Lea and Febiger, Philadelphia, pp. 1959–1979.

Lance, J. W. and Hinterberger, H. (1976): Symptoms of pheochromocytoma, with particular reference to headache, correlated with catecholamine production. Arch. Neurol. 33:281–288.

Lashley, K. S. (1941): Patterns of cerebral integration indicated by the scotomas of migraine. Arch. Neurol. Psychiatry 46:331–339.

Leão, A. A. P. (1944): Spreading depression of activity in cerebral cortex. J. Neurophysiol. 7:359–390.

Liebig, J. (1846): Baldriansäure und ein neuer Körper aus Käsestoff. Ann. d. Chem. 57:127–129.

Lin, M. T. (1979): Effects of brain serotonin alterations on prostaglandin E_1-induced bradycardia in rats. J. Pharmacol. Exp. Ther. 208:232–235.

Lord, G. D. A., Duckworth, J. W. and Charlesworth, J. A. (1977): Complement activation in migraine. Lancet 1:781–782.

Lorenz, W. and Doenicke, A. (1978): Histamine release in clinical conditions. Mt. Sinai J. Med. 45:357–386.

MacMillan, A. L. and Hockaday, J. (1967): The effect of migraine and ergot upon reflex vasodilatation to radiant heating. In Proc. 4th European Conf. Microcirculation. Karger, Basel/New York, pp. 343–347.

Manku, M. S., Mtabaji, J. P. and Horrobin, D. F. (1977): Effects of prostaglandins on baseline pressure and responses to noradrenaline in a perfused rat mesenteric artery preparation: PGE_1 as an antagonist of PGE_2. Prostaglandins 13:701–709.
Marshall, W. H. (1959) Spreading cortical depression of Leão. Physiol. Rev. 39:239–279.
McCauley, R. and Racker, E. (1973): Separation of two monoamine oxidases from bovine brain. Mol. Cell. Biochem. 1:73–81.
McCulloch, J. and Harper, A. M. (1979): Factors influencing the response of the cerebral circulation to phenylethylamine. Neurology 29:201–207.
McLoughlin, J. C., Buchanan, K. D. and Ardill, J. E. (1978): Entero-pancreatic hormones in migraine. Ir. J. Med. Sci. 147:151–155.
Merskey, H. (1975): Psychiatric aspects of migraine. In Modern Topics in Migraine, ed. J. Pearce. Wm. Heinemann, London, pp. 52–61.
Merskey, H. and Boyd, D. (1978): Emotional adjustment and chronic pain. Pain 5:173–178.
Millichap, G. (1978): Recurrent headaches in 100 children. Child's Brain 4:95–105.
Moffett, A. M., Swash, M. and Scott, D. F. (1972): Effect of tyramine in migraine: a double-blind study. J. Neurol. Neurosurg. Psychiatry 35:496–499.
Moffett, A. M., Swash, M. and Scott, D. F. (1974): Effect of chocolate in migraine: a double-blind study. J. Neurol. Neurosurg. Psychiatry 37:445–448.
Morley, S. (1977): Migraine: a generalized vasomotor dysfunction? A critical review of evidence. Headache 17:71–74.
Murphy, D. L. (1978): Substrate-selective monoamine oxidases — inhibitor, tissue, species and functional differences. Biochem. Pharmacol. 27:1889–1893.
Needleman, P. and Kaley, G. (1978): Cardiac and coronary prostaglandin synthesis and function. N. Engl. J. Med. 298:1122–1128.
Needleman, P., Marshall, G. R. and Douglas, J. R., Jr. (1973): Prostaglandin release from vasculature by angiotensin II: dissociation from lipolysis. Eur. J. Pharmacol. 66:316–319.
Olivecrona, H. (1974): Notes on the surgical treatment of migraine. Acta Med. Scand. (suppl.) 196:229–238.
Ostfeld, A. M., Chapman, L. F., Goodell, H. and Wolff, H. G. (1957): Studies in headache: summary of evidence concerning a noxious agent active locally during migraine headache. Psychosom. Med. 19:199–208.
Ostfeld, A. M., Reis, D. J., Goodell, H. and Wolff, H. G. (1955): Headache and hydration. Arch. Intern. Med. 96:142–152.
Ostfeld, A. M. and Wolff, H. G. (1955): Arteronol (norepinephrine) and vascular headache of the migraine type. Arch. Neurol. Psychiatry 14:131–136.
Parbtani, A. and Cameron, J. S. (1978): Platelets, serotonin, migraine, and immune complex disease. Lancet 2:679.
Parsonage, M. (1975): Electroencephalographic studies in migraine. In Modern Topics in Migraine, ed. J. Pearce. Wm. Heinemann, London, pp. 72–84.
Paton, W. D. M. (1951): Compound 48/80: a potent histamine liberator. Br. J. Pharmacol. 6:499–508.
Paulson, O. B., Lassen, N. A. and Skinhøj, E. (1970): Regional cerebral blood flow in apoplexy without arterial occlusion. Neurology 20:125–138.
Pearce, J. (1971): Insulin-induced hypoglycemia in migraine. J. Neurol. Neurosurg. Psychiatry 34:154–156.
Pearce, J. (1977): Migraine: a psychosomatic disorder. Headache 17:125–128.
Pickering, G. W. (1933): Observations on the mechanism of headache produced by histamine. Clin. Sci. 1:77–101.
Pickering, G. W. (1939): Experimental observations on headache. Br. Med. J. 1:907–912.
Pilc, A. and Nowak, J. Z. (1979): Inffluence of histamine on the serotonergic system of rat brain. Eur. J. Pharmacol. 55:269–272.
Piper, P. and Vane, J. (1971): The release of prostaglandins from lung and other tissues. Ann. N.Y. Acad. Sci. 180:363–385.
Rao, N. S. and Pearce, J. (1971): Hypothalamic-pituitary-adrenal axis studies in migraine with special reference to insulin sensitivity. Brain 94:289–298.
Raskin, N. H. and Knittle, S. C. (1976): Ice cream headache and orthostatic symptoms in patients with migraine. Headache 16:222–225.

Ray, B. S. and Wolff, H. G. (1940): Experimental studies on headache. Pain-sensitive structures of the head and their significance in headache. Arch Surg. 41:813–856.

Rees, W. L. (1971): Psychiatric and psychological aspects of migraine. In Background to Migraine, 4th Migraine Symposium, ed. J. N. Cumings. Springer-Verlag, New York, pp. 45–54.

Sabelli H. C., Borison, R. L., Diamond, B. I. and Havdala, H. S. (1978): Phenylethylamine and brain function. Biochem. Pharmacol. 27:1729–1730.

Sakai, F. and Meyer, J. S. (1978): Regional cerebral hemodynamics during migraine and cluster headaches measured by the Xe¹³³ inhalation method. Headache 18:122–132.

Sakai, F. and Meyer, J. S. (1979): Abnormal cerebrovascular reactivity in patients with migraine and cluster headache. Headache 19:257–266.

Sandler, M. (1975): Monoamines and migraine: a path through the wood? In Vasoactive Substances Relevant to Migraine, eds. S. Diamond, D. J. Dalessio, J. R. Graham, and J. L. Medina. Charles C Thomas, Springfield, Ill., pp. 3–18.

Sandler, M. (1977): Transitory platelet monoamine oxidase deficit in migraine: some reflections. Headache 17:153–158.

Sandler, M., Youdim, M. B. H. and Hanington, E. (1974): A phenylethylamine-oxidising defect in migraine. Nature 250:335–337.

Schumacher, G. A. and Wolff, H. G. (1941): Experimental studies on headache. Arch. Neurol. Psychiatry 45:199–214.

Schweitzer, J. W., Friedhoff, A. J. and Schwartz, R. (1975): Chocolate, β-phenylethylamine and migraine re-examined. Nature 257:256.

Selby, G. and Lance, J. W. (1960): Observations on 500 cases of migraine and allied vascular headache. J. Neurol. Neurosurg. Psychiatry 23:23–32.

Shaw, S. W. J., Johnson, R. H. and Keogh, H. J. (1977): Metabolic changes during glucose tolerance tests in migraine attacks. J. Neurol. Sci. 33:51–59.

Shaw, S. W. J., Johnson, R. H. and Keogh, H. J. (1978): Oral tyramine in dietary migraine sufferers. In Current Concepts in Migraine Research, ed. R. Greene. Raven Press, New York, pp. 31–39.

Shinohara, M., Dollinger, B., Brown, G., Rapoport, S. and Sokoloff, L. (1979): Cerebral glucose utilization: local changes during and after recovery from spreading cortical depression. Science 203:188–190.

Sicuteri, F. (1963): Mast cells and their active substances. Their role in the pathogenesis of migraine. Headache 3:86–92.

Sicuteri, F. (1967): Vasoneuractive substances and their implication in vascular pain. Res. Clin. Stud. Headache 1:6–45.

Sicuteri, F. (1972): 5-Hydroxytryptamine in the prophylaxis of migraine. Pharmacol. Res. Commun. 4:213–218.

Sicuteri, F., Buffoni, F., Anselmi, B. and Delbianco, P. L. (1972): An enzyme (MAO) defect on the platelets in migraine. Headache 3:245–251.

Sicuteri, F., Testi, A. and Anselmi, B. (1961): Biochemical investigations in headache: increase in hydroxyindole acetic acid excretion during migraine attacks. Int. Arch. Allergy Appl. Immunol. 19:55–58.

Simard, D. and Paulson, O. B. (1973): Cerebral vasomotor paralysis during migraine attack. Arch. Neurol. 29:207–209.

Sjaastad, O. (1975): Is histamine of significance in the pathogenesis of headache? In Vasoactive Substances Relevant to Migraine, eds. S. Diamond, D. J. Dalessio, J. R. Graham and J. L. Medina. Charles C Thomas, Springfield, Ill., pp. 45–66.

Skinhøj, E. (1973): Hemodynamic studies within the brain during migraine. Arch. Neurol. 29:95–98.

Smith, I., Gordon, A. J., Hanington, E., Marsh, S. E. and Wilkinson, M. I. P. (1973): Studies of tyramine metabolism in migraine patients and control subjects. In Background to Migraine, 5th Migraine Symposium, ed. J. N. Cumings. Springer-Verlag, New York, pp. 34–39.

Smith, I., Kellow, A. H. and Hanington, E. (1970): A clinical and biochemical correlation between tyramine and migraine headache. Headache 10:43–52.

Smith, I., Mullen, P. E. and Hanington, E. (1971): Dietary migraine and tyramine metabolism. Nature 230:246–248.

Sneddon, J. (1973): Blood platelets as a model for monoamine-containing neurones. Progr. Neurobiol. 1:153–198.

Somerville, B. W. (1976): Platelet-bound and free serotonin levels in jugular and forearm venous blood during migraine. Neurology 26:41–45.

Spector, S., Melmon, K., Lovenberg, W. and Sjoerdsma, A. (1963): The presence and distribution of tyramine in mammalian tissues. J. Pharmacol. Exp. Ther. 140:229–235.

Spira, P. J., Mylecharane, E. J., Misbach, J., Duckworth, J. W. and Lance, J. W. (1978): Internal and external carotid vascular responses to vasoactive agents in the monkey. Neurology 28:162–173.

Stone, E. A. (1975): Stress and catecholamines. In Catecholamines and Behavior, Vol. 2, ed. A. J. Friedhoff. Plenum Press, New York, pp. 31–72.

Taggart, P., Carruthers, M. and Somerville, W. (1973): Electrocardiogram, plasma catecholamines and lipids, and their modification by oxyprenolol when speaking before an audience. Lancet 2:341–346.

Vardi, Y., Röbeg, I. M., Streifler, M., Schwartz, A., Lindner, H. R. and Zor, U. (1976): Migraine attacks: alleviation by an inhibitor of prostaglandin synthesis and action. Neurology 26:447–450.

Waters, W. E. (1971): Migraine: intelligence, social class, and familial prevalence. Br. Med. J. 2:77–80.

Weiss, H. J. (1975): Platelet physiology and abnormalities of platelet function. N. Engl. J. Med. 293:531–541, 580–588.

Weiss, H. J. (1978): Anti-platelet therapy. N. Engl. J. Med. 298:1344–1347, 1403–1406.

Welch, K. M. A., Chabi, E., Nell, J., Bartosh, K., Meyer, J. S. and Mathew, N. T. (1978): Similarities in biochemical effects of cerebral ischemia in patients with cerebrovascular disease and migraine. In Current Concepts in Migraine Research, ed. R. Greene. Raven Press, New York, pp. 1–9.

Welch, K. M. A., Gaudet, R., Wang, T. P. F. and Chabi, E. (1977): Transient cerebral ischemia and brain serotonin: relevance to migraine. Headache 17:145–147.

Welch, K. M. A. and Lance, J. W. (1975): Prostaglandins in migraine syndrome (letter). Neurology 25:33–34A.

Welch, K. M. A., Spira, P. J., Knowles, L. and Lance, J. W. (1974a): The effect of serotonin and prostaglandins on internal and external carotid blood flow measured simultaneously in the monkey. Arch. Neurobiol. 37:253–279.

Welch, K. M. A., Spira, P. J., Knowles, L. and Lance, J. W. (1974b): Effects of prostaglandins on the internal and external carotid blood flow in the monkey. Neurology 24:705–710.

Wennerholm, M. (1961): Postural vascular reactions in cases of migraine and related vascular headaches. Acta Med. Scand. 169:131–139.

Wolff, H. G. (1937): Personality features and reactions of subjects with migraine. Arch. Neurol. Psychiatry 37:895–921.

Youdim, M. B. H., Bonham-Carter, S., Sandler, M., Hanington, E. and Wilkinson, M. (1971): Conjugation defect in tyramine-sensitive migraine. Nature 230:127–128.

CHAPTER 4

MIGRAINE: TREATMENT AND CLINICAL PHARMACOLOGY

Approximately 90 per cent of patients with migrainous attacks can be helped substantially, but because of our incomplete understanding of the pathogenesis of migraine there is at present no complete and permanent cure. In general, the management of migraine consists of the removal or modification of precipitating factors whenever possible, the provision of an adequate support system to lessen the severity and shorten the duration of individual attacks, and the prevention of recurring attacks. Several nonpharmacologic treatments have been advocated in recent years, but only a small minority of patients derive significant benefit from these techniques. The mainstay of therapy is the judicious use of one or more of the many drugs that are relatively specific for migraine. The relief of pain with appropriate analgesics, if other means fail, can almost always be provided, and on occasion may be the only modality that has an impact on the attacks. The treatment of migraine strikingly exemplifies the need for individualized approaches to management.

Therapy begins with the initial interview, careful physical examination, and in particular the assurance that the physician and patient derive from the knowledge that everything possible has been done to exclude the presence of alternative causes of headache. At times this kind of reassurance may require CAT scanning but, as a rule of thumb, a recurring headache disorder with migrainous features of more than three years' duration is not at all likely to be the manifestation of a cerebral neoplasm. Coned-down views of the sella turcica may be important to exclude the possibility of a

111

pituitary adenoma. Plain skull x-rays offer little reassurance if negative, and are of negligible value.

MODIFICATION OF TRIGGER FACTORS

Many patients will have already discovered certain circumstances that provoke headache but will have observed that the avoidance of these has had little impact on their problem. Some confuse the precipitation of attacks by certain factors with causation, and conclude that because their attacks continue despite the modification of these factors they are irrelevant. Furthermore, some trigger factors, such as menses or modest levels of physical exertion, cannot be modified effectively. Attention to easily corrected precipitants is worthwhile; these include dental problems, refractive errors, irregular sleep habits, skipped meals and excessive coffee intake. Oral contraception, if suspect, should be discontinued for at least six months to assess its implication in the headache problem at hand; if this is not feasible, a low estrogen preparation is a reasonable compromise. For the woman in her menopausal years, the presence or absence of supplementary estrogen should be assessed carefully, with attention to the dosage and type of preparation in use or about to be used.

Any medication being taken for a concurrent medical problem should be carefully assessed and eliminated or changed if any doubt exists. Many drugs have the capacity to exacerbate migraine; the commonest are nitroglycerin, hydralazine, reserpine, vitamin A, clomiphene and indomethacin, but there are many others. Exogenous thyroid should be stopped unless it is unequivocally necessary. Attention to the lighting conditions at the patient's place of work may be important; if fluorescent lighting cannot be altered, the wearing of tinted or polarized lenses indoors as well as outdoors may be quite effective in some cases. For those who are sensitive to hunger, smoothing out the normal fluctuations of plasma glucose with a high-protein, low-carbohydrate multiple feeding schedule is worth a trial (Dexter et al, 1978). Attention to inadequate blood pressure control in a patient with essential hypertension may be fruitful in lessening the frequency and/or severity of headaches (see Chapter 1).

DIETARY FACTORS

In general, the modification of patients' diets has not been very helpful in lessening headache attacks (Medina and Diamond, 1978). Nevertheless, the exceptions prove the rule, and it is worthwhile to inform patients of the common food and beverage precipitants of headache attacks, tabulated in Chapter 2. For those who have clear-cut food-provocation, a radical dietary revision occasionally may render them headache-free and is worth seriously considering, especially for the individual with frequent or daily headaches. In this latter instance, the patient cannot possibly correlate what he eats or drinks with headache, and all exogenous chemicals are sus-pect. It has been the authors' practice to suggest a very simple, somewhat distasteful diet comprising foodstuffs to which no chemicals have been added and which have either rarely, or never, been implicated as precipitants of migrainous attacks. If a patient reports that he has continued to experience headache during a period of relative starvation, such as the interval following a surgi-cal procedure, it may not be necessary to assess dietary factors any further. The diet must be adhered to for a period that varies with the frequency of headache attacks. Distilled water (for cooking, drinking and brushing the teeth), lettuce, cauliflower, carrots, boiled or baked potatoes, cottage cheese and chicken are permitted; corn or olive oil and distilled white vinegar may be used for salads without added seasoning or condiments. No other foodstuffs, bever-ages or medications (including vitamins) are permitted. If the head-ache pattern is unaffected, no further efforts are necessary toward examining exogenous factors; the air has been cleared, usually within two weeks, and food diaries collected over a period of months to years will not be relevant. The yield, as noted above, in pursuing these rather stringent dietary measures is very small; how-ever, once or twice per year, sometimes wholly unexpectedly, a pa-tient's headache disorder has been substantially improved, and the offending factors have then been tracked down by adding only one foodstuff per week, and continually surveying and recording head-ache frequency and severity.

STRESS AND ANXIETY

There is no evidence that patients with migraine are subject to more stress than headache-free subjects; overresponsiveness to stress appears to be the issue at hand (see Chapters 2 and 3). Occa-sionally, a patient may be able to rearrange his life so that sources of anxiety are lessened, and sometimes psychotherapy may be im-plemented to accomplish this end (Hunter and Ross, 1960), espe-cially if he is trapped in a situation in which all apparent solutions are compromising, such as marital difficulties and dissatisfaction with work achievements. However, for the vast majority, the stresses of everyday living cannot be eliminated, and dealing with these by learning to relax, using various techniques, has been shown to be helpful for many patients, so long as these methods are practiced continually. They include yoga, transcendental meditation, hypnosis (Anderson et al, 1975), and a variety of conditioning techniques (Warner and Lance, 1975; Fahrion, 1978; Cohen, 1978). Controlled studies have shown that the production of benefit is independent of peripheral skin temperature changes (Mullinix et al, 1978; Largen et al, 1978; Blanchard et al, 1978) or any other biologic alteration that occurs during the conditioning process (Price and Tursky, 1976), and it appears likely that patient expectation and suggestibility are important factors common to the various relaxation techniques that have been studied for the treatment of migraine. Any treatment that enlists the enthusiasm of the therapist and which convinces the patient that he is being cared for will probably be of benefit. Achieving psychologic and physical relaxation may be helpful to some individuals, and we have found the simple relaxation exercises recommended by Lance (1978a) to be as helpful as any other method and to have the advantages of requiring no instrumentation and costing nothing.

Friedman (1975) has observed, after 30 years of evaluating a large number of patients who underwent formal psychotherapy and psychoanalysis, that the results were disappointing and do not justify use of this approach. A supportive physician–patient relationship, permitting emotional contact, dependency–need gratification and reassurance, probably has the greatest impact in the modification of the anxiety that may both trigger and arise from migrainous attacks.

PHARMACOTHERAPY IN MIGRAINE

The drugs that have been proved effective in aborting individual attacks, as well as in preventing them, have been employed for empirical reasons or for actions that subsequently have been shown to be unrelated to the benefits observed clinically. These agents traditionally have been classified according to their actions in other conditions for which an effect outside the central nervous system has usually been implicated. Included in this group are the extracranial vasoconstrictors (ergotamine, dihydroergotamine and caffeine), the serotonin antagonists (methysergide, cyproheptadine), a beta-adrenergic blocker (propranolol), a tricyclic antidepressant (amitriptyline), a monoamine oxidase inhibitor (phenelzine) and a vasodilator (papaverine). However, there is evidence (see below) that the beneficial· effect of propranolol is mediated by an action other than, or in addition to, peripheral beta-receptor antagonism, and similarly that the actions of amitriptyline and papaverine in migraine probably are not as antidepressant and vasodilator. Although it is certainly possible that some of these actions are relevant to the effectiveness of these drugs in migraine, the lack of some common property among them has frustrated the development of new agents, and has discouraged investigators of scientific persuasion from entering a field rife with such apparent empiricism.

It has not been generally appreciated that there is *substantial evidence that almost all of these drugs (including caffeine), through somewhat different mechanisms, depress the firing rate of serotonergic neurons within the brain stem* (see below). Since there is evidence that migraine may be a central disorder and no compelling evidence militating against this possibility, the role of these agents in altering the neurotransmitter function of serotonin will be examined in some detail in this chapter.

TREATMENT OF THE ACUTE ATTACK

The earlier the acute migrainous attack is dealt with, the greater is the probability that it will be aborted. If feasible, a useful adjunct for most patients, whatever else is done, is to recline in a dark room with a cold pack applied to the forehead or temple(s) and try to sleep. The immediate ingestion of a simple analgesic, such as aspirin, dextropropoxyphene (Hakkarainen et al, 1978) or codeine (Somerville, 1976), is superior to placebo and may be all that is necessary to abort an attack. For others, a meperidine tablet may be required to accomplish the same end. Isometheptene, a vasoconstrictor, is available only in combination with acetaminophen and dichloralphenazone (Midrin), and has been shown to be more effective than placebo for mild-to-moderately severe attacks (Yuill et al, 1972; Diamond, 1976). Generally, two to three capsules should be taken at once, and two further capsules 45 minutes later if regression of head pain has not begun. For a great many patients these relatively simple measures will suffice; as a general principle, whichever agent is chosen an adequate dosage should be used at the onset of the attack. If additional medication is required in 30 to 60 minutes because the symptoms return or have not abated, the initial dosage should be increased for subsequent attacks. The inhalation of 100 per cent oxygen through a tight-fitting mask at a flow rate of 8 liters per minute for 15 to 60 minutes has been reported to produce complete relief in over 40 per cent of patients so treated (Alvarez and Mason, 1940). The weak constrictor effect of oxygen on cerebral arteries may be relevant to its benefit in migraine; however, the important rate-limiting step in the synthesis of brain serotonin is dependent on molecular oxygen, and there is evidence that rats administered 100 per cent oxygen greatly increase their brain levels of serotonin (Costa and Meek, 1974), which perhaps explains the beneficial effects of oxygen. However, oxygen inhalation is not practicable for most patients. Acupuncture has been shown to be generally ineffectual (Levine et al, 1976).

DRUG ABSORPTION DURING MIGRAINOUS ATTACKS

The absorption of salicylates has been studied during migrainous attacks, and an impairment in the rate of absorption has been found (Volans, 1978). Delayed absorption occurs in the absence of nausea, and is related to the severity of the attack and not to its duration (Table 4–1). Two lines of evidence suggest that reduced gastrointestinal motility is an important mechanism of impaired drug absorption. Gastric stasis and prolonged gastric emptying time have been demonstrated radiologically after barium meals were taken during attacks, and when the same patients were headache-free repeat studies showed normal gastrointestinal function (Kaufman and Levine, 1936; Carstairs, 1958; Kreel, 1973). Metoclopramide, a drug known to accelerate gastrointestinal motility and gastric emptying in man (Nimmo, 1976), injected intramuscularly ten minutes before the ingestion of aspirin by migrainous patients, normalized the absorption of aspirin and did not affect the absorption of aspirin in control subjects (Volans, 1975). There is preliminary evidence that ergotamine absorption is also impaired during migrainous attacks (Volans, 1978), so that there may be impaired gastrointestinal absorption of many drugs. The neurotransmitter function of serotonin within the synapses of the myenteric plexus has been implicated in the regulation of gastrointestinal motility (Gershon, 1968; Costa and Furness, 1979). It is possible that the gastric stasis that accompanies migrainous attacks is a reflection of an alteration of these gastrointestinal serotonergic circuits. However, diminished gastrointestinal motility may also result from alterations in brain serotonin turnover (Saller and Stricker, 1978), so that a central mechanism is also a possibility.

TABLE 4–1. PLASMA SALICYLATE LEVELS AFTER INGESTION OF 900 mg ASPIRIN*

| | No. | MEAN PLASMA SALICYLATE (mg%) | |
		30 Min	60 Min
Control Subjects	20	7.9 ± 0.4**	8.2 ± 0.3
Migrainous Subjects	42		
During attack		4.8 ± 0.4	6.6 ± 0.6
Interictal period		7.0 ± 0.6	7.6 ± 0.9

*Modified from Volans, 1978.
**S.E.M.

It is not yet clear when, in the course of a migraine attack, gastrointestinal motility diminishes, but the timing of this phenomenon may explain, at least in part, why it is important to ingest oral medications immediately, as soon as the earliest symptoms appear. Delayed absorption probably is not the only mechanism accounting for the ineffectiveness of agents administered too late, since parenterally administered drugs, given after an attack crescendoes, usually produce poor results also.

The impaired absorption of oral agents as well as the frequent occurrence of vomiting in migrainous attacks have led to the usage of medications in forms other than oral tablets. Rectal suppositories are especially useful (unless diarrhea accompanies an attack), and it is well to recall that aspirin and acetaminophen are available in this formulation; codeine can be prepared as a suppository by many pharmacists, and the potent analgesic, hydromorphone, is available as a 3-mg suppository. Thus, the entire range of analgesics may be administered in a form that is likely to be absorbed and retained during an attack, and when all else fails this technique may avoid a trip to the emergency room.

ERGOTAMINE TARTRATE

The abortion of migrainous attacks is accomplished most effectively and reproducibly, especially for patients with severe attacks, by ergotamine. The original source of ergotamine was the sclerotium of the fungus *Claviceps purpurea*, which is known commonly as ergot because of its spurlike shape and is a parasite of the head of rye stalks. The contamination of edible grain by ergot during the

Figure 4-1.

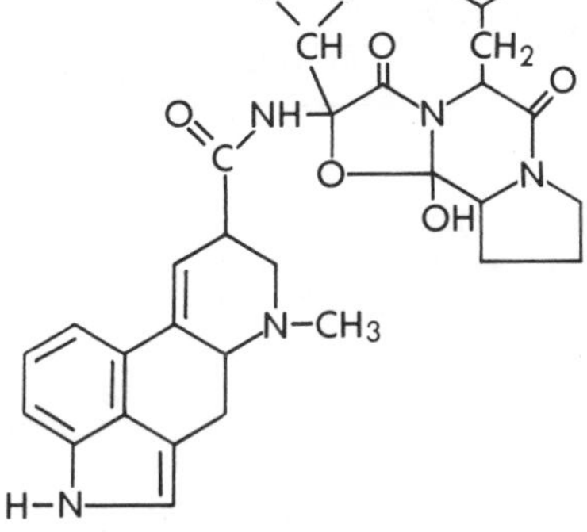

ERGOTAMINE

Middle Ages led to epidemics of gangrene called "holy fire" or "Saint Anthony's fire" in honor of the patron saint of a religious order founded for the purpose of caring for the victims of ergotism. Convulsions were also recognized as a symptom of ergotism during this period; by the 17th century the cause of ergotism was finally recognized and since then only sporadic outbreaks have occurred (Hofmann, 1978).

The first mention of fluid extracts of ergot for the treatment of migraine was made toward the end of the 19th century by Eulenberg in Germany and Thomson in the United States. Thomson (1894) suggested that the ergot extract should be taken by mouth as soon as the early symptoms of an attack were noted, and that if vomiting occurred the drug should be taken as an enema; he observed that the drug only rarely failed to stop the progression of migrainous attacks. However, probably because of the inconsistent effects of crude extracts, the ergot therapy of migraine was largely forgotten for 30 years. In 1918, ergotamine was isolated from extracts of its fungal source and was introduced to medicine as an oxytocic agent. In 1925 migraine was believed to be caused by heightened sympathetic activity, and, since ergotamine was then known to produce sympathetic blockade, the subcutaneous injection of the drug was suggested by Rothlin (1955). A number of studies in Europe subsequently established the drug as an effective agent in the arrest of migrainous attacks.

In the United States, studies soon appeared, exemplified by that of Lennox (1938) in Table 4-2, showing that parenteral ergotamine was dramatically effective in 90 per cent of patients, whereas orally administered ergotamine was considerably less effective. Eventually, controlled studies demonstrated that oral ergotamine, given in a·single 5-mg dose, was significantly more effective than placebo (Ostfeld, 1961); studies carred out with lower oral doses produced results not significantly better than placebo (Waters,

TABLE 4-2.   EFFECT OF ERGONOVINE AND ERGOTAMINE ON MIGRAINOUS HEADACHE IN 218 PATIENTS[*]

DRUG	DOSE	No. Patients	PERCENTAGE Headache-free	Improved
Ergotamine	0.5 mg IV	140	89	5
	2 mg/hr PO up to 8 mg	56	41	27
Ergonovine	0.2–0.5 mg IV	54	39	40
	0.5–1 mg/hr PO up to 4 mg	42	43	24

[*]Modified from Lennox, 1938.

TABLE 4–3. DISTRIBUTION OF TRITIATED ERGOTAMINE IN THE RAT°

| | TIME AFTER ADMINISTRATION | | | |
| | 2 hrs | | 8 hrs | |
TISSUE	IV	PO	IV	PO
Blood	0.09	0.02	0.02	0.02
Liver	1.36	0.37	0.52	0.26
Lung	1.09	0.04	0.44	0.02
Kidney	0.74	0.09	0.17	0.07
Heart	0.26	0.03	0.03	0.02
Brain	0.05	0.02	0.01	0

Tritiated ergotamine tartrate was administered at a dosage of 1 mg/kg body weight. The results are expressed as microgram equivalents of ergotamine per gram of fresh tissue.

°Modified from Eckert et al, 1978.

1970). Moreover, a controlled study of the inhalational aerosol formulation of ergotamine showed it to be significantly better than placebo (Crooks et al, 1964). In an analysis of 263 patients and their response to ergotamine in oral, sublingual, rectal or injectable formulations, Selby and Lance (1960) found that 47 per cent promptly became headache-free, and that an additional 34 per cent reported that some of their attacks were completely aborted or that headache of diminished severity continued.

The oral absorption of ergotamine is rapid, with an absorption half-time of 30 minutes, although only two-thirds of the oral dosage is absorbed. Peak plasma concentrations are reached two hours after ingestion. Its metabolic disposition occurs in two phases, one with a half-life of two hours and another with a half-life of 20 hours (Aellig and Nüesch, 1977); the longer half-life correlates with the duration of the drug's clinical effects. These pharmacokinetic data are based on studies in which isotopically-labeled metabolites were measured together with the unchanged drug. Orton and Richardson (1978) and Ala-Hurula et al. (1979), using a specific radioimmunoassay, have shown in control subjects without headache that higher plasma levels are achieved after the administration of rectal suppositories of ergotamine than after the ingestion of oral tablets.

Tritiated ergotamine is distributed primarily to the liver, lung and kidney, but also is present in brain (Table 4–3). Only 0.1 to 0.01 per cent of an intravenous dose of ergotamine can be identified in the urine as the pharmacologically active drug or as metabolites; bile is its main excretory pathway (Nimmerfall and Rosenthaler, 1976). The products of ergotamine metabolism are largely unknown.

Caffeine was originally added to ergotamine formulations to enhance the vasoconstrictive activity of the drug (Moyer et al, 1952),

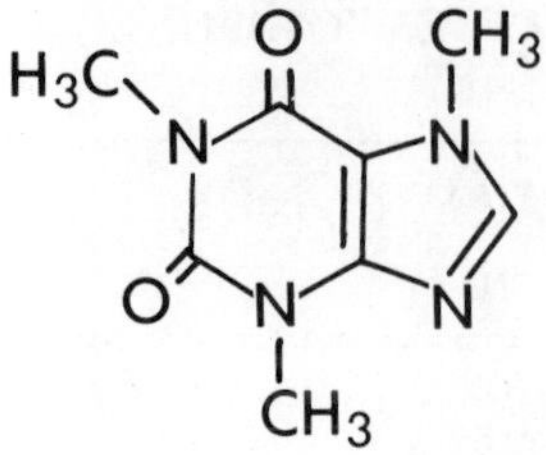

Figure 4-2.

CAFFEINE

and subsequently was shown also to enhance the intestinal absorption of ergotamine (Schmidt and Fanchamps, 1974), probably by altering its solubility (Berde et al, 1970). Although controlled studies have not been done regarding the benefit added to ergotamine by caffeine, there is widespread agreement that caffeine is of value (Friedman and von Storch, 1951). In this regard, it is useful to know that the caffeine content of tea and coffee is quite variable (Bunker and McWilliams, 1979). In a study of samples of tea and coffee prepared at the homes of volunteers, the range of caffeine concentrations of 46 coffee samples was 29 to 176 mg per cup; the median concentration was 74 mg per cup. Coffee prepared by drip or filter methods contained higher caffeine concentrations (median = 112 mg per cup), whereas instant coffee contained lower concentrations (median = 66 mg per cup) (Gilbert et al, 1976).

MECHANISMS OF ACTION OF ERGOTAMINE

Evidence that ergotamine constricts branches of the external carotid artery that are dilated during a migrainous attack was first put forth by Graham and Wolff (1938). These authors administered ergotamine intravenously to patients after their first focal neurologic symptoms had subsided and headache had just begun. Pulsations of the temporal or occipital arteries were recorded by means of tambours placed over the vessels. In 16 out of 20 migrainous subjects, the injection of ergotamine was followed by a decrease in amplitude of the pulsations of scalp arteries that bore a close relationship to the decline in the intensity of headache; if the pulse amplitude decreased slowly, headache diminished slowly; precipitous declines in pulse amplitude were paralleled by a prompt cessation of headache. *However, in four subjects a correlation was not evident.* These findings, taken together with other evidence suggesting that dampening of arterial pulsations by pharmacologic or physical means often ameliorated migrainous headaches, led to general acceptance of the conclusion that the beneficial effects of ergotamine were mediated by vasoconstriction of the extracranial arterial bed. Subsequent experiments have established that powerful and selective constriction of the external carotid artery and its branches is produced by ergotamine (Saxena, 1972; Lance et al, 1978). Only slight α-adrenergic blockade occurs at the doses used clinically, and there is evidence that the vasoconstrictor effect of ergotamine is mediated by a direct effect on arterial serotonin receptors (Müller-Schweinitzer, 1978; Hardebo et al, 1978).

The effect of ergotamine on arterial tone depends on the pre-existing resistance of the vascular bed; when the vascular resistance is low, ergotamine acts as a constrictor, but when the vascular resistance is increased it may produce vasodilatation (Aellig and Berde, 1969). This action may explain how ergotamine may prevent either phase of a migrainous attack (Barrie et al, 1968). Regional CBF studies performed during both the focal neurologic and headache phases of migrainous attacks after the administration of ergotamine have shown no constrictor effects on the internal carotid circulation (see Chapter 2, Hemiplegic Migraine). However, Sakai and Meyer (1978) have recently shown that hyperemia in the basilar artery distribution was markedly reduced by therapeutically effective doses of ergotamine, suggesting the possibility that the pain-sensitive arteries at the base of the brain at least contribute to the pain of headache attacks. Johnston and Saxena (1978) have demonstrated that an additional effect of ergotamine is the closure of cephalic arteriovenous shunts that open during migrainous attacks. However, it is uncertain whether this action is related to the therapeutic effects of the drug.

It seems likely that extracranial arterial constriction is important to the benefits conferred by ergotamine with regard to the cessation of migrainous attacks; however, this may not be the primary site of the drug's effect. Ergotamine has significant effects on serotonin turnover in brain (Sofia and Vassar, 1975), and several ergot alkaloids have been studied and found to depress the firing rate of central serotonergic neurons (Aghajanian and Wang, 1978). There is evidence that central serotonergic neurons participate in the regulation of the systemic circulation (Chalmers and Wing, 1975; Smits and Struyker-Boudier, 1976; Cabot et al, 1979), and in view of the less-than-perfect correlation between scalp artery constriction and headache relief, it is possible that the abortion of attacks by ergotamine is secondary to a central rather than a peripheral action. Pichler et al (1956) made the following observations on 13 subjects who were given ergotamine tartrate: (1) blood pressure elevation during the cold pressor response was not prevented; (2) carotid sinus reflex sensitivity was unaltered; (3) reflex bradycardia occurred during infusions of norepinephrine; and (4) cranial vasoconstriction was as evident in two subjects who had undergone cervical sympathectomy as in the other 11 patients. This evidence was interpreted as supporting a peripheral vascular action of ergotamine and rendering unlikely a primary central action. However, the anatomic projections of central serotonergic neurons are diverse and greatly overlapping throughout the neuraxis (Moore et al, 1978), and there is evidence that there is little or no involvement of the autonomic nervous system in the centrally-modified circulatory response to serotonin (Lambert et al, 1978). Therefore, the preservation of reflex responses after ergotamine administration, and the failure of sympathectomy to inhibit vasoconstriction, neither confirm nor deny a central locus of action for ergotamine.

CLINICAL USE OF ERGOTAMINE

A number of preparations of ergotamine are available (Table 4–4) — oral and sublingual tablets, an aerosol, rectal suppositories and injectable preparations, in ascending order of efficacy. Two principles regarding dosage are important for achieving optimal results with ergotamine. First, an adequate dose should be taken as soon as possible and not divided into half-hourly or hourly supplements; if the initial dose fails, subsequent doses usually fail also. Second, a subnauseating dose must be determined. Patients' sensitivities to ergotamine vary over a broad dosage range; a dose that provokes nausea or vomiting — probably a centrally-mediated side-effect (Loew et al, 1978) — is too high and may even intensify a migrainous attack. The mechanism underlying this apparently paradoxical effect may be through the blockade of arterial serotonin receptors that occurs with high doses of ergotamine (Hardebo et al, 1978), resulting in arterial dilatation instead of constriction. Therefore, whichever route of administration of ergotamine is chosen, the appropriate dosage for a given patient must be arrived at by titrating his capacity to tolerate ergotamine, preferably during a headache-free period. For example, it is the authors' practice, upon prescribing the 2-mg rectal suppository form of ergotamine, to instruct patients to perform the following experiment during a headache-free evening: slice the suppository into thirds, and insert each third at 60-minute intervals; if nausea appears at any stage, then the accumulated dose is too high for that patient. If nausea occurs after the second third, the appropriate dose for a migrainous attack is between one-third and one-half; if nausea does not appear at all, the entire 2-mg suppository should be used as the initial dosage. The average dosage for the ergotamine suppository, determined in this way, is 1 mg; however, a few individuals are very sensitive to the drug and require only 0.25 to 0.5 mg for an optimal response. For these patients, suppositories containing only 1 mg (Table 4–4) are more practicable.

TABLE 4–4. ERGOT-CONTAINING DRUGS

Brand and Generic Names	Route	Ergot Alkaloid	Caffeine	Belladonna	Other
Bellergal	PO	Ergotamine 0.3 mg		0.1 mg	Phenobarbital 20 mg
Bellergal-S	PO	Ergotamine 0.6 mg		0.2 mg	Phenobarbital 40 mg
Cafergot	PO	Ergotamine 1 mg	100 mg		
Cafergot	PR	Ergotamine 2 mg	100 mg		
Cafergot-PB	PO	Ergotamine 1 mg	100 mg	0.125 mg	Pentobarbital 30 mg
Cafergot-PB	PR	Ergotamine 2 mg	100 mg	0.25 mg	Pentobarbital 60 mg
D.H.E. 45	IM/IV	Dihydroergotamine mesylate 1 mg/ml			
Ergomar	SL	Ergotamine 2 mg			
Ergonovine	PO	Ergonovine 0.2 mg			
Ergostat	SL	Ergotamine 2 mg			
Ergotamine	SC/IM	0.25 mg/0.5 ml or 0.5 mg/1 ml			
Ergotamine	INHAL.	0.36 mg/puff			
Ergotamine	PO	1 mg			
Ergotrate	PO	Ergonovine 0.2 mg			
Gynergen	PO	Ergotamine 1 mg			
Medihaler Ergotamine Aerosol	INHAL.	Ergotamine 0.36 mg/puff			
Migral	PO	Ergotamine 1 mg	50 mg		Cyclizine 25 mg
Wigraine	PO	Ergotamine 1 mg	100 mg	0.1 mg	Phenacetin 130 mg
Wigraine	PR	Ergotamine 1 mg	100 mg	0.1 mg	Phenacetin 130 mg

A lack of appreciation of the variability of the dosage of ergot-amine is an important reason for the drug's apparent failure for many patients. Because of the delayed absorption of orally adminis-tered agents and the high frequency of vomiting that accompanies migrainous attacks, the ergotamine suppository is most frequently prescribed by the authors. Suppositories should be stored in the refrigerator if the ambient temperature becomes high enough to soften them. The vast majority of patients who use suppositories need also some other ergotamine formulation that can be carried on their person.

The dosage range for the subcutaneous administration of ergot-amine is from 0.125 to 0.5 mg, and on occasion, if other formula-tions of ergotamine are ineffectual, patients can easily be taught to self-administer the drug. However, for the vast majority, this route will be neither feasible nor desirable. The usual well-tolerated and effective dosage is 0.25 mg.

Ergotamine tartrate aerosol (0.36 mg per inhalation, 50 doses per cartridge) is composed of a fine powder of ergotamine which is not in solution with the vehicle contained in the canister; therefore, patients must be instructed to shake the canister vigorously before each inhalation. The mouthpiece of the canister should be held close to but not inserted into the open mouth (Connolly, 1975); a deep inhalation should commence after complete exhalation, and once an inward air flow is established the puff should be produced by pressing the device on the canister. The inhalation should be continued to maximum capacity and held for as long as possible; the breath may then be released through semiclosed lips. The usual initial dose is 1 to 2 puffs. A disadvantage of the aerosol is the bulk-iness of the canister; for many patients it is not feasible to carry this device with them so that it may be used as soon as possible.

An uncoated, pulverized formulation of ergotamine is marketed as a preparation for sublingual usage, and probably is more effec-tive than the coated tablets used orally (Crooks et al, 1964). Impor-tant advantages of this form of ergotamine are that a glass of water is not required for its administration and the tablets are individually wrapped for easy carriage. Studies of the absorption of ergotamine across the buccal mucosa have shown that only a small fraction of a dose is absorbed in five minutes (Sutherland et al, 1974). It appears likely that this more easily disintegrated form of ergotamine is help-ful in migrainous attacks when saliva containing the drug is swal-lowed. It has been the authors' practice to instruct patients to chew the tablet(s) and then maneuver the bits to a sublingual position. The usual dosage is 1 to 1½ tablets (2 to 3 mg).

The coated tablet of ergotamine for oral administration is the least expensive and probably the least effective mode of using the drug. It is most effective for patients with clear-cut premonitory symptoms several minutes before a headache begins. The usual dose is 2 to 3 mg, with a range of 1 to 4 mg.

The ergot alkaloids are light-sensitive (Rutschmann and Stadler, 1978) and have a short shelf-life, especially the parenteral formulations. An occasional cause of a poor response to ergotamine is the use of an outdated preparation.

ERGOTAMINE TOXICITY

The broad latitude of human sensitivity to ergotamine is illustrated by the many documented instances in which patients have used massive daily dosages for years without ill effects (Friedman et al, 1959). At the other end of the spectrum, there have been a few patients with high sensitivity to ergotamine in whom myocardial infarction (Goldfischer, 1960), renal arterial stenosis (Fedotin and Hartman, 1970) or cerebral infarction (Senter et al, 1976) developed after relatively brief exposures to modest doses of the drug. A predisposition to enhanced vasoconstriction outside the external carotid artery distribution appears to result from several conditions which include sepsis, hyperthyroidism, malnutrition, pregnancy, renal and hepatic diseases, and pre-existing coronary artery or peripheral vascular disease. The concurrent administration of triacetyloleandomycin has been reported to precipitate peripheral vasoconstriction also (Griffith et al, 1978). Therefore, it is essential to warn patients to severely restrict their use of ergotamine during intervals of intercurrent illness; analgesics with potencies appropriate to the problem should be substituted, and, in general, are nearly as effective as ergotamine.

Abdominal cramps, vertigo, muscle cramps (usually in the lower limbs), diarrhea and distal paresthesias are the commonest side-effects when subnauseating doses are used, and arise in about 5 per cent of patients. Less commonly, syncope, tremor, dyspnea, angina pectoris and limb claudication may occur; the latter two symptoms call for an immediate curtailment or cessation of the drug. Serious side-effects probably arise in less than 0.01 per cent of patients (von Storch, 1938). The vast majority tolerate the drug well, and its benefits far outweigh the risks when dosage and frequency of use are monitored. Problems with ergotamine may begin when the drug is used daily and continuously in doses that exceed 20 mg per week, especially in the suppository formulation (Hokkanen et al, 1978). Ergot toxicity less frequently results from abuse of oral ergotamine; however, one instance of bilateral ischemic optic neuropathy has been reported as a consequence of chronic oral ergotamine use at a daily dosage of 6 to 8 mg (Gupta and Strobos, 1972).

The commonest of the potential serious side-effects of ergotamine is gangrene of the limbs, which for historical reasons continues to be referred to as "ergotism." Whereas convulsions were part of the clinical manifestations of the intoxication that resulted from ingesting fungus-contaminated rye, convulsions have been reported only rarely (Carliner et al, 1974) following the excessive ingestion of ergotamine. Serious vasoconstriction usually preferentially affects the lower limbs bilaterally and symmetrically, and almost always is heralded by the symptoms of distal paresthesia (at first transient, then fixed), coldness of the digits and exertional pain in the calves or heels. All patients who are to use ergotamine should be apprised of these symptoms and should stop taking the drug immediately should any appear. The vast majority of reported cases of serious ergot-induced arterial insufficiency of the limbs have occurred when *patients continued to use ergotamine after claudication pain had become evident.*

There is a characteristic angiographic appearance of ergot-induced arterial insufficiency: the configuration of the main arteries is normal, but at the lower third of the leg they fade out to a point; a collateral circulation is usually apparent around the vasospastic segment (Bagby and Cooper, 1972). Intense vasoconstriction with secondary occlusion and thrombosis of medium and small arteries has been the mechanism of gangrene, in the few cases studied. Many vascular beds have been constricted by ergotamine, including the mesenteric, cerebral, renal, coronary and ophthalmic circulations (Senter et al, 1976). Peroneal nerve palsies have also occurred, probably caused by constriction of the vasa nervorum (Merhoff and Porter, 1974; Perkin, 1974).

The appearance of cyanosis of the limbs may be a forewarning of gangrene, so that active therapy at this stage is judicious, although many patients will recover simply by stopping the use of ergotamine. There is persuasive evidence that sodium nitroprusside, a direct-acting vasodilator (Tinker and Michenfelder, 1976), is the treatment of choice for this condition (Carliner et al, 1974; Andersen et al, 1977; Eurin et al, 1978). Infusion of the drug, titrated to between 0.5 and 2 μg/kg/min and maintained until sufficient ergotamine metabolism has occurred (usually between 10 and 20 hours), has produced dramatic reversal of vasoconstriction in several patients. Alternative treatment methods — low molecular weight dextran, corticosteroids, anticoagulation, hydralazine and sympathetic blockade — have had disappointing or equivocal results.

Tolerance to ergotamine develops at a variable rate and to a broad dose range of the drug (Friedman et al, 1955). Physical dependence on ergotamine (and caffeine) generally parallels the tolerance phenomenon and often is expressed symptomatically by a worsening of a headache disorder (Peters and Horton, 1951; Rowsell et al, 1973; Andersson, 1975; Pearce, 1976). This occurs in patients using ergotamine daily in oral doses of 2 to 10 or more mg; the cycle is perpetuated because cessation of ergotamine results in severe withdrawal headache, whereas continued elevation in dosage produces transient improvement. The development of ergot dependence usually requires hospitalization during which the ergotamine dose is rapidly tapered over three to four days; heavy sedation and analgesic support are usually necessary to support a patient through this difficult experience. The peak intensity of the withdrawal headache that occurs if ergotamine is ceased abruptly, without tapering, is reached during the first two days, and then lessens over the ensuing one to three days. Tapering the ergotamine dose usually prolongs the withdrawal process to six to seven days, but is less unpleasant for the patient and simpler to manage. The daily use of opiates and other analgesics occasionally may result in a tolerance–dependence cycle identical to that encountered with ergotamine (Medina and Diamond, 1977), and must be dealt with in a similar manner; the efficacy of propranolol in opiate withdrawal (Grosz, 1972) lends itself well as an adjunct in this latter circumstance.

The daily use of ergotamine at times may render a patient headache-free; if this can be achieved with 1 or 2 mg (rectally), it is an option that may be worth at least a short-term trial for a few months until a better pharmacologic solution to the problem is found, so long as the patient is informed of the danger signals. Some reduction in the pressure head of the limb arteries occurs in over 15 per cent of those who use daily ergotamine (Dige-Petersen et al, 1977); there is no correlation between the dose of ergotamine and the magnitude of this effect, again underlining the variable individual susceptibility to ergotamine.

Ergotamine is also a potent venoconstrictor (Brooke and Robinson, 1970), and (rarely) varicose veins have become painful and thrombophlebitis has occurred, usually after single doses of the drug (Carter, 1958). There is no evidence that hypertension is a contraindication to the use of ergotamine, despite widespread impressions to the contrary. Normotensive subjects respond to parenteral doses of 0.25 to 0.5 mg with increases of up to 20 mm Hg in systolic and diastolic pressure that lasts for approximately one hour (Pool et al, 1936; Lennox, 1938); in hypertensive patients, modest reductions in blood pressure take place (Immerwahr, 1927; Lennox, 1938).

PREGNANCY AND ERGOTAMINE

Although Wainscott et al (1978) have reported that the frequency and type of congenital abnormalities in babies born to women who used ergotamine during the first trimester of pregnancy was no greater than in a control population, there is substantial evidence of the detrimental effects of ergotamine on animal fetuses, so that its use is best avoided if pregnancy is contemplated. Increased fetal death, postnatal mortality, lenticular cataracts, abortion, delayed skeletal ossification, cleft palate, and shortened phalanges and digits have been reported after large doses of ergotamine were administered to mice, rats and rabbits during early pregnancy (Griffith et al, 1978). The dosage of ergotamine required to produce these defects, however, is massive, usually over 10 mg/kg by mouth. There is only minimal transplacental passage of ergotamine; an important mechanism underlying its embryotoxicity is probably the interruption of uterine blood flow. The relevance of these animal data to the problem of migrainous women contemplating pregnancy stems from a possibly heightened sensitivity of some women to ordinary or low doses of the drug.

DOSAGE GUIDELINES

Daily or weekly limits on the use of ergotamine have been derived arbitrarily. There have been occasional patients with striking sensitivities to the drug so that myocardial infarction has resulted after a 2-mg oral dose was followed by 0.5 mg intramuscularly (Goldfischer, 1960); renal arterial spasm has been produced after 10 mg was used rectally over three days (Fedotin and Hartman, 1970). On the other hand, most patients have high thresholds to ergotamine, as evidenced by the many reports of the long-term usage of large doses of the drug without untoward effects (Friedman et al, 1959). Of those who have developed toxic side-effects from ergotamine, the vast majority have been those who were using the drug daily at moderate-to-high dosage for several months (Hokkanen et al, 1978). As a rule of thumb, when 1 or 2 mg of ergotamine daily no longer completely controls a headache disorder, some other therapeutic avenue should be pursued. For patients who use ergotamine periodically, daily maximums of 8 mg orally, 4 mg rectally or 0.5 mg subcutaneously are probably safe limits, but if attacks begin to occur more often than once weekly, and the maximal dosage is required for each attack, it is time to attempt prophylaxis (see below).

PREVENTIVE TREATMENT

The decision to employ continuous medication to prevent migrainous attacks should be based on the frequency, duration and severity of the attacks, and the degree of success in aborting each one.

Some patients on average experience only one attack monthly, but the attacks are unaffected by ergotamine, last three or four days and cause the patient to take to bed and miss work. In such circumstances, preventive medication is reasonable, although in general an attack rate that exceeds two to three per month is the usual indication to consider this option seriously.

Before commitment to this approach is made, it is prudent to re-examine the possibility that removable or ameliorable trigger factors may be present. If the attack rate has recently increased, the possibility that ergotamine or opiate-dependence has developed should be considered.

A preliminary report of the successful prophylaxis of migrainous attacks with aspirin at a dosage of 650 mg twice daily (O'Neill and Mann, 1978) is generally contrary to our experience; aspirin used this way has usually been ineffectual. There are several drugs that are effective in preventing migrainous attacks with varying degrees of success (Tables 4–5, 4–6), for most of which there may be a latency of several days or weeks at optimal dosage before benefits become evident. Furthermore, the probability of success with any one of these drugs is less than 70 per cent, so that if one drug is assessed each month there may be an interval of one to several months before effective prophylaxis is achieved. The drugs have long half-lives and, in general, need not be taken more often than twice daily. During this period it is usually necessary to provide the patient with an effective method for dealing with those headache attacks that continue; the two approaches are not mutually exclusive, and ergotamine tartrate or analgesics should be provided for this contingency.

There is, at present, no evidence that ergotamine-responsiveness

TABLE 4–5.   PREVENTIVE TREATMENT OF MIGRAINE: COMPARATIVE RESPONSIVENESS TO DRUGS*

| DRUG | PERCENTAGE OF PATIENTS | | No. PATIENTS |
	Headache-free	>50% Improved	
Methysergide	22	35	325
Cyproheptadine	15	31	100
Ergotamine–phenobarbital–belladonna	10	24	174
Amitriptyline	57**	15	110
Propranolol	3	31	40
Papaverine	32	26	19
Phenelzine	28	52	25
Placebo	2	18	50

*Data drawn from Curran and Lance, 1964; Lance et al, 1965; Anthony and Lance, 1969; Couch et al, 1976; Forssman et al, 1976; Sillanpää and Koponen, 1978.
**80% improved.

TABLE 4-6. INTERVAL THERAPY OF MIGRAINOUS ATTACKS –
PRESCRIBING INFORMATION

Drug	Tablet Size(s)	Daily Dose Range	Commonest Side-Effects
Ergonovine	0.2 mg	0.4–2.0 mg	Nausea, abdominal pain, leg "tiredness"
Amitriptyline	10,25,50 mg	10–175 mg	Sedation, dry mouth
Propranolol	10,20,40,80 mg	40–320 mg	Lethargy, insomnia, constipation, lightheadedness
Papaverine	150,300 mg	300–900 mg	Nausea
Cyproheptadine	4 mg	12–32 mg	Sedation, weight gain
Ergotamine– phenobarbital– belladonna	tabs	1–4 tablets	Nausea, sedation
Phenelzine	15 mg	15–75 mg	Insomnia, lightheadedness, constipation
Methysergide	2 mg	2–8 mg	Nausea, abdominal pain, muscle cramps, insomnia, weight gain, edema, peripheral vasoconstriction

has predictive value regarding responsiveness to drugs of a similar structure, such as ergonovine or methysergide (Curran and Lance, 1964). Methysergide is the most effective agent in the prevention of migrainous attacks and has the greatest chance of rendering a patient headache-free; however, it also has the most serious potential toxic effects, connective tissue proliferation that may compromise renal, cardiac or pulmonary function, so that it is more reasonable to begin interval therapy with less effective drugs for which there are very low or negligible risk factors. In the authors' experience, 90 per cent of patients are successfully managed with the sequential monthly use of amitriptyline, propranolol and ergonovine. Should each of these three drugs fail to produce substantial benefit, cyproheptadine, papaverine, and an ergotamine–phenobarbital–belladonna combination (Steig, 1977) are then sequentially employed; if nonresponsiveness continues, methysergide or phenelzine are prescribed as a last resort. Only seldom is it necessary to prescribe the latter two drugs. Once effective prophylaxis is achieved, the drug is continued for three to four months and then slowly tapered to assess the continued need for it. Although there is no clear evidence that these drugs alter the natural history of the disorder, many patients are able to discontinue medication completely after six months or so, and experience fewer and less severe attacks for long periods. At the very least, these drugs act in a suppressive fashion, containing the mechanism that disposes patients to frequent and/or severe attacks of migraine.

PUTATIVE MECHANISMS OF ACTION OF PROPHYLACTIC DRUGS

Several lines of evidence suggest that a common mode of action of the antimigrainous drugs is the suppression of the firing rate of the serotonergic neurons that are located in the brain stem. Whereas the peripheral actions of some of these drugs on receptor sites in arterial walls may contribute to their beneficial effects in migraine, all of them are known to cross the blood–brain barrier, so that their central actions are potentially therapeutically important also. Their dual actions centrally and peripherally are not mutually exclusive. To put forth the central actions clearly, we must briefly review the physiology and pharmacology of serotonergic synapses and the metabolism of serotonin within the central nervous system.

Synapses and neurotransmitters. Transmission occurs in only one direction at synapses, the sites of interneuronal communication. There is good evidence that at almost all vertebrate synapses transmission is chemically mediated (Fig. 4–3). Some of the chemical messengers, or neurotransmitters, at these junctions within the CNS have been identified, and include acetylcholine, norepinephrine and

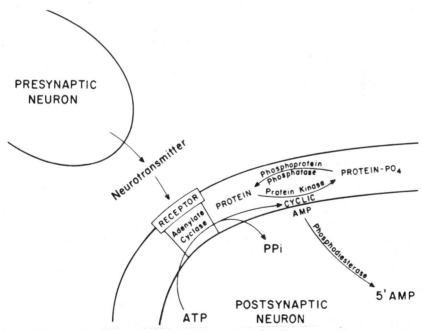

Figure 4–3. Components of a cyclic AMP-mediated synapse. Neurotransmitter released from presynaptic nerve terminal vesicles binds to the postsynaptic membrane receptor, activating adenylate cyclase and the synthesis of cyclic AMP. (*From* Greengard, P., 1975: Adv. Cyclic Nucleotide Res. 5:585–602. Reproduced by permission of Raven Press, New York.)

serotonin (Cooper et al, 1978). Nerve terminals at the synapse are packed with spherical vesicles that contain the neurotransmitter(s). The secretion of these transmitters into the synaptic cleft is usually induced by the depolarization of the nerve terminal by an action potential. When the transmitter is released from its storage site, it then binds to a particular site on the postsynaptic membrane which is designated as a receptor. The receptor–transmitter complex produces either excitatory or inhibitory postsynaptic potentials, depending on the nature of the receptor. Presynaptic nerve terminals contain the enzymes necessary to synthesize the transmitters mentioned above *de novo* from amino acid precursors in the extracellular fluid spaces; furthermore, nerve terminals have the capacity to reaccumulate the transmitter they release. This re-uptake process is energy-dependent and, therefore, is called "active" re-uptake. Drugs that selectively inhibit the re-uptake mechanism can prolong the survival of the chemical transmitter near its receptor before it is eventually metabolized. Other drugs may prolong the survival of a transmitter by inhibiting its catabolism or by increasing its synthesis; still others, receptor agonists, may mimic the effect of a transmitter by acting on the receptor directly — these latter drugs usually contain chemical moieties that resemble the configuration of the transmitter.

Another mechanism by which drugs may affect synaptic transmission is altering the turnover of adenosine 3', 5'-monophosphate (cyclic AMP), a substance that mediates some of the postsynaptic effects of certain neurotransmitters that probably include serotonin (Nathanson, 1977). Cyclic AMP is formed from adenosine 5'-triphosphate (ATP) by activation of the membrane-bound enzyme adenylate cyclase, which may be intimately associated with the postsynaptic membrane receptor. The effects of cyclic AMP on synaptic transmission may be terminated by its hydrolysis which is catalyzed by cyclic nucleotide phosphodiesterase (PDE). Inhibition of PDE increases the intracellular levels of cyclic AMP, which has the effect of activating the synaptic pathway and potentiating the effect of the transmitter on the postsynaptic receptor.

Serotonergic synapses.   It has become clear that brain serotonin is contained within specific nerve circuits, and functions as an inhibitory neurotransmitter (Gerschenfeld et al, 1978; Aghajanian and Wang, 1978). Serotonin-containing neuronal cell bodies are principally those located in the midline or raphe regions of the brain stem; axons of the rostral cell groups project to a large portion of the cerebrum (Moore et al, 1978), whereas the more caudal cell groups project to the medulla and spinal cord. Thus, nerve terminals containing serotonin are found throughout the CNS (Saavedra, 1977). Neuronal receptors of serotonergic nerve terminals are affected by serotonin in a fashion that mimics the stimulation of the brain stem raphe system; drugs that simulate the effects of serotonin on postsynaptic receptors also simulate the response to electrical stimulation of the raphe system, or to serotonin applied directly into the immediate spatial environment of the raphe neurons (microiontophoresis).

The predominant synaptic action of serotonin is inhibitory; a depression of cerebral neuronal firing rates occurs postsynaptically after stimulation of the raphe nuclei electrically. There appear to be both presynaptic and postsynaptic serotonin receptors, since iontophoretically-applied serotonin to the raphe nuclei presynaptically inhibits the spontaneous firing rate of these serotonin-containing neurons, as well as the firing rate of (postsynaptic) neurons surrounded by serotonergic nerve terminals in the cerebrum (Haigler and Aghajanian, 1977). Thus, the brain stem serotonergic neurons are called *autoreceptors*, which are conceived to be neurons with receptors generally distributed over their surfaces that are sensitive to the transmitter secreted by that neuron. This mechanism allows for presynaptic modulation of the release of serotonin.

The serotonin-antagonist drugs, pharmacologically so-classified on the basis of actions on *peripheral* receptor systems, do not generally block the inhibitory effects of serotonin within the CNS (Aghajanian and Wang, 1978). Indeed, these drugs that resemble serotonin structurally, and include the ergot alkaloids and cyproheptadine, *mimic the actions of serotonin* centrally by depressing the firing rate of serotonergic neurons, more so presynaptically than postsynaptically (Haigler and Aghajanian, 1974, 1977). Methysergide, cyproheptadine, and probably ergotamine and ergonovine also, have central actions most aptly described as *serotonin agonism*.

There appears to be a relationship between the firing rate of serotonergic neurons and the metabolic turnover of serotonin. For example, electrical stimulation of the raphe nuclei increases the synthesis and turnover of serotonin postsynaptically in the cerebrum. In general, an elevation of the intrasynaptic neurotransmitter level depresses the firing rate and synthetic activity of the presynaptic secretory neuron, suggesting the possibility that serotonin receptors are a link in a feedback loop that regulates the rate of firing of raphe neurons (Aghajanian, 1972). Stimulation of the receptor by a neurotransmitter agonist also results in a depression of the raphe neuron firing rate. Conversely, blockade of the neurotransmitter receptor produces an increase in the firing rate and release of transmitter by the presynaptic neuron (Jacoby et al, 1978). These observations are consistent with the reciprocal relationship between synaptic serotonin levels or availability and serotonergic neuronal activity. Thus, amitriptyline, a drug that blocks serotonin re-uptake more than other tricyclic drugs (Table 4–7), produces sustained higher intrasynaptic concentrations of the transmitter and a reduced firing rate of the raphe neurons (Fuller and Wong, 1977). Similarly, phenelzine, a monoamine oxidase inhibitor, blocks the primary route of brain serotonin (a

TABLE 4-7. COMPARATIVE EFFECTS OF TRICYCLIC DRUGS ON
BLOCKADE OF RE-UPTAKE OF SEROTONIN AND NOREPINEPHRINE[*]

DRUG	SEROTONIN	NOREPINEPHRINE
Amitriptyline	4+	0
Nortriptyline	2+	2+
Imipramine	3+	2+
Desipramine	0	4+

[*] Modified from Maas, 1978.

monoamine) catabolism, resulting in elevations of intrasynaptic serotonin and a depression in the firing rate of the raphe neurons (Aghajanian, 1972).

There is some evidence, although not compelling at present, that
the effects of serotonin at its receptor sites are mediated by cyclic
AMP (Fig. 4-3; Nathanson, 1977). Both caffeine (Butcher and Sutherland, 1962) and papaverine (Markwardt and Hoffman, 1970; Lugnier
et al, 1972) inhibit phosphodiesterase, the enzyme catalyzing the
degradation of cyclic AMP. There is evidence that PDE inhibition in
cyclic AMP-mediated postsynaptic potentials results in a potentiation
of the effects of the neurotransmitter in activating the postsynaptic
receptor. Caffeine substantially increases brain stem serotonin levels
(Berkowitz and Spector, 1971) and decreases brain serotonin turnover
(Valzelli and Bernasconi, 1973); the effects of papaverine on serotonin
turnover have not been studied. The effects of papaverine and caffeine on the firing rate of serotonergic neurons have not been examined either, so that the putative central mechanism of action of these
drugs (Table 4-8), although based on sound biologic principles, is
speculative.

$$\text{L-tryptophan} \rightarrow \text{5-OH tryptophan} \rightarrow \text{serotonin}$$
$$\text{melatonin} \swarrow \searrow \text{5-HIAA}$$

The above schema outlines the metabolic pathway of serotonin
within the CNS. L-tryptophan, an essential amino acid derived from
dietary sources, crosses the blood–brain barrier by an active energy-
dependent process (Fernstrom, 1978); the rate of synthesis of brain
serotonin has been shown to increase almost immediately after the
parenteral or oral administration of L-tryptophan. This linkage of the
rate of serotonin synthesis in brain to the availability of its precursor is
explicable by the observation that tryptophan hydroxylase, the rate-
limiting enzyme in the conversion of tryptophan to serotonin, is not
saturated by the levels of tryptophan normally present in brain; therefore, the concentration of tryptophan in brain plays a determinant role
in the rate of serotonin synthesis. The highest activities of brain

tryptophan hydroxylase are found within the midbrain raphe system (Saavedra, 1977), so that serotonin synthesized from L-tryptophan is relatively selectively located within serotonergic neurons. Consistent with these observations, the rate of firing of serotonergic neurons is markedly depressed after injections of L-tryptophan into laboratory animals (Aghajanian, 1972). Moreover, in a preliminary controlled study in which eight patients with migraine were given 2 gm of L-tryptophan daily, four of the eight experienced less frequent and less severe headaches (Kangasniemi et al, 1978).

Molecular oxygen is required for the hydroxylation of tryptophan to 5-hydroxytryptophan, the rate-limiting step in serotonin synthesis. The inhalation of 100 per cent oxygen by rats substantially increases brain serotonin synthesis, and hypoxia has the opposite effect (Costa and Meek, 1974). The expansion of the metabolic pool of brain serotonin may explain the action of oxygen in migraine, but neuronal firing rates after oxygen administration have not been measured.

Several lines of evidence suggest that there is an interaction between central adrenergic and serotonergic neuronal circuits. The pharmacologic evidence includes a correlation between the capacity of certain drugs to depress the brain stem serotonergic neuronal firing rate and central adrenergic blocking efficacy (Keller et al, 1973). Propranolol has been shown to weakly depress the firing rate of the raphe neurons when administered systemically, but not when applied microiontophoretically to serotonergic neurons (Gallager and Aghajanian, 1976). Thus, these drug effects are probably indirect, secondary to effects on a central adrenergic system that in turn influences the serotonergic neuronal circuit. The localization of this adrenergic system is not known at present.

Propranolol also produces an elevation of the level of serotonin in the pineal gland, by preventing the formation of melatonin, a reaction

TABLE 4–8. PUTATIVE MECHANISMS OF ACTION AT
SEROTONERGIC SYNAPSES OF THE MIGRAINE DRUGS

DRUGS	MECHANISMS OF ACTION
Methysergide, cyproheptadine, ergonovine, ergotamine	Serotonin agonism at presynaptic autoreceptor and/or postsynaptic receptor.
Amitriptyline	Inhibition of synaptic re-uptake of serotonin
Papaverine, caffeine	Inhibition of phosphodiesterase, cyclic AMP activation
Phenelzine	Inhibition of serotonin catabolism
Propranolol	Inhibition of adrenergic influence upon serotonergic neurons; ? prevention of serotonin release from synaptic cleft; ? inhibition of synaptic re-uptake of serotonin; inhibition of conversion of serotonin to melatonin.
Oxygen	Activation of tryptophan hydroxylase, increase in serotonin level

that occurs in no other organ (Zatz et al, 1978). The pineal gland is located at the dorsal surface of the thalamus, is innervated by the superior cervical sympathetic ganglion, and contains the highest concentration of serotonin in the brain. In fact, although in juxtaposition to the brain, the pineal is biologically isolated from it, in that it is on the "other" side of the blood–brain barrier. Environmental lighting and the daily light–dark cycle have profound effects on the level of serotonin in the pineal; this rhythmicity and light sensitivity, in addition to its involvement in the modulation of gonadal and pituitary activity, raises the possibility that the pineal may somehow be involved in the mechanism of migraine. However, it is uncertain whether the effect of propranolol on pineal serotonin turnover is relevant to its beneficial actions in migraine.

On a speculative note, several studies have shown propranolol to be a potent inhibitor of the uptake of serotonin by human platelets, both *in vivo* and *in vitro* (Grobecker et al, 1973; Lingjaerde, 1977). The platelet may be applicable as a model for the presynaptic nerve terminal owing to striking similarities in the manner in which both tissues transport, store and metabolize serotonin (Sneddon, 1973). Amitriptyline, for example, inhibits platelet serotonin uptake as well as the re-uptake of serotonin at central synapses; the effect of propranolol on platelet serotonin uptake may reflect a similar central action, although there is no evidence that supports this possibility. Similarly, the recent observation that the epinephrine-induced release of serotonin from duodenal enterochromaffin cells was blocked specifically by d,1-propranolol but not by d-propranolol or metoprolol, another beta-adrenergic blocking agent (Pettersson et al, 1978), may also be relevant to the action of propranolol in migraine. If the enterochromaffin cell is assumed to be a model for synaptic vesicles, the inhibition of sporadic releases of serotonin from the synaptic cleft, a putative mechanism of migraine (see below), may be a mode of action of propranolol.

HYPOTHESIS: THE PATHOPHYSIOLOGY OF MIGRAINE

The evidence presented above suggests that a depression of the activity of serotonergic brain stem neurons may be the common mode of action of drugs effective in migraine. By serotonin agonism, by prolonging the biologic half-life of serotonin in the synaptic cleft (through blockade of its re-uptake or metabolic degradation or an increase in its synthesis), or by activation of cyclic AMP (Table 4–8), a unitary expression for the action of these drugs can be formulated which is corroborated, for the most part, by direct measurement of serotonergic neuronal firing rates. What, then, is the basic abnormality that produces migrainous attacks? Two hypothetic possibilities that immediately arise are: (1) that defective regulation of raphe neurons produces sporadically high firing rates; and (2) that the modulation of transmitter release is defective, resulting in sporadically low synaptic serotonin levels and secondarily increased neuronal firing rates. The second possibility is more consistent with the bulk of the available evidence. How a derangement of serotonergic transmission can account for the dramatic circulatory alterations that accompany migrainous attacks can only be inferred at present from evidence imputing participation of the serotonergic circuit in the central regulation of the circulation (Chalmers and Wing, 1975; Smits and Struyker-Boudier, 1976; Lambert et al, 1978; Cabot et al, 1979). It is certainly possible that serotonin dysmodulation also occurs in the myenteric plexus of the intestinal walls, thus explaining the gastrointestinal motility alterations that often take place during migrainous attacks by a local mechanism.

Many of the phenomena of migraine, not well-explained by prior theories, may be rationalized by the hypothesis under discussion. For example, the administration of reserpine to migrainous subjects that results in the reproduction of migrainous attacks in the majority (Curzon et al, 1969) is as close as we have come thus far to an experimental

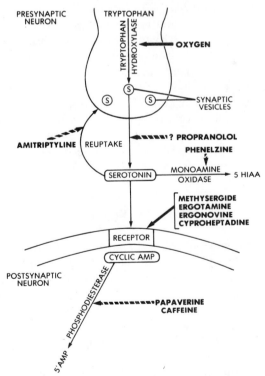

Figure 4-4. The actions of drugs effective in migraine at brain stem serotonergic synapses. The solid arrows indicate stimulative or agonist properties and the segmented arrows indicate inhibitory properties.

model of migraine in man. The mechanism of reserpine is probably related to a release of serotonin from neurons and nerve terminals, resulting in a depletion of brain serotonin to negligible levels; the released serotonin is exposed to the degradative action of monoamine oxidase, producing concomitant increases in 5-hydroxyindoleacetic acid (5-HIAA), the principal metabolite of serotonin, which appears in the urine (Sanders-Bush and Massari, 1977). Reduction of synaptic serotonin in patients whose synaptic levels are already low, or whose compensatory mechanisms for responses to changes in serotonin release are defective, might be expected to result in a greater increase in raphe neuronal firing rates than in nonmigrainous subjects; it is also understandable that control subjects may experience mild headaches after reserpine administration. Moreover, the previous administration of methysergide has been shown to prevent reserpine-induced headaches in migrainous subjects as well as in control subjects (Carroll and Hilton, 1973), without preventing the release of serotonin from its stores. This phenomenon is now explicable; the mechanism of action of methysergide appears to be as a serotonin agonist, affecting receptor sites directly, so that the biologic consequences of inadequate synaptic serotonin may be reversed by its action.

The implication of the serotonergic raphe cells in pain suppression (Fields and Basbaum, 1978), the regulation of sleep (Morgane and Stern, 1978), thermoregulation (Myers and Waller, 1978), endocrine regulation (Krieger, 1978) and stress (Bliss et al, 1972; Yuwiler, 1979) parallels the protean clinical manifestations and precipitants of migrainous attacks, conferring plausibility to the hypothesis. Furthermore, the hypothesis lends itself to an animal model of migraine, so that it may be tested in a controlled laboratory setting. This dysmodulation of synaptic serotonin hypothesis is an extension and modification of the general proposal put forth by Sicuteri et al (1974) that migraine may be a disorder of the pain modulation system in which the turnover of serotonin is defective.

METHYSERGIDE

Sicuteri (1959) was prompted to carry out the first clinical trial of methysergide (1-methyl-D-lysergic acid butanolamide) in migraine because of speculation at the time that serotonin was involved in the mechanism of migraine, and the observation that methysergide blocked the edema provoked by serotonin in the rat's paw with more potency than 16 other lysergic acid derivatives (Doepfner and Cerletti, 1958). Methysergide had been developed as one among many semisynthetic ergot alkaloid compounds derived from the naturally occurring ergonovine, and in due course was found to be a potent antagonist of many other peripheral actions of serotonin (Müller-Schweinitzer and Weidmann, 1978). The eventual designation of methysergide as the most effective drug in the prevention of migraine was the impetus for subsequent investigations of serotonin metabolism during migrainous attacks. There is now serious question whether the benefits conferred by methysergide to migrainous patients depend on the drug's peripheral serotonin-blocking actions.

Methysergide enters the systemic circulation after oral administration with a half-time of 23 minutes (Meier and Schreier, 1976); as is true of all ergot alkaloids, its disappearance from plasma occurs in two phases, a fast one with a half-life of about three hours and a longer one with a half-life of ten hours. Methysergide enters the brain, and its distribution to the tissues of experimental animals is similar to that of ergotamine (Doepfner, 1962; Bianchine, 1968). The kidneys are an important excretory pathway for methysergide, in contrast to ergotamine, over 50 per cent of the drug and its metabolites eventually appearing in the urine (Eckert et al, 1978). Methylergonovine is its principal metabolite; detailed information regarding its metabolic fate is not available. The CSF concentration of the drug is approximately 15 per cent of the plasma concentration.

Methysergide has resulted in substantial and sustained improvement in over 50 per cent of 376 patients to whom it was administered for 30 months before their final evaluation (Curran et al, 1967). About 20 per cent of those who have used methysergide have been rendered headache-free (Lance et al, 1965). The dosage is from 2 to 8 mg per day; occasional patients require 10 mg daily for an optimal effect. The usual dosage is 4 to 6 mg daily. Methysergide is usually ineffectual for the treatment of an acute migrainous attack, but some patients have found that an attack may be aborted by the early ingestion of a methysergide tablet. Strictly nocturnal headache may be optimally controlled with bedtime medication only (Curran et al, 1967).

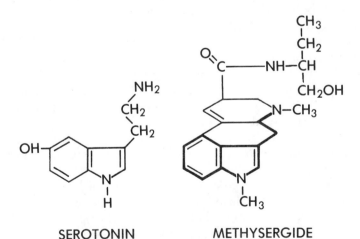

SEROTONIN   METHYSERGIDE

Figure 4-5. The similarities in the configurations of methysergide and serotonin are indicated by the darkened lines of the structure of methysergide.

TABLE 4-9.   METHYSERGIDE: SIDE-EFFECTS°

GASTROINTESTINAL	NEUROLOGIC
Nausea, vomiting	Drowsiness
Abdominal pain	Vertigo, giddiness
Diarrhea	Insomnia, vivid dreams
Constipation	Anxiety, poor concentration
	Confusion, sense of unreality
	Limb paresthesias
	Visual obscurations
	Asthenia, depression
CARDIOVASCULAR	
Peripheral vasoconstriction	
Palpitations	MISCELLANEOUS
Angina pectoris	
	Hair loss
	Sensation of swollen tongue
MUSCULOSKELETAL	Weight gain
	Pedal edema
Muscle cramps	Nasal congestion
Arthralgia	Flushing
Joint stiffness	Sweating

° Modified from Curran et al, 1967.

When full maintenance doses are begun, about 30 per cent of patients experience side-effects such as nausea, muscle cramps or abdominal pain; these usually subside over a period of days to weeks, and can be considerably lessened if the drug is begun at a 2-mg daily dosage and gradually increased, if well tolerated, to the optimal maintenance dosage. The beneficial effects usually become evident within seven to ten days, but occasionally there may be a latency of three or four weeks before improvement is noted. Once this occurs, many patients can reduce the daily dose gradually to a minimal dosage that confers continuous suppression of the migrainous mechanism. Many note that the effect of ergotamine on those headaches that continue to recur is much greater while they are regularly using methysergide; some who obtained no relief from ergotamine at all prior to methysergide are able effectively to abort their headaches after prophylaxis is instituted (Curran et al, 1967).

The side-effects of methysergide are presented in Table 4-9. Nausea, abdominal pain, pedal edema, weight gain and peripheral arterial insufficiency are the commonest; about 10 per cent of patients cannot tolerate methysergide, usually because of limb claudication. The latter appears to be dose-related, developing more often in those using doses of 8 mg or more daily; dosage reduction or, if the symptoms are mild, the addition of a peripheral vasodilator have successfully overcome these untoward effects (Curran and Lance, 1964). Angina pectoris has occurred only rarely. The vast majority of patients who experience side-effects develop them on the first or second day of therapy, often after only one or two tablets of the drug.

FIBROTIC DISORDERS

Graham (1967) and his colleagues (Graham et al, 1967; Bana et al, 1974) have summarized the evidence regarding the development of retroperitoneal fibrosis, pleuropulmonary fibrosis with effusion, and/or endocardial fibrosis in about 100 patients of the 500,000 who had been treated with methysergide before the recognition of the fibrotic complications of the drug. Lance et al (1970) encountered two patients with a fibrotic syndrome out of 1,000 treated with methysergide during the same period; in both instances, fibrosis receded upon the cessation of the drug. These disorders developed from seven to 79 months after methysergide was instituted; whereas a few patients developed a fibrotic disorder after as little as 2 mg daily, the vast majority of those affected had used 8 mg or more daily. The greatly decreased frequency of these complications of methysergide therapy in recent years (Griffith et al, 1978) may be a reflection of the dosage conservatism that has been practiced. However, in 1967 it was also recommended that prolonged methysergide therapy should be interrupted periodically by one-month drug holidays based on the hope, rather than data, that such drug-free interludes might lessen the frequency of fibrotic complications. The number of patients who have been willing to discontinue methysergide periodically and sustain what may be a month of total disability is not clear. In the authors' view, the general practice of using the minimally effective dosage of methysergide is probably the more important factor in reducing the frequency of the fibrotic disorders.

The fact that methysergide is causally linked to fibrotic disorders is firmly established; the diseases almost always regress when the drug is stopped and may recur if it is reinstituted. Recent reports of retroperitoneal fibrosis in patients who had not received methysergide but had consumed large amounts of analgesics, especially phenacetin, suggest that other pharmacologic factors may bear on this uncommon disorder (MacGregor et al, 1973; Lewis et al, 1975). Similarly, ergotamine tartrate usage has also been linked, albeit rarely, to retroperitoneal fibrosis (Graham et al, 1967; Griffith et al, 1978).

Retroperitoneal fibrosis producing ureteral obstruction, the commonest of the fibrotic complications of methysergide therapy, has been reported in over 50 patients. Once recognized and established as such a complication, it was no longer reported, so that the number of those who developed it is probably much larger. Retroperitoneal fibrosis usually is clinically silent, requiring intravenous pyelography for its detection; ureteral narrowing generally is apparent between the

TABLE 4-10. CARDIAC MURMURS ASSOCIATED WITH
METHYSERGIDE THERAPY IN 47 PATIENTS°

Systolic murmurs		22
Mitral	17	
Aortic	5	
Systolic and diastolic murmurs		19
Diastolic murmurs, aortic and/or		
mitral, alone		6

°Modified from Bana et al, 1974.

levels of the third lumbar and first sacral vertebrae (Elkind et al, 1968). On occasion, flank pain, fever and an elevation of the erythrocyte sedimentation rate may be the symptomatic expression of the disorder.

Endocardial fibrosis has been reported in 48 patients treated with methysergide, nine of whom also developed retroperitoneal fibrosis (Bana et al, 1974). The development of murmurs, systolic and/or diastolic, reflecting involvement of the left heart valves (Table 4–10) is the major clinical manifestation of this complication, which ultimately may result in congestive heart failure. Pathologic specimens have been examined in four patients, and the findings are very similar to those noted in association with the carcinoid syndrome (Roberts and Sjoerdsma, 1964), except that in the latter condition the right heart valves are usually involved. Collagen deposition upon otherwise normal heart valves and endocardial ventricular surfaces are the cardinal pathologic features of methysergide-induced endocardial fibrosis; mast cells are characteristically present in the valvular collagen deposition.

Pleuropulmonary fibrosis has occurred with a frequency about one-half that of endocardial fibrosis (Graham, 1967). Chest pain, dyspnea and fever have occasionally called attention to the pleural effusions and friction rubs that eventually were identified. Chest x-rays occasionally have shown posterior, tumor-like nodules that have been identified at operation as fibrotic areas that involved the pleura, chest wall and lung.

Rare examples of constrictive pericarditis (Orlando et al, 1978), rectosigmoid strictures (Gelford and Cromwell, 1968) and constriction of the great vessels (Regan and Poletti, 1968) have also been reported. Therefore, for patients who use methysergide for six months or longer, periodic intravenous pyelography and x-rays of the chest, in addition to careful cardiac auscultation, are important for the early detection of these now rare, generally reversible fibrotic complications. Furthermore, Graham and his colleagues (Bana et al, 1974) have interrupted the use of methysergide for one to four weeks during each 12-month period in addition to using the minimal dosage necessary, and have observed no new fibrotic complications in over 300 patients treated with the drug.

Mechanisms of fibrotic complications.   Substantial efforts have been made to establish an animal model for methysergide-induced fibrosis. However, despite the use of seven different animal species, periods of drug administration up to 2½ years, and contrivances such as fibrosis provocation and induced hormone imbalance, lesions corresponding to those in humans have not been produced (Griffith et al, 1978). No differences in the metabolism of methysergide have been found in migrainous patients (Bianchine and Eade, 1969) or in three individuals who had previously developed retroperitoneal fibrosis caused by methysergide (Bianchine and Friedman, 1970).

The development of retroperitoneal, pleuropulmonary and endocardial fibrosis in patients with serotonin-secreting carcinoid tumors (Thompson, 1977; Feldman, 1978) suggests the possibility that the effects of methysergide may be mediated through an interaction with serotonin or serotonin receptors. Injections of serotonin into animals have failed to produce fibrosis (Bianchine et al, 1968; Bianchine and Eade, 1969; Spatz, 1969), but there is good evidence that serotonin participates in the modulation of collagen synthesis, possibly by an effect on fibroblast receptors (Boucek, 1977). Furthermore, fibrotic lesions are characteristically produced by those parasites that contain high concentrations of serotonin — in schistosomiasis (Schiller and Haese, 1973) and fascioliasis (Bartlett, 1968). It is worth noting in this context that serotonin is probably a neurotransmitter in schistosomes, and methysergide exerts profound effects on the motility of these organisms (Hillman et al, 1974).

The ground substance components of connective tissue are invariably initiated by an accumulation of mast cells (Asboe-Hansen, 1973). Mast cells are degranulated following serotonin administration (Asboe-Hansen and Wegelius, 1956), as are basophilic leukocytes by methysergide (Shelley and Resnick, 1964); the release of potent amines by tissue mast cells in response to serotonin or methysergide is a possible mechanism of the fibrotic complications of carcinoid and methysergide. Moreover, methysergide can pass through the ureteral wall *in vitro* (Bianchine and Eade, 1969); it is possible that mast cell degranulation or activation of the putative fibroblastic serotonin receptors in the retroperitoneal area by a transudate of methysergide may result in retroperitoneal fibrosis.

West (1962) was unable to detect any toxic effects of methysergide on the rat fetus, and there is no evidence that the drug is harmful during pregnancy (Curran et al, 1967). However, the observations that methysergide inhibits the secretion of growth-hormone and prolactin (Bivens et al, 1973; Mendelson et al, 1975; Krulich et al, 1978) suggest that the hormonal milieu of a developing fetus may not be optimally influenced by methysergide. None of the preventive migraine drugs are safe enough for a developing fetus to warrant use during pregnancy.

When simpler measures fail, methysergide is well worth considering, especially for patients with severe and frequent headaches.

Since the most serious potential side-effects of the drug require several months for their development, the risk–benefit ratio may be better evaluated after a one-month trial of the drug at optimal dosage. For the patient rendered headache-free, the rare and preventable risks of methysergide are then in a clearly focused perspective.

EFFECTS ON THE CRANIAL VASCULATURE

Methysergide blocks the vasoconstrictor effect of serotonin, more so in the internal than in the external carotid circulation; the drug itself has only a mild and transient vasoconstrictor effect and it also potentiates the constrictor effects of norepinephrine (Welch et al, 1974; Spira et al, 1976). The direct constrictor effect of methysergide appears to be unrelated to its norepinephrine-potentiating effect (Saxena, 1974). Methysergide also antagonizes the dilator effects of serotonin on cranial arteries noncompetitively (Edvinsson et al, 1978); it has no effect on the vasodilator responses to histamine, bradykinin or prostaglandin E_1. Some of these peripheral vascular effects may be relevant, at least in part, to the therapeutic action of methysergide in migraine; blockade of arterial serotonin receptors and/or potentiation of the vasoconstrictor effects of endogenous norepinephrine are the actions likeliest to be beneficial.

CONTRAINDICATIONS

The high incidence of peripheral vasoconstriction as a side-effect of methysergide suggests extreme caution or avoidance of the drug in patients with peripheral vascular disease or coronary artery disease. As is true of all the ergot alkaloids, methysergide is a potent venoconstrictor (Aellig, 1976), so that those with previous experiences of thrombophlebitis ought not to be treated with the drug. Activation of peptic ulcers has occurred often with methysergide (Curran et al, 1967), which probably is explained by the drug's capacity to double gastric acid secretion (Resnick et al, 1962).

CYPROHEPTADINE

The demonstration that serotonin, in addition to histamine, may be released in certain allergic reactions gave rise to studies of the serotonin-blocking actions of various antihistaminic agents. Cyproheptadine was found to be the most active peripheral serotonin antagonist of all the antihistaminics studied (Stone et al, 1961). It bears some resemblance to the phenothiazine antihistaminics, and also to the ergot alkaloids in possessing an N-substituted heterocyclic ring.

Figure 4-6.

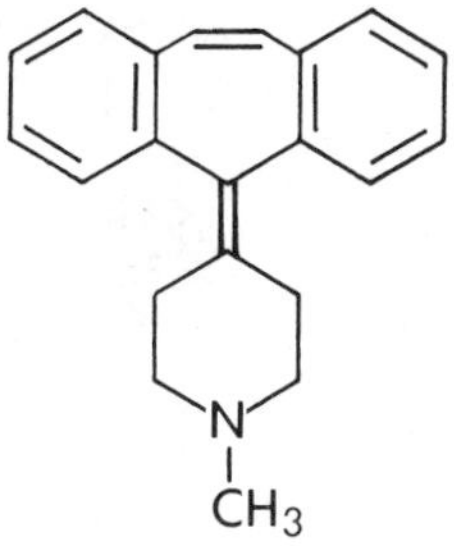

CYPROHEPTADINE

The drug is rapidly absorbed and accumulates in tissues, entering brain, with only low concentrations remaining in plasma (Wold and Fischer, 1972). Very little is known of its metabolic fate; its main metabolic urinary product is a glucuronidase-sensitive conjugate involving only the nitrogen of the parent drug (Porter et al, 1975).

The central serotonin-agonist effects of cyproheptadine are quite similar to those of methysergide (Haigler and Aghajanian, 1977; Jacoby et al, 1978), and the amelioration of the diarrhea that accompanies the carcinoid syndrome is also common to both drugs (Brown, 1977). However, the peripheral effects of cyproheptadine on the cranial vasculature are quantitatively less than those of methysergide; it only weakly antagonizes the vasoconstrictor effects of serotonin (Fozard, 1975; Hardebo et al, 1978). The effects of norepinephrine are not potentiated by cyproheptadine. These peripheral vascular actions are not likely to be relevant to the drug's benefits in migraine. It is possible that its platelet anti-aggregating properties are important to its therapeutic effect in migraine (Ambrus et al, 1977).

The usual dosage of cyprohepatadine is 12 to 24 mg daily, given in two doses, with occasional patients requiring 32 mg for an optimal effect. Sedation and weight gain are the commonest side-effects; dry mouth, nausea, lightheadedness, pedal edema, aching legs and diarrhea also occur occasionally. The over-all effect in migraine patients is less than that of methysergide (Curran and Lance, 1964; Lance et al, 1965, 1970). When the effects of either methysergide or cyproheptadine alone are less than substantial, the use of both drugs concurrently has sometimes been dramatically effective, in the authors' experience.

Pizotifen (B.C.-105, Sandomigran), not available at present in the United States, resembles cyproheptadine structurally and possesses similar serotonin-blocking actions peripherally (Carroll et al, 1974). Like the ergot alkaloids it is a potent venoconstrictor (Aellig, 1978). Its central actions have not been studied. It appears to be more effective than cyproheptadine in the treatment of migraine (Speight and Avery, 1972; Mikropoulos, 1978).

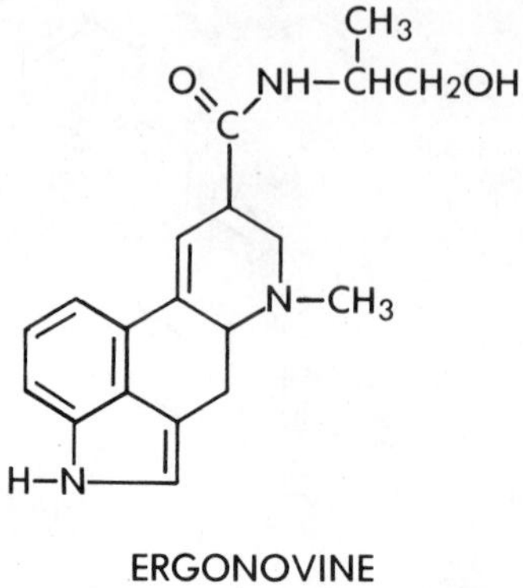

CH₃ O NH—CHCH₂OH N—CH₃ H—N

Figure 4-7.

ERGONOVINE

ERGONOVINE

The introduction of ergotamine to medicine for the treatment of acute migrainous attacks led to the testing of other ergot alkaloids for their effects in migraine. Ergonovine (D-lysergic acid propanolamide), also known as ergometrine, has greater oxytocic effects than ergotamine but lacks significant peripheral vasoconstrictor properties (Haley et al, 1954; Klingenberg, 1973). Although early studies demonstrated a beneficial effect toward aborting migrainous attacks (Table 4–2), with a much lower incidence of nausea and vomiting (Lennox, 1938), its therapeutic action was disappointingly inferior to that of ergotamine, and ergonovine was largely forgotten. However, Barrie et al (1968) in a controlled study showed that ergonovine probably prevented vascular headaches, but was inferior to the two other preventive drugs studied, methysergide and ergotamine.

The structure of ergonovine is very similar to that of methysergide and to the latter's principal metabolite, methylergonovine. The peripheral serotonin-blocking effects of ergonovine are greater than those of ergotamine and less than those of methysergide (Cerletti and Doepfner, 1958; Bunag and Walaszek, 1962). It is almost as potent as ergotamine as a peripheral venoconstrictor (Brooke and Robinson, 1970). Ergonovine has potent central pharmacologic effects (Longo and Loizzo, 1978), and there is evidence that it possesses both agonist and antagonist properties toward central dopamine receptors (Loew et al, 1978), but studies of its effects on serotonin receptors have not been performed.

If one assumes that pharmacokinetic data derived from studies with methylergonovine approximate the biologic behavior of ergonovine, approximately 60 per cent of an oral dose reaches the systemic circulation and peak plasma levels are evident within 30 minutes (Mäntylä et al, 1978). Only 3 per cent of an oral dose appears in the urine as the parent drug or its metabolites, probably reflecting primary hepatic metabolic clearance, similar to the biologic fate of ergotamine. There is a prolonged clinical response of the uterus to ergonovine, lasting several hours (Roth-Brandel et al, 1970), that correlates poorly with its rapid disappearance from plasma.

The drug is unusually well tolerated. Its most common side-effects are nausea, abdominal pain, and aching or tiredness of the legs. Only rarely does constriction of the peripheral or coronary arteries occur. Recently, ergonovine has beem employed in intravenous doses of 0.05 to 0.2 mg as a provocative diagnostic test for Prinzmetal's angina (Curry, 1978; Heupler et al, 1978; Curry et al, 1979), a variant form of angina pectoris that occurs at rest in association with transient electrocardiographic S–T segment elevation, and appears to be mediated by coronary artery spasm (Hillis and Braunwald, 1978). Intravenous 0.2-mg doses of ergonovine result in plasma levels eight to 16 times higher than those reached after oral doses (Mäntylä et al, 1978); the provocation of angina pectoris is fairly specific for Prinzmetal's angina, with no positive responses observed in control subjects and only rare positive responses in those with coronary artery disease (Cipriano et al, 1979). In over ten years of extensive use of the drug in over 2,000 patients, only one instance of angina pectoris has occurred after a single 0.2-mg tablet of the drug was taken by an individual with no previous history of chest pain (Raskin, unpublished observations).

Several additional effects of ergonovine render it inappropriate for use during pregnancy or for women who are planning to become pregnant. Strong and lasting stimulation of fallopian tube motility is produced by oral doses of the drug (Coutinho et al, 1976); this effect may impair the transport of an ovum through the tube, thus exerting a contraceptive effect. Like methysergide, ergonovine inhibits prolactin secretion (Shane and Naftolin, 1974), and more importantly there is evidence that it, like LSD, can induce chromosomal aberrations in cultured human lymphocytes (Kato and Jarvik, 1969).

The only clear contraindications to the use of ergonovine are Prinzmetal's angina, peripheral venous disease, and anticipated or *de facto* pregnancy.

PROPRANOLOL

The original observation that propranolol was effective in preventing migrainous attacks was made fortuitously. Rabkin et al (1966),

Figure 4-8.

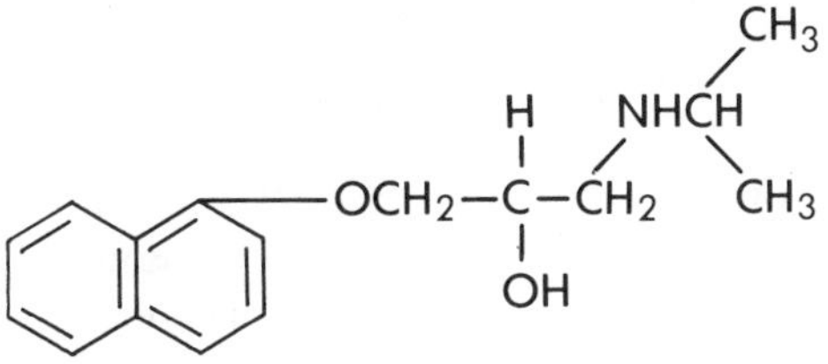

PROPRANOLOL

during a study of the value of this drug in preventing angina pectoris, noted that one of the 20 treated patients, a 59-year-old man, was promptly relieved of his longstanding vascular headaches as well as angina pectoris; his headaches returned during the crossover to placebo medication. Wykes (1968), noting this observation, treated four patients who had both angina pectoris and migraine headaches with propranolol, and reported that two of them experienced relief from both the headaches and the chest pain. Thereafter, controlled studies established the value of propranolol in the treatment of migraine (Weber and Reinmuth, 1972; Diamond and Medina, 1976; Forssman et al, 1976 — review of six studies). Because of its effectiveness and very low incidence of side-effects, the drug has had a major impact in migraine therapy. The beta-adrenergic blocking properties of propranolol, important for its therapeutic action in patients with cardiac arrhythmias, led to the inference that this was its mode of action in migraine. However, subsequent data cast considerable doubt that beta-blockade is important to its action in migraine.

Norepinephrine, the principal neurotransmitter at peripheral sympathetic synapses, evokes responses that vary in different tissues. The adrenergic receptors have been divided into alpha and beta types, suggested by Ahlquist (1948) as a basis for classifying the different actions of norepinephrine as well as those of sympathetic agonists and antagonists. Agonists vary only quantitatively in their capacity to stimulate both receptors, but the inhibitors are specific for one or the other. Alpha-receptors are abundant in the resistance vessels of the skin, mucosa, intestine and kidney, and when stimulated they result in vasoconstriction. Beta-receptors predominate in the heart (β_1), the arteries of skeletal muscle, and the bronchi (β_2), subserving myocardial excitation, vasodilatation and bronchodilatation (Kunos, 1978).

$$\text{stimulated adrenergic} \atop \text{receptors} \left\{ \begin{array}{l} \alpha - \text{vasoconstriction} \\ \beta_1 - \text{myocardial excitation} \\ \beta_2 - \text{vasodilatation, bronchodilatation} \end{array} \right.$$

Thus, blockade of peripheral vasodilator beta-receptors, preventing the vasodilatation that underlies the headache phase of a migraine attack, was put forth as a possible mode of action of the drug; however, no convincing evidence of beta-adrenergic regulation of intra- or extracerebral arteries has been found.

Studies in animals as well as in man have shown that propranolol produces no significant alterations of either CBF or the cerebral metabolic rate (Olesen et al, 1978; Berntman et al, 1978). The dilator effect that a low concentration of serotonin produces on cerebral arteries and arterioles is blocked by propranolol (Edvinsson et al, 1975, 1978). The clinical relevance of this finding is uncertain.

The various beta-blockers now available in most of the world

(Table 4–11) differ quantitatively in potency, beta-receptor selectivity, agonist activity and membrane stabilizing actions. A number of these beta-blockers, in addition to propranolol, have been studied for their possible benefits in migraine — including prindolol (Sjaastad and Stensrud, 1972; Anthony et al, 1972; Ekbom, 1975a), a much more potent beta-blocker than propranolol (Clark and Saameli, 1970); alprenolol (Ekbom, 1975b), equal in potency to propranolol (Brown et al, 1978); oxprenolol (Ekbom and Zetterman, 1977); and acebutolol (Nanda et al, 1978). Although some patients may have benefited from these drugs, in none of these studies were results obtained that differed significantly from placebo; it is safe to conclude that all are inferior to propranolol in the prevention of migrainous attacks.

An ingenious study was formulated in which the effects of the dextro(d-)optical isomer of propranolol were compared to the usually prescribed drug, which is one-half d-propranolol and one-half levo(l)-propranolol, in the treatment of patients with migraine. Both produced results significantly better than placebo (Stensrud and Sjaastad, 1976), although the results with racemic(dl-)propranolol were more striking. Both the d- and l-isomers enter brain almost immediately; about 65 per cent of the propranolol contained in plasma crosses the blood–brain barrier in a single passage through the brain (Olesen et al, 1978), approximating the extraction rate of water. However, beta-adrenergic receptors are differentially inhibited more by l-propranolol than by d-propranolol in various tissues studied by a factor of 100 to 1,000 (Brown et al, 1978); clinically, the d-isomer is almost devoid of beta-blocking activity (Howitt et al, 1968). Therefore, substantial evidence renders it very unlikely that peripheral beta-blockade is the mode of action of propranolol in migraine. This conclusion is hardly unprecedented since several other beneficial effects of the drug, including its antihypertensive action (Klevans et al, 1976; Tuttle and McCleary, 1978; Sharma et al, 1979) and its effects on essential tremor (Young et al, 1975) also are probably mediated by effects of the drug on the CNS (Koch-Weser, 1975).

*TABLE 4–11.   PROPERTIES OF SOME β-ADRENERGIC BLOCKING DRUGS**

	β-STIMULATION (AGONIST ACTIVITY)	MEMBRANE STABILIZATION	CARDIOSELECTIVE, β_1-INHIBITION
Propranolol	−	+	−
Acebutolol	−	+	+
Oxprenolol	+	+	−
Alprenolol	+	+	−
Practolol	+	−	+
Prindolol	+	+	−

*Modified from Ekbom, 1975a.

The therapeutically effective dosage range of propranolol is one of the broadest of all the drugs effective in migraine; it varies from 40 to 320 mg per day, and need not be given more often than three times daily since its half-life is 3.5 to 6 hours (Routledge and Shand, 1979). For many patients a twice-daily dosage regimen suffices, especially for those using 240 mg or more daily, and enables them to comply with the drug program better. Propranolol is completely absorbed from the GI tract and is virtually completely metabolized in the liver. In addition to its hepatic metabolism the drug is avidly extracted from the plasma by the liver, so that hepatic blood flow is an important factor regarding its elimination (Kornhauser et al, 1978). The plasma concentrations of the drug that can saturate this hepatic extraction mechanism are quite variable, and account for the observation that plasma levels of the drug among patients receiving the same oral dosage differ by factors that may be as large as 20 (Shand, 1974). Several metabolites of propranolol have been identified, some of which are pharmacologically active and may contribute to the effects of propranolol in man (Walle and Gaffney, 1972).

Because of the varying dose response from patient to patient, it is reasonable to begin treatment with 20 mg three times daily, and progressively to increase the dosage at weekly intervals until an optimal effect is achieved. The average effective dosage is 120 mg daily. Occasional patients have noted a worsening of their headache disorder when propranolol is begun; this paradoxical effect sometimes subsides and headaches may then be controlled.

Congestive heart failure and asthma are absolute contraindications to propranolol therapy. Renal insufficiency is also a contraindication to its use because of recent evidence that the glomerular filtration rate is depressed by the drug (Bauer and Brooks, 1979). The use of propranolol by patients with diabetes mellitus who do not require insulin is generally safe (Wright et al, 1979); however, those with brittle diabetes should avoid the drug because of its rare provocation of hypoglycemia (Skinner and Misbin, 1979; Lager et al, 1979). Fatigue and gastrointestinal symptoms (flatulence, diarrhea, constipation) are the commonest side-effects; orthostatically-induced lightheadedness may also occur. Tolerance to these side-effects is often acquired over a period of weeks, so that their appearance need not call for immediate cessation of the drug. An association has been noted between the use of propranolol and the fibrotic disorder of the penile shaft, Peyronie's disease (Pryor and Khan, 1979); however, whether the drug is the cause of fibrous tissue growth is uncertain. A single report has been made of severe peripheral vasoconstriction that appeared to be caused by the concurrent use of propranolol and ergotamine (Baumrucker, 1973). However, this must be an exceedingly rare adverse interaction, since it has not been noted in any of the propranolol studies, nor in the authors' experience with the concurrent use of propranolol and ergotamine. Significantly smaller infants are born to pregnant rats treated with high doses of propranolol (Schoenfeld et al, 1978), suggesting that this drug should be avoided for women contemplating pregnancy (Rosen et al, 1979).

A withdrawal syndrome may occur after the sudden cessation of propranolol therapy; it comprises tachycardia and tremulousness, headache, ventricular arrhythmia, severe angina pectoris, myocardial infarction and even death (Shand and Wood, 1978). Among patients using propranolol for the control of angina pectoris, the incidence of this withdrawal syndrome is approximately 5 per cent; however, severe withdrawal symptoms must be very rare among migrainous patients who suddenly stop using it. Prudence dictates caution; a tapering period of fourteen days minimizes the magnitude of a potential, but rare, hazard of the cessation of propranolol (Nattel et al, 1979).

AMITRIPTYLINE

There are two lines of reasoning that led to the introduction of amitriptyline for the treatment of migraine. First, the demonstration in the early 1960s that carbamazepine, an analogue of imipramine, was remarkably effective in the suppression of trigeminal neuralgia, led to informal empirical trials of imipramine itself as well as other tricyclic drugs in the therapy of a variety of painful states. Second, because patients with chronic headache disorders often become depressed (Couch et al, 1975), pain in this setting was believed to be an expression of depression that might be expected to be alleviated by the administration of a drug with antidepressant properties. However, the beneficial effect of amitriptyline in migraine probably occurs independent of its antidepressant action (Gomersall and Stuart, 1973; Couch et al, 1976), and although formal studies have not been done there is a consensus that drugs with equivalent antidepressant actions, such as imipramine, have been relatively ineffectual in the treatment of migraine. The sparse literature regarding the effectiveness of amitriptyline is remarkable, given the drug's successful use throughout the world.

Amitriptyline is completely absorbed, and with regular daily dos-

Figure 4-9.

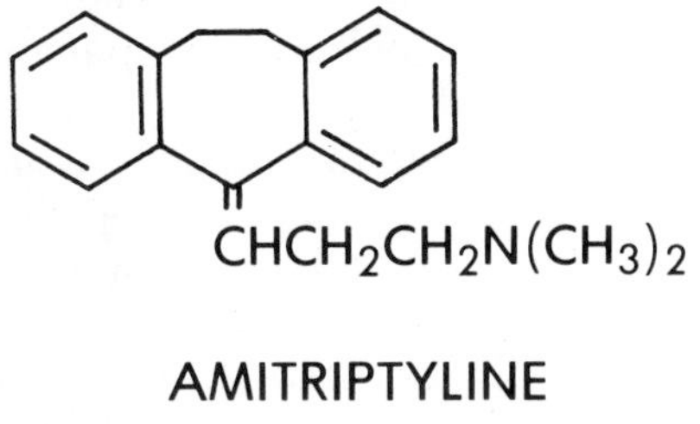

$CHCH_2CH_2N(CH_3)_2$

AMITRIPTYLINE

ing the plasma concentration increases progressively until a steady plasma concentration is reached, usually within two to three days. Amitriptyline tissue levels are much higher than are steady-state plasma levels; plasma concentrations of the drug may vary as much as thirtyfold among patients given the same dose of the drug (Ziegler et al, 1977; Coppen et al, 1978). The plasma half-life of amitriptyline varies from eight to 16 hours, with a mean of 13 hours (Rogers et al, 1978), so that it usually need be taken only once daily. Amitriptyline is extensively extracted from plasma by the liver, similar to but of lesser magnitude than the case of propranolol (see above); its degradation is complete and occurs in the liver also (Sjöqvist, 1975). Variations in the saturability of the hepatic extraction mechanism probably account for the wide plasma level fluctuations and the broad range of effective doses of the drug, similar to the dosage principles discussed above for propranolol. Amitriptyline is demethylated to nortriptyline *in vivo*; plasma levels of the parent drug are approximately the same or slightly higher than those of its pharmacologically active metabolite (Coppen et al, 1978). It is possible that some of the pharmacologic properties of amitriptyline are mediated by nortriptyline; indeed, on many occasions the authors have found that, for patients who tolerate amitriptyline poorly, nortriptyline may be better tolerated and appears to be effective in the prevention of migrainous attacks.

The effective dosage of amitriptyline has varied from 10 to 175 mg daily; 90 per cent of patients achieve an optimal effect with 50 to 75 mg per day. The authors have found it most useful to begin therapy with 25 mg taken at bedtime, and progressively to increase the daily dosage in 25-mg increments weekly up to 100 mg. If, after six weeks' treatment, there is no benefit at all, there is no point in further increasing the dosage. Two-thirds of patients who derive benefit from amitriptyline note improvement within seven days, but the range for the time of onset of improvement varies from one to 42 days (Couch et al, 1976).

Excessive sedation is by far the commonest side-effect of the drug. It may be countered in many patients by reducing the initial dosage to 10 mg, and slowing the progression of the dosage increments over several weeks to allow for tolerance to the sedating properties of the drug, which usually does occur. Some patients tolerate amitriptyline better when it is taken in two divided doses. Dry mouth is also common but rarely interdicts therapy. Constipation, orthostatic hypotension, palpitations, perspiration and weight gain occur occasionally, and urinary retention rarely.

The sometimes prominent actions of amitriptyline on the cardiovascular system (Raisfeld, 1972) preclude its use in patients disposed to cardiac arrhythmias or congestive heart failure. Prostatism or other causes of bladder insufficiency are additional relative contraindications to the use of the drug.

Several lines of evidence suggest that amitriptyline exerts its central effects principally through actions on serotonergic systems and not through actions on noradrenergic systems (Maas and Garver, 1975; de Montigny and Aghajanian, 1978; Maas, 1978). Indeed, compared to the other tricyclic drugs, amitriptyline appears to be the most potent regarding its capacity to block the re-uptake of serotonin at central synapses (Table 4–7). Other than the potentiation of the pressor effects of norepinephrine (Cairncross, 1965), there are no known effects of amitriptyline on cerebral arteries that might explain its actions in the treatment of migraine.

PHENELZINE

The rationale for the sole study of phenelzine therapy in migraine (Anthony and Lance, 1969) was based on the formulation that the platelet release of serotonin known to accompany migrainous attacks might result in arterial dilatation by virtue of the withdrawal of a vasoconstrictor influence from the circulation. The metabolic degradation of serotonin, a monoamine, would be predictably blocked in the presence of phenelzine, an inhibitor of monoamine oxidase (MAO), resulting in the elevation of plasma and tissue levels, thus preventing uncontrolled vasodilatation.

In Anthony and Lance's (1969) study of 25 patients with severe migraine, 14 had been treated previously with both cyproheptadine and methysergide, three had received cyproheptadine alone and eight had been treated with ergotamine alone — all without benefit. Phenelzine was administered at a daily dosage of 45 mg for a period that ranged from five to 24 months. At the end of the study, seven patients were headache-free, seven were improved by 75 per cent, six improved by 50 per cent, and five unimproved — compared to the previous 12 months, which served as the control for these patients. The trial was otherwise uncontrolled, but these results are far beyond an anticipated placebo response of 30 to 40 per cent. Platelet serotonin levels had been determined serially before and during phenelzine therapy. Whereas the levels generally rose during drug treatment, there was no correlation between the magnitude of the elevations and clinical responses; for example, a patient with only a modest rise in platelet serotonin had remained headache-free, whereas another with the highest elevations was unimproved.

$$\text{Benzene ring}-CH_2-CH_2-NH-NH_2$$

Figure 4–10.

PHENELZINE

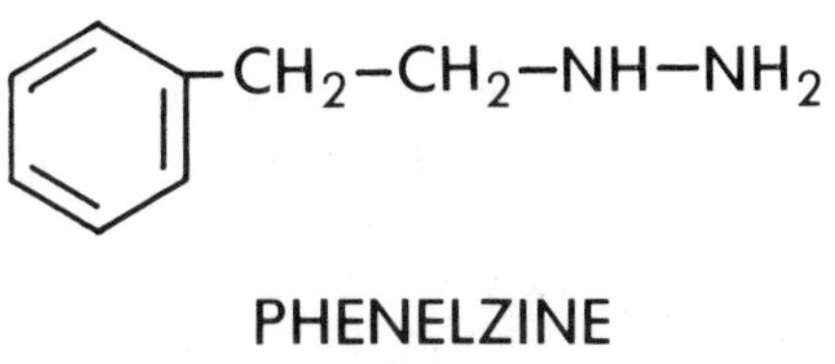

TABLE 4-12. SOME INHIBITORS AND SUBSTRATES OF BRAIN—
MONOAMINE OXIDASE TYPES A AND B[*]

| | MONOAMINE OXIDASE | |
	Type A	Type B
Preferred substrates	Serotonin Norepinephrine Normetanephrine	2-Phenylethylamine Dopamine
Relatively specific inhibitors	Clorgyline Harmaline	Deprenyl Pargyline '
Nonspecific substrates	Tyramine Tryptamine	
Nonspecific inhibitors	Phenelzine Iproniazid Tranylcypromine Nialamide	

[*]Modified from Neff and Fuentes, 1976; Murphy, 1978.

Recently, these authors' hypothesis for the mode of action of phenelzine in migraine was supported by the observation that pretreatment of baboons with tranylcypromine, a potent MAO inhibitor, markedly potentiated the intracerebral vasoconstrictor effect of intraarterially administered serotonin (Eidelman et al, 1978). Phenelzine is well absorbed, but direct assay of plasma levels has not been feasible because of its low concentration and the drug's irreversible binding to intracellular monoamine oxidase. Patients treated with the drug have been monitored with measurements of platelet MAO activity and serotonin levels; maximal MAO inhibition and elevation of serotonin occur within one to three weeks of the initiation of therapy (Robinson et al, 1978; Marshall et al, 1978). Phenelzine metabolism appears to be dose-dependent; higher doses result in a longer elimination half-life. Its metabolic fate is uncertain.

Monoamine oxidase is localized to the mitochondria of most human tissues, and is present in highest concentrations in the GI tract and liver. The enzyme probably functions in the degradation of intracellular biogenic amines; in contrast to other monoamines degraded by MAO, norepinephrine and dopamine, for example, the metabolic disposition of serotonin depends almost entirely on oxidation by MAO. Moreover, there are probably two forms of MAO, based on differential responsiveness to specific inhibitors (Table 4-12), referred to as types A and B, that are relatively substrate-selective (Murphy, 1978). The enzyme variants are not distributed in constant proportion in different tissues, but vary among cell types. In human platelets and the pineal gland the B form predominates, and brain contains the A and B forms in a ratio of 20:80. Peripheral sympathetic neurons contain mainly type A. In human brain, dopamine is predominantly oxidized by type B (Glover et al, 1977). Serotonin is consistently an MAO-A preferred substrate. Although much remains unknown, the balance of evidence suggests that these two forms of MAO, each with distinctive properties, exist separately in some tissues and together in others. Whether they are different conformations of the same enzyme or distinct enzymes is uncertain. The MAO inhibitors in clinical use are nonspecific inhibitors of both forms of MAO (Table 4–12); the fact that newer therapeutic agents with greater specificity can be derived from this better understanding of the biology of MAO is illustrated by the potential usefulness of the MAO type B inhibitor, deprenyl, in the treatment of parkinsonism (Birkmayer et al, 1975).

The commonest side-effects noted with phenelzine are orthostatic hypotension, constipation, insomnia and perspiration; less commonly, there is inhibition of ejaculation or of bladder tone. Hepatotoxicity was an unfortunately common problem with the early MAO inhibitors in clinical use, such as iproniazid and isocarboxazid, but there is no evidence that phenelzine is hepatotoxic. As to the hypertensive interactions between MAO inhibitors and certain foodstuffs, mainly cheese (Table 4–13), a problem of the 1960s that resulted in the abandonment of MAO inhibitors by many physicians, the risk of these rare reactions in patients using phenelzine was one-fifth that associated with tranylcypromine, a more potent MAO inhibitor (Blackwell et al, 1967). The surges of hypertension that resulted in cerebral hemorrhage in several cases were probably caused by the ingestion of large amounts of a pressor amine, tyramine in most instances, that escaped oxidative deamination in the gut and liver; the intestinal absorption of tyramine does not normally occur without inhibition of intestinal wall MAO (Marley, 1977). Over one-half of the affected patients had previously eaten the implicated foodstuff on many occasions without experiencing adverse effects; the wide variation of tyramine concentrations within food groups is undoubtedly a

TABLE 4–13. FOODSTUFF PRECIPITANTS OF REACTIONS IN 83 PATIENTS TREATED WITH MONOAMINE OXIDASE INHIBITORS*

FOODSTUFF	NO. PATIENTS
Cheese	67
Alcohol	5
Yeast products	3
Cream	3
Broad beans	2
Pickled herring	2
Chocolate	1

*From Blackwell et al, 1967.

factor that at least partially accounts for this apparent inconsistency. Only four out of 14 samples of cheddar cheese contained enough tyramine to potentially provoke hypertension in patients using MAO inhibitors (Blackwell and Mabbitt, 1965).

There is evidence that the affected patients did not metabolize MAO inhibitors more slowly than nonaffected patients (Blackwell et al, 1967). The dosage of phenelzine used by the affected patients was often considerably higher than 60 mg daily; furthermore, there is evidence that the interval between the last dose of drug before the ingestion of food is an important determinant as to whether a hypertensive response will occur, suggesting that a proportion of gut MAO recovers rapidly. Indeed, a high rate of recovery of MAO has been found in biopsies of human intestinal mucosa within 18 hours of the last dose of drug (Levine and Sjoerdsma, 1963); in mice, after a single dose of tranylcypromine, gut enzyme inhibition is maximal in one to two hours, but by four hours MAO activity is 80 per cent of control activity at a time hepatic MAO activity is 70 per cent inhibited (Natoff, 1965). Thus, the considerable variation in tyramine content of foods, and the degree of inhibition of intestinal (and possibly hepatic) MAO at the time of ingestion of the culpable food, are probably the most important variables that explain why most patients who consume cheese or other foods that have been incriminated in the hypertensive crises of the past remain asymptomatic.

Since the publication of lists of foods that should be avoided when using MAO inhibitors (Marley and Blackwell, 1970) the incidence of hypertensive reactions has been exceedingly low. Indeed, Lance (1978b) has used phenelzine extensively in the treatment of migraine for over ten years and regards the drug as completely safe; none of his patients have developed a hypertensive episode. The highest levels of tyramine are found in ripened cheeses such as cheddar, emmenthaler, gruyere, stilton, brie and camembert; cottage, cream cheese and yogurt contain barely detectable amounts of tyramine. Chicken liver, canned figs, pickled herring, alcoholic beverages, broad beans, yeast, chocolate, coffee and caviar (Isaac et al, 1977) should be avoided, or eaten in small amounts; narcotic analgesics and drugs with potential sympathomimetic effects such as nasal decongestants and bronchodilators should similarly be avoided (Marley, 1977).

For patients who do not experience difficulties in sleeping with phenelzine, the ingestion of the entire daily dose at bedtime may be an important safeguard in preventing food-induced hypertension, since an overnight fast of eight hours is probably long enough for gut MAO activity to recover to a degree that minimizes the risk of tyramine entering the circulation.

The admonition regarding the use of an MAO inhibitor such as phenelzine concurrent with amitriptyline has probably been overstated. There is evidence supporting the relative safety of amitriptyline and phenelzine in laboratory animals (Loveless and Maxwell, 1965) that has been confirmed by clinical experience (Shuckit et al, 1971; Pare, 1976; Spiker and Pugh, 1976). The negligible effects of amitriptyline on noradrenergic nerve endings (Nybäck et al, 1975), in contrast to the other tricyclic drugs, is probably the single most important factor accounting for its relative safety when used with phenelzine. Therefore, the waiting period of 10 to 14 days after cessation of amitryptyline therapy before phenelzine is begun probably should be adhered to, but if phenelzine is started at 15 mg daily for the first two weeks the risks are likely to be negligible.

PAPAVERINE

Poser (1974) treated 20 migrainous patients, all of whom regularly experienced focal neurologic symptoms preceding the development of headache, with papaverine, 300 mg daily, and reported that 18 of them became completely headache-free. The rationale for this therapeutic program was that the intracerebral vasoconstrictive phase of a migrainous attack may be an obligatory part of the mechanism, and its prevention with a vasodilator drug, therefore, may block the appearance of attacks. Although disputed in the past, it is clear that oral papaverine can result in a modest increase (10 per cent) in CBF which is probably due to a reduction in cerebrovascular resistance since systemic blood pressure is uninfluenced by the drug. Poser's (1974) hypothesis is further supported by the observation that the higher the cerebrovascular resistance before administration of papaverine, the greater is the increase in CBF produced by the drug (Wang and Obrist, 1976).

Subsequently, a controlled, double-blind study of papaverine was carried out among 37 children with migraine (Sillanpää and Koponen, 1978), and a substantial therapeutic effect of the drug was documented in children with, as well as without, focal neurologic symptoms accompanying their attacks (Table 4–5). Vijayan (1977) treated seven patients with complicated migraine with papaverine, and observed that four became headache-free and the remaining three were markedly improved. Although there may be a particular sensitivity to papaverine among patients with striking focal neurologic symptoms,

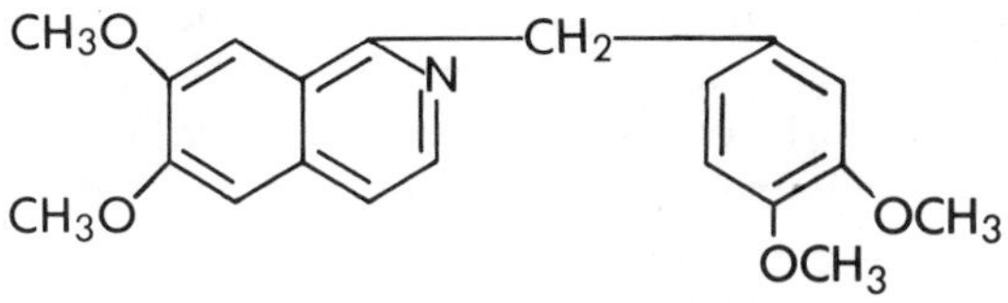

PAPAVERINE

Figure 4-11.

the authors have found the drug to be effective in many of those without such symptoms. Further studies will be necessary to clarify this issue.

The absorption of papaverine is rapid and complete. Peak plasma levels are reached in one to two hours, and the biologic half-life of the drug is 90 to 120 minutes. This short half-life has led to the production of sustained release preparations that also are rapidly absorbed and result in plasma levels of the drug that are sustained for 10 to 12 hours (Miller et al, 1978). The drug crosses the blood–brain barrier rapidly and is distributed more or less uniformly throughout the tissues, with highest concentrations found in the liver. The drug is completely metabolized, predominantly in the liver, to glucuronide conjugates of phenolic metabolites and formaldehyde (Axelrod et al, 1958). The smooth muscle-relaxing properties of papaverine may be mediated by its potent inhibition of cyclic nucleotide PDE resulting in increased levels of cyclic AMP. The latter has been implicated as a possible mediator of β-adrenergic relaxation of smooth muscle (Andersson et al, 1975).

OTHER DRUGS

A bewildering number of drugs have been suggested over the years as having merit in the prophylaxis of migrainous attacks. Some, like *clonidine*, have been studied carefully, utilizing the double-blind controlled format; initial statistically significant benefit (Shafar et al, 1972; Sjaastad and Stensrud, 1971) has not been confirmed in several subsequent studies (Mondrup and Møller, 1977; Boisen et al, 1978). The authors have not observed a single patient derive benefit from this drug out of approximately 100 to whom it was administered, and regard it as of little to no value in migraine prophylaxis.

On the other hand, a carefully controlled study has managed to overlook the beneficial effects of methysergide in migraine (South-well et al, 1964), illustrating the variability of the natural history of the disorder, the difficulties in overcoming a high placebo response rate, and (an important issue that does not often come to light) the use of patients who are treatment failures in studies of new drugs. This latter factor may produce a study population that is relatively drug-resistant, and more likely than not to have especially severe migrainous attacks. In view of these large obstacles to obtaining statistical significance in double-blind trials, there are few precedents for the checkered history of clonidine. It is worth examining the other side of the coin, those drugs that have not been found to be effective in studies, the sample size and design of which could have resulted in important therapeutic benefits being overlooked (Freiman et al, 1978).

Phenytoin may be a representative of this category. An adequate-ly controlled study utilizing this drug in migraine has never been published. The remarkably high uncontrolled success rate in treating migrainous children (Millichap, 1978) has led to the drug's widespread use in younger patients for many years. Dramatic responses of several adult patients to either phenytoin or primidone (Swanson and Vick, 1978) suggests that there is a subpopulation of adult migraineurs sensitive to these agents. If the subpopulation is a small proportion of migrainous patients, a study comprising several hundred individuals may be necessary to overcome a placebo response rate of 30 to 40 per cent. The persisting anecdotal reports of the effects of phenytoin over the past 30 years (Fields and Raskin, 1976) are difficult to discount. No other unestablished drug has enjoyed this kind of empirical usage over such an extended period. It is the authors' view that *phenytoin* and *primidone* probably have a role in the prophylaxis of migraine, and that their effects may be mediated independent of their anticonvulsant properties via effects on serotonergic synapses (Chadwick et al, 1978; Quattrone et al, 1978; Essman, 1978). On the other hand, another anticonvulsant drug, *carbamazepine*, has been disappointing in open studies (Anthony et al, 1972), and experiential data supporting the drug are virtually nonexistent.

Intravenous *histamine* (Butler and Thomas, 1945) given in three weekly infusions has produced results that do not appear to exceed those that would be expected of placebo infusions (Selby and Lance, 1960). Intravenous and inhalational *heparin* in very low dosage has been claimed to provide relief in uncontrolled studies (Thonnard-Neumann, 1977); the authors have used the suggested intravenous heparin regimen in six otherwise unsuccessfully treated patients without apparent benefits. Intravenous *reserpine* has been administered at a dosage of 0.2 mg every two to three days for six to eight weeks, with substantial improvement reported (Nattero et al, 1976; Fog-Møller et al, 1976); there are no other reports of this apparently paradoxical therapeutic avenue. *Bromocriptine* has been given to seven women with menstrual migraine at a dosage of 3 mg per day at four-day intervals over 15 menstrual cycles; striking reduction of weight gain, breast discomfort and premenstrual mood alteration was observed during the treatment period, as well as modest improvement in migrainous attacks (Hockaday et al, 1976).

INTRACTABLE MIGRAINE

There is a small proportion of patients who, despite all efforts, continue to have migraine attacks. Some of these enter a stage of progressively worsening headache that remains at a high level of intensity for days to weeks, and occasionally months, so-called "status migrainosus." It is generally best to hospitalize such patients, withdraw all vasoactive medication and support them through what is usually a self-limited exacerbation. There is no evidence that any particular measure shortens the natural history of such cycles; it is possible that the provision of relaxing sleep with sedating drugs is the mechanism by which a short-term hospitalization often appears to terminate an otherwise seemingly endless siege. Because the firing rate of the brain stem serotonergic neurons is inhibited by thioridazine, and not by comparable drugs such as chlorpromazine and haloperidol (Gallager and Aghajanian, 1976), the authors have used thioridazine and amobarbital in doses that enhance relaxation and provide eight to ten hours of daily sleep. Corticosteroids have been shown to provide at least temporary respite from migrainous headaches (Graham, 1950), perhaps through an activation of tryptophan hydroxylase (Costa and Meek, 1974), so that for patients with especially severe and intractable problems the authors on occasion have administered dexamethasone, 8 mg intravenously, twice daily for three or four days. At times, an abrupt and marked improvement in headache has occurred concurrent with steroid administration, but the variable natural history of these cycles makes it difficult to assess the impact of any therapeutic agent. Hospitalization with analgesic support alone may well be as effective as any other measures employed; there are no controlled studies regarding the management of this difficult aspect of migraine.

REFERENCES

Aellig, W. H. (1976): Influence of ergot compounds on compliance of superficial hand veins in man. Postgrad. Med. J. 52(suppl. 1):21–23.

Aellig, W. H. (1978): Clinical pharmacological experiments with pizotifen (Sandomigran) on superficial hand veins in man. In Current Concepts in Migraine Research, ed. R. Greene. Raven Press, New York, pp. 53–62.

Aellig, W. H. and Berde, B. (1969): Studies of the effect of natural and synthetic polypeptide type ergot compounds on a peripheral vascular bed. Br. J. Pharmacol. 36:561–570.

Aellig, W. H. and Nüesch, E. (1977): Comparative pharmacokinetic investigations with tritium-labeled ergot alkaloids after oral and intravenous administration in man. Int. J. Clin. Pharmacol. 15:106–112.

Aghajanian, G. K. (1972): Influence of drugs on the firing of serotonin-containing neurons in brain. Fed. Proc. 31:91–96.

Aghajanian, G. K. and Wang, R. Y. (1978): Physiology and pharmacology of central serotonergic neurons. In Psychopharmacology: A Generation of Progress, eds. M. A. Lipton, A. DiMascio and K. F. Killam. Raven Press, New York, pp. 171–183.

Ahlquist, R. P. (1948): A study of the adrenotropic receptors. Am. J. Physiol. 153:586–600.

Ala-Hurula, V., Myllylä, V. V., Arvela, P. et al (1979): Systemic availability of ergotamine tartrate after oral, rectal and intramuscular administration. Eur. J. Clin. Pharmacol. 15:51–55.

Alvarez, W. C. and Mason, A. Y. (1940): Results obtained in the treatment of headache with the inhalation of pure oxygen. Mayo Clin. Proc. 15:616–618.

Ambrus, J. L., Ambrus, C. M. and Thurber, L. (1977): Study of platelet aggregation in vivo. V. Effect of the antiserotonin agent cyproheptadine. J. Med. 8:317–320.

Andersen, P. K., Christensen, K. N., Hole, P. et al (1977): Sodium nitroprusside and epidural blockade in the treatment of ergotism. N. Engl. J. Med. 296:1271–1273.

Anderson, J. A. D., Basker, M. A. and Dalton, R. (1975): Migraine and hypnotherapy. Int. J. Clin. Exp. Hypn. 23:48–58.

Andersson, P. G. (1975): Ergotamine headache. Headache 15:118–121.

Andersson, R., Nilsson, K., Wikberg, J. et al (1975): Cyclic nucleotides and the contraction of smooth muscle. Adv. Cyclic Nucleotide Res. 5:491–518.

Anthony, M. and Lance, J. W. (1969): Monoamine oxidase inhibition in the treatment of migraine. Arch. Neurol. 21:263–268.

Anthony, M., Lance, J. W. and Somerville, B. (1972): A comparative trial of prindolol, clonidine, and carbamazepine in the interval therapy of migraine. Med. J. Aust. 1:1343–1346.

Asboe-Hansen, G. (1973): The mast cell in health and disease. Acta Derm. Venereal. (Stockh.) (suppl.) 73:139–148.

Asboe-Hansen, G. and Wegelius, O. (1956): Serotonin and connective tissues. Nature 178:262.

Axelrod, J., Shofer, R., Inscoe, J. K. et al (1958): The fate of papaverine in man and other mammals. J. Pharmacol. Exp. Ther. 124:9–15.

Bagby, R. J. and Cooper, R. D. (1972): Angiography in ergotism. Am. J. Roentgenol. 116:179–186.

Bana, D. S., MacNeal, P. S., LeCompte, P. M., Shah, Y. and Graham, J. R. (1974): Cardiac murmurs and endocardial fibrosis associated with methysergide therapy. Am. Heart J. 88:640–655.

Barrie, M. A., Fox, W. R., Weatherall, M. and Wilkinson, M. I. P. (1968): Analysis of symptoms of patients with headaches and their response to treatment with ergot derivatives. Q. J. Med. 37:319–336.

Bartlett, A. L. (1968): 5-hydroxytryptamine and enterochromaffin cells in the ovine biliary mucosa during fascioliasis. Br. J. Pharmacol. 33:408–412.

Bauer, J. H. and Brooks, C. S. (1979): The long-term effect of propranolol therapy on renal function. Am. J. Med. 66:405–410.

Baumrucker, J. F. (1973): Drug interaction — propranolol and Cafergot. N. Engl. J. Med. 288:916–917.

Berde, B., Cerletti, A., Dengler, H. J. and Zoglio, M. A. (1970): Studies of the interaction between ergot alkaloids and xanthine derivatives. In Background to Migraine, 3rd Migraine Symposium, ed. A. L. Cochrane. Springer-Verlag, New York, pp. 80–102.

Berkowitz, B. A. and Spector, S. (1971): The effect of caffeine and theophylline on the disposition of brain serotonin in the rat. Eur. J. Pharmacol. 16:322–325.

Berntman, L., Carlsson, C. and Siesjo, B. K. (1978): Influence of propranolol on cerebral metabolism and blood flow in the rat brain. Brain Res. 151:220–224.

Bianchine, J. R. (1968): Metabolism of methysergide in the rabbit and man. Fed. Proc. 27:238.

Bianchine, J. R. and Eade, N. R. (1969): Vasoactive substances and fibrosis. Res. Clin. Stud. Headache 2:60–85.

Bianchine, J. R. and Friedman, A. P. (1970): Metabolism of methysergide and retroperitoneal fibrosis. Arch. Intern. Med. 126:252–254.

Bianchine, J. R., Macaraeg, P. V. J. and Brandes, D. (1968): Serotonin and fibrosis. Arch. Intern. Med. 122:167–170.

Birkmayer, W., Riederer, P., Youdim, M. B. H. and Linauer, W. (1975): The potentiation of the anti-kinetic effect after L-dopa treatment by an inhibitor of MAO-B. J. Neural Trans. 36:303–326.

Bivens, C. H., Lebovitz, H. E. and Feldman, J. M. (1973): Inhibition of hypoglycemic-induced growth hormone secretion by the serotonin antagonists cyproheptadine and methysergide. N. Engl. J. Med. 289:236–239.

Blackwell, B. and Mabbitt, L. A. (1965): Tyramine in cheese related to hypertensive crises after monoamine oxidase inhibition. Lancet 1:938–940.

Blackwell, B., Marley, E., Price, J. and Taylor, D. (1967): Hypertensive interactions between monoamine oxidase inhibitors and foodstuffs. Brit. J. Psychiatry 113:349–365.

Blanchard, E. B., Theobald, D. E., Williamson, D. A., Silver, B. V. and Brown, D. A. (1978): Temperature biofeedback in the treatment of migraine headaches. Arch. Gen. Psychiatry 35:581–588.

Bliss, E. L., Thatcher, W. and Ailion, J. (1972): Relationship of stress to brain serotonin and 5-hydroxyindole-acetic acid. J. Psychiatr. Res. 9:71–80.

Boisen, E., Deth, S., Hübbe, P. et al (1978): Clonidine in the prophylaxis of migraine. Acta Neurol. Scand. 58:288–295.

Boucek, R. J. (1977): Serotonin and collagen metabolism. In Serotonin in Health and Disease, Vol. 4, ed. W. B. Essman. Spectrum, New York, pp. 1–39.

Brooke, O. G. and Robinson, B. F. (1970): Effect of ergotamine and ergometrine on forearm venous compliance in man. Br. Med. J. 1:139–142.

Brown, E. M., Spiegel, A. M., Gardner, J. D. and Aurbach, G. D. (1978): Direct identification and characterization of β-adrenergic receptors and functional relationship of adenylyl cyclase. Receptors Horm. Act. 3:101–131.

Brown, H. (1977): Serotonin-producing tumors. In Serotonin in Health and Disease, Vol. 4, ed. W. B. Essman. Spectrum, New York, pp. 393–423. .

Buñag, R. D. and Walaszek, E. J. (1962): Blockade of depressor responses to serotonin and tryptamine by lysergic acid derivatives in the chicken. Arch. Int. Pharmacodyn. Ther. 135:142–151.

Bunker, M. L. and McWilliams, M. (1979): Caffeine content of common beverages. J. Am. Dietetic Assoc. 74:28–32.

Butcher, R. W. and Sutherland, E. W. (1962): Adenosine 3′,5′-phosphate in biological materials. J. Biol. Chem. 237:1244–1250.

Butler, S. and Thomas, W. A. (1945): Intravenous histamine in the treatment of migraine. J.A.M.A. 128:173–175.

Cabot, J. B., Wild, J. M. and Cohen, D. H. (1979): Raphe inhibition of sympathetic preganglionic neurons. Science 203:184–186.

Cairncross, K. D. (1965): On the peripheral pharmacology of amitriptyline. Arch. Int. Pharmacodyn. Ther. 154:438–448.

Carliner, N. H., Denune, D. P., Finch, C. S., Jr. and Goldberg, L. I. (1974): Sodium nitroprusside treatment of ergotamine-induced peripheral ischemia. J.A.M.A. 227:308–309.

Carroll, J. D. and Hilton, B. P. (1975): The effects of reserpine injection on methysergide treated control and migrainous subjects. In Background to Migraine, 5th Migraine Symposium, ed. J. N. Cumings. Springer-Verlag, New York, pp. 122–133.

Carroll, P. R., Ebeling, P. W. and Glover, W. E. (1974): The responses of the human temporal and rabbit ear artery to 5-hydroxytryptamine and some of its antagonists. Aust. J. Exp. Biol. Med. Sci. 52:813–823.

Carstairs, L. S. (1958): Headache and gastric emptying time. Proc. R. Soc. Med. 51:790–791.

Carter, E. R. (1958): Bilateral thrombophlebitis after a single dose of ergotamine tartrate for migraine. Br. Med. J. 2:1452–1453.

Cerletti, A. and Doepfner, W. (1958): Comparative study on the serotonin antagonism of amide derivatives of lysergic acid and of ergot alkaloids. J. Pharmacol. Exp. Ther. 122:124–136.

Chadwick, D., Gorrod, J. W., Jenner, P., Marsden, C. D. and Reynolds, E. H. (1978): Functional changes in cerebral 5-hydroxytryptamine metabolism in the mouse induced by anticonvulsant drugs. Br. J. Pharmacol. 62:115–124.

Chalmers, J. P. and Wing, L. M. H. (1975): Central serotonin and cardiovascular control. Clin. Exp. Pharmacol. Physiol. (suppl.) 2:195–200.

Cipriano, P. R., Guthaner, D. F., Orlick, A. E. et al (1979): The effects of ergonovine maleate on coronary arterial size. Circulation 59:82–89.

Clark, B. and Saameli, K. (1970): Pharmacological properties of a new beta-receptor blocking agent. Triangle 9:300–308.

Cohen, M. J. (1978): Psychophysiological studies of headache: is there similarity between migraine and muscle contraction headaches? Headache 18:189–196.

Connolly, C. K. (1975): Method of using pressurized aerosols. Br. Med. J. 3:21.

Cooper, J. R., Bloom, F. E. and Roth, R. H. (1978): Cellular foundations of neuropharmacology. In The Biochemical Basis of Neuropharmacology, 3rd ed. Oxford University Press, New York, pp. 9–46.

Coppen, A., Ghose, K., Montgomery, S. et al (1978): Amitriptyline plasma concentration and clinical effect. Lancet 1:63–66.

Costa, E. and Meek, J. (1974): Regulation of biosynthesis of catecholamines and serotonin in the CNS. Annu. Rev. Pharmacol. 14:491–511.

Costa, M. and Furness, J. B. (1979): On the possibility that an indoleamine is a neurotransmitter in the gastrointestinal tract. Biochem. Pharmacol. 28:565–571.

Couch, J. R., Ziegler, D. K. and Hassanein, R. S. (1975): Evaluation of the relationship between migraine headache and depression. Headache 15:41–50.

Couch, J. R., Ziegler, D. K. and Hassanein, R. S. (1976): Amitriptyline in the prophylaxis of migraine. Neurology 26:121–127.

Coutinho, E. M., Maia, H. and Nascimento, L. (1976): The response of the human fallopian tube to ergonovine and methylergonovine in vivo. Am. J. Obstet. Gynecol. 126:48–54.

Crooks, J., Stephen, S. A. and Brass, W. (1964): Clinical trial of inhaled ergotamine tartrate in migraine. Br. Med. J. 1:221–224.

Curran, D. A., Hinterberger, H. and Lance, J. W. (1967): Methysergide. Res. Clin. Stud. Headache 1:74–122.

Curran, D. A. and Lance, J. W. (1964): Clinical trial of methysergide and other preparations in the management of migraine. J. Neurol. Neurosurg. Psychiatry 27:463–469.

Curry, R. C. (1978): Prinzmetal's angina. Provocative test and current therapy. J.A.M.A. 240:677–680.

Curry, R. C., Pepine, C. J., Sabom, M. B. and Conti, C. R. (1979): Similarities of ergonovine-induced and spontaneous attacks of variant angina. Circulation 59:307–312.

Curzon, G., Barrie, M. and Wilkinson, M. I. P. (1969): Relationships between headache and amine changes after administration of reserpine to migrainous patients. J. Neurol. Neurosurg. Psychiatry 32:555–561.

Dexter, J. D., Roberts, J. and Byer, J. A. (1978): The five hour glucose tolerance test and effect of low sucrose diet in migraine. Headache 18:91–94.

Diamond, S. (1976): Treatment of migraine with isometheptene, acetaminophen, and dichloralphenazone combination: a double-blind, crossover trial. Headache 15:282–287.

Diamond, S. and Medina, J. L. (1976): Double blind study of propranolol for migraine prophylaxis. Headache 16:238–245.

Dige-Petersen, H., Lassen, N. A., Noer, I., Tønnesen, K. H. and Olesen, J. (1977): Subclinical ergotism. Lancet 2:65–66.

Doepfner, W. (1962): Biochemical observations on LSD-25 and Deseril. Experientia 18:256–257.

Doepfner, W. and Cerletti, A. (1958): Comparison of lysergic acid derivatives and anti-histamines as inhibitors of the edema provoked in the rat's paw by serotonin. Int. Arch. Allergy Appl. Immunol. 12:89–97.

Eckert, H., Kiechel, J. R., Rosenthaler, J., Schmidt, R. and Schrier, E. (1978): Biopharmaceutical aspects. In Ergot Alkaloids and Related Compounds, Handbook of Experimental Pharmacology, Vol. 49, eds. B. Berde and H. O. Schild. Springer-Verlag, New York, pp. 719–803.

Edvinsson, L., Hardebo, J. E., MacKenzie, E. T. and Stewart, M. (1975): Dual action of serotonin on pial arterioles in situ and the effect of propranolol on the response. Blood Vessels 14:366–371.

Edvinsson, L., Hardebo, J. E. and Owman, C. (1978): Pharmacological analysis of 5-hydroxytryptamine receptors in isolated intracranial and extracranial vessels of cat and man. Circ. Res. 42:143–151.

Eidelman, B. H., Mendelow, A. D., McCalden, T. A. and Bloom, D. S. (1978): Potentiation of the cerebrovascular response to intra-arterial 5-hydroxytryptamine. Am. J. Physiol. 234:H300–H304.

Ekbom, K. (1975a): Adrenergic beta-receptor blockers. In Vasoactive Substances Relevant to Migraine, eds. S. Diamond, D. J. Dalessio, J. R. Graham and J. L. Medina. Charles C Thomas, Springfield, Ill., pp. 19–24.

Ekbom, K. (1975b): Alprenolol for migraine prophylaxis. Headache 15:129–132.

Ekbom, K. and Zetterman, M. (1977): Oxprenolol in the treatment of migraine. Acta Neurol. Scand. 56:181–184.

Elkind, A. H., Friedman, A. P., Bachman, A. et al (1968): Silent retroperitoneal fibrosis associated with methysergide therapy. J.A.M.A. 206:1041–1044.

Essman, W. B. (1978): Serotonin in seizures and seizure disorders. In Serotonin in Health and Disease, Vol. 3, ed. W. B. Essman. Spectrum, New York, pp. 317–401.

Eurin, B., Samii, K., Rouby, J-J. and Glaser, P. (1978): Ergot and sodium nitroprusside. N. Engl. J. Med. 298:632–633.

Fahrion, S. L. (1978): Autogenic biofeedback treatment for migraine. Res. Clin. Stud. Headache 5:47–71.

Fedotin, M. S. and Hartman, C. (1970): Ergotamine poisoning producing renal arterial spasm; case report. N. Engl. J. Med. 283:518–520.

Feldman, J. M. (1978): Serotonin metabolism in patients with carcinoid tumors: incidence of 5-hydroxytryptophan-secreting tumors. Gastroenterology 75:1109–1114.

Fernstrom, J. D. (1978): Brain serotonin and nutrition. In Serotonin in Health and Disease, Vol. 3, ed. W. B. Essman. Spectrum, New York, pp. 1–49.

Fields, H. L. and Basbaum, A. I. (1978): Brainstem control of spinal pain-transmission neurons. Annu. Rev. Physiol. 40:217–248.

Fields, H. L. and Raskin, N. H. (1976): Anticonvulsants and pain. Clin. Neuropharmacol. 1:173–184.

Fog-Møller, F., Bryndum, B., Dalsgaard-Nielsen, T. et al (1976): Therapeutic effect of reserpine on migraine syndrome: relationship to blood amine levels. Headache 15:275–278.

Forssman, B., Henricksson, K-G., Johannson, V., Lindvall, L. and Lundin, H. (1976): Propranolol for migraine prophlaxis. Headache 16:238–245.

Fozard, J. P. (1975): The animal pharmacology of drugs used in the treatment of migraine. J. Pharm. Pharmacol. 27:297–321.

Freiman, J. A., Chalmers, T. C., Smith, H., Jr. and Kuebler, R. R. (1978): The importance of beta, the type II error and sample size in the design and interpretation of the randomized control trial. N. Engl. J. Med. 299:690–694.

Friedman, A. P. (1975): Migraine: an overview. In Modern Topics in Migraine, ed. J. Pearce, Wm. Heinemann, London, pp. 159–167.

Friedman, A. P., Brazil, P. and von Storch, T. J. C. (1955): Ergotamine tolerance in patients with migraine. J.A.M.A. 157:881–884.

Friedman, A. P. and von Storch, T. J. C. (1951): Recent advances in treatment of migraine. J.A.M.A. 145:1325–1329.

Friedman, A. P., von Storch, T. J. C. and Araki, S. (1959): Ergotamine tartrate: its history, action, and proper use in the treatment of migraine. N.Y. State J. Med. 59:2359–2366.

Fuller, R. W. and Wong, D. T. (1977): Inhibition of serotonin reuptake. Fed. Proc. 36:2154–2158.

Gallager, D. W. and Aghajanian, G. K. (1976): Effect of antipsychotic drugs on the firing of dorsal raphe cells. I. Role of adrenergic system. Eur. J. Pharmacol. 39:341–355.

Gelford, G. J. and Cromwell, D. K. (1968): Methysergide, retroperitoneal fibrosis and rectosigmoid strictures. Am. J. Roentgenol. 104:566–570.

Gerschenfeld, H. M., Hamon, M. and Paupardin-Tritsch, D. (1978): Release of endogenous serotonin from two identified serotonin-containing neurons and the physiological role of serotonin re-uptake. J. Physiol. 274:265–278.

Gershon, M. D. (1968): Serotonin and the motility of the gastrointestinal tract. Gastroenterology 54:453–456.

Gilbert, R. M., Marshman, J. A., Schweider, M. and Berg, R. (1976): Caffeine content of beverages as consumed. Can. Med. Assoc. J. 114:205–208.

Glover, V., Sandler, M., Owen, F. and Riley, G. J. (1977): Dopamine is a monoamine oxidase B substrate in man. Nature 265:80–81.

Goldfischer, J. D. (1960): Acute myocardial infarction secondary to ergot therapy. Report of a case and review of the literature. N. Engl. J. Med. 262:860–863.

Gomersall, J. D. and Stuart, A. (1973): Amitriptyline in migraine prophylaxis. J. Neurol. Neurosurg. Psychiatry 36:684–690.

Graham, J. (1950): The effect of cortisone and ACTH on migraine. Trans. Am. Clin. Climatol. Assoc. 62:181–190.

Graham, J. (1967): Cardiac and pulmonary fibrosis during methysergide therapy for headache. Am. J. Med. Sci. 254:1–12.

Graham, J. R., Suby, H. I., LeCompte, P. M. and Sadowsky, N. L. (1967): Inflammatory fibrosis associated with methysergide therapy. Res. Clin. Stud. Headache 1:123–164.

Graham, J. R. and Wolff, H. G. (1938): Mechanism of migraine headache and action of ergotamine tartrate. Arch. Neurol. Psychiatry 39:737–763.

Greengard, P. (1975): Cyclic nucleotides, protein phosphorylation, and neuronal function. Adv. Cyclic Nucleotide Res. 5:585–602.

Griffith, R. W., Grauwiler, J., Hodel, Ch., Leist, K. H. and Matter, B. (1978): Toxicologic considerations. *In* Ergot Alkaloids and Related Compounds, Handbook of Experimental Pharmacology, Vol. 49, eds. B. Berde and H. O. Schild. Springer-Verlag, New York, pp. 805–851.

Grobecker, H., Lemmer, B., Hellenbrecht, D. and Wiethold, G. (1973): Inhibition by antiarrhythmic and β-sympatholytic drugs of serotonin uptake by human platelets: experiments *in vitro* and *in vivo*. Eur. J. Clin. Pharmacol. 5:145–150.

Grosz, H. J. (1972): Narcotic withdrawal symptoms in heroin users treated with propranolol. Lancet 2:564–566.

Gupta, D. R. and Strobos, R. J. (1972): Bilateral papillitis associated with Cafergot therapy. Neurology 22:793–797.

Haigler, H. J. and Aghajanian, G. K. (1974): Peripheral serotonin antagonists: failure to antagonize serotonin in brain areas receiving a prominent serotonergic input. J. Neural Trans. 35:257–273.

Haigler, H. J. and Aghajanian, G. K. (1977): Serotonin receptors in the brain. Fed. Proc. 36:2159–2164.

Hakkarainen, H., Gustafsson, B. and Stockman, O. (1978): A comparative trial of ergotamine tartrate, acetyl salicylic acid and a dextropropoxyphene compound in acute migraine attacks. Headache 18:35–39.

Haley, T. J., Andem, M. R. and Liebig, C. (1954): Comparison between capillary effects produced by topical application and intravenous action of ergot alkaloids. Arch. Int. Pharmacodyn. Ther. 98:373–378.

Hardebo, J. E., Edvinsson, L., Owman, Ch. and Svendgaard, N-Aa. (1978): Potentiation and antagonism of serotonin effects on intracranial and extracranial vessels. Neurology 28:64–70.

Heupler, F. A., Proudfit, W. L., Razavi, M. et al (1978): Ergonovine maleate provocative test for coronary arterial spasm. Am. J. Cardiol. 41:631–640.

Hillis, L. D. and Braunwald, E. (1978): Coronary-artery spasm. N. Engl. J. Med. 299:695–702.

Hillman, G. R., Olsen, N. J. and Senft, A. W. (1974): Effect of methysergide and dihydroergotamine on *Schistosoma mansoni*. J. Pharmacol. Exp. Ther. 188:529–535.

Hockaday, J. M., Peet, K. M. S. and Hockaday, T. D. R. (1976): Bromocriptine in migraine. Headache 16:109–114.

Hofmann, A. (1978): Historical view on ergot alkaloids. Pharmacology 16(suppl.1):1–11.

Hokkanen, E., Waltimo, O. and Kallanranta, T. (1978): Toxic effects of ergotamine used for migraine. Headache 18:95–98.

Howitt, G., Husaini, M., Rowlands, D. J. et al (1968): The effect of the dextro isomer of propranolol on sinus rate and cardiac arrhythmias. Am. Heart J. 76:736–745.

Hunter, R. A. and Ross, I. P. (1960): Psychotherapy in migraine. Br. Med. J. 1:1084–1088.

Immerwahr, P. (1927): Über die Wirkung des Ergotamin auf Puls, Blutdruck and Blutzucker und ihre Beeinflussung durch Atropin. Med. Klin. 23:1–3.

Isaac, P., Mitchell, B. and Grahame-Smith, D. G. (1977): Monoamine oxidase inhibitors and caviar. Lancet 2:816.

Jacoby, J. H., Poulakos, J. J. and Bryce, G. F. (1978): On the central antiserotoninergic actions of cyproheptadine and methysergide. Neuropharmacology 17:299–306.

Johnston, B. M., and Saxena, P. R. (1978): The effect of ergotamine on tissue blood flow and the arterio-venous shunting of radio active microspheres in the head. Br. J. Pharmacol. 63:541–549.

Kangasniemi, P., Falck, B., Långvik, V-A. and Hyyppä, M. T. (1978): Levotryptophan treatment in migraine. Headache 18:161–166.

Kato, T. and Jarvik, L. F. (1969): LSD-25 and genetic damage. Dis. Nerv. Syst. 30:42–46.

Kaufman, J. and Levine, I. (1936): Acute gastric dilatation of the stomach during attack of migraine. Radiology 27:301–302.

Keller, H., Bartholini, G. and Pletscher, A. (1973): Increase of 3-methoxy-4-hydroxyphenylethylene glycol in rat brain by neuroleptic drugs. Eur. J. Pharmacol. 23:183–186.

Klevans, L. R., Kovacs, J. L. and Kelly, R. (1976): Central effects of beta-adrenergic blocking agents on arterial blood pressure. J. Pharmacol. Exp. Ther. *196*:389–395.

Klingenberg, I. (1973): Measurement of uterine blood flow in non-pregnant women by electromagnetic flowmeter. Acta Obstet. Gynecol. Scand. 52:317–321.

Koch-Weser, J. (1975): Non-beta-blocking actions of propranolol. N. Engl. J. Med. *293*:988–989.

Kornhauser, D. M., Wood, A. J. J., Vestal, R. E. et al (1978): Biological determinants of propranolol disposition in man. Clin. Pharmacol. Ther. *23*:165–174.

Kreel, L. (1973): The use of metoclopramide in radiology. Postgrad. Med. J. *49* (suppl.):42–45.

Krieger, D. T. (1978): Endocrine processes and serotonin. In Serotonin in Health and Disease, Vol. 3, ed. W. B. Essman. Spectrum, New York, pp. 51–67.

Krulich, L., Coppings, R. J., McCann, S. M. and Mayfield, M. A. (1978): Inhibition of prolactin secretion by direct effect of methysergide on the pituitary lactotrophs in the rat. Life Sci. *23*:1665–1674.

Kunos, G. (1978): Adrenoreceptors. Annu. Rev. Pharmacol. Toxicol. *18*:291–311.

Lager, I., Blohmé, G. and Smith, U. (1979): Effect of cardioselective and non-selective β-blockade on the hypoglycaemic response in insulin-dependent diabetics. Lancet *1*:458–462.

Lambert, G. A., Friedman, E., Buchweitz, E. and Gershon, S. (1978): Involvement of 5-hydroxytryptamine in the central control of respiration, blood pressure and heart rate in the anesthetized rat. Neuropharmacology *17*:807–813.

Lance, J. W. (1978a): Mechanism and Management of Headache, 3rd ed. Butterworths, Boston, pp. 123–128.

Lance, J. W. (1978b): Mechanism and Management of Headache, 3rd ed. Butterworths, Boston, pp. 182–207.

Lance, J. W., Anthony, M. and Somerville, B. (1970): Comparative trial of serotonin antagonists in the management of migraine. Br. Med. J. 2:327–330.

Lance, J. W., Curran, D. A. and Anthony, M. (1965): Investigations into the mechanism and treatment of chronic headache. Med. J. Aust. 2:909–914.

Lance, J. W., Spira, P. J., Mylecharane, E. J., Lord, G. D. A. and Duckworth, J. W. (1978): Evaluation of drugs applicable to treatment of migraine in the cranial circulation of the monkey. Res. Clin. Stud. Headache 6:13–18.

Largen, J. W., Mathew, R. J., Dobbins, K., Meyer, J. S. and Claghorn, J. L. (1978): Skin temperature self-regulation and non-invasive regional cerebral blood flow. Headache *18*:203–210.

Lennox, W. G. (1938): Ergonovine versus ergotamine as a terminator of migraine headaches. Am. J. Med. Sci. *195*:458–468.

Levine, J. D., Gormley, J. and Fields, H. L. (1976): Observations on the analgesic effects of needle puncture (acupuncture). Pain 2:149–159.

Levine, R. J. and Sjoerdsma, A. (1963): Estimation of MAO activity in man: techniques and applications. Ann. N.Y. Acad. Sci. *107*:966–974.

Lewis, C. T., Molland, E. A., Marshall, V. R., Tresidder, G. C. and Blandy, J. P. (1975): Analgesic abuse, ureteric obstruction, and retroperitoneal fibrosis. Br. Med. J. 2:76–78.

Lingjaerde, O. (1977): Platelet uptake and storage of serotonin. In Serotonin in Health and Disease, Vol. 4, ed. W. B. Essman. Spectrum, New York, pp. 139–199.

Loew, D. M., van Deusen, E. B. and Meier-Ruge, W. (1978): Effects on the central nervous system. In Ergot Alkaloids and Related Compounds, Handbook of Experimental Pharmacology, Vol. 49, eds. B. Berde and H. O. Schild. Springer-Verlag, New York, pp. 421–531.

Longo, V. G. and Loizzo, A. (1978): Evaluation of the central effects of ergot alkaloids by means of electroencephalography. Pharmacology *16* (suppl. 1):189–192.

Loveless, A. H. and Maxwell, D. R. (1965): A comparison of the effects of imipramine, trimipramine, and some other drugs in rabbits treated with a monoamine oxidase inhibitor. Br. J. Pharmacol. 25:158–170.

Lugnier, C., Bertrand, Y. and Stoclet, J. C. (1972): Cyclic nucleotide phosphodiesterase inhibition and vascular smooth muscle relaxation. Eur. J. Pharmacol. *19*:134–136.

Maas, J. W. (1978): Clinical and biochemical heterogeneity of depressive disorders. Ann. Intern. Med. 88:556–563.

Maas, J. W. and Garver, D. (1975): Linkages of basic neuropharmacology and clinical pharmacology. *In* American Handbook of Psychiatry, eds. D. A. Hamburg and H. K. H. Brodie. Basic Books, New York, pp. 427–459.

MacGregor, G. A., Jones, N. F., Barraclough, M. A. et al (1973): Ureteric stricture with analgesic nephropathy. Br. Med. J. *2*:271–272.

Mäntylä, R., Kleimola, T. and Kanto, J. (1978): Methylergometrine (methylergonovine) concentrations in the human plasma and urine. Int. J. Clin. Pharmacol. *16*:254–257.

Markwardt, F. and Hoffman, A. (1970): Effects of papaverine derivatives on cyclic AMP phosphodiesterase of human platelets. Biochem. Pharmacol. *19*:2519–2520.

Marley, E. (1977): Monoamine oxidase inhibitors and drug interactions. *In* Drug Interactions, ed. D. G. Grahame-Smith. University Park, Baltimore, pp. 171–194.

Marley, E. and Blackwell, B. (1970): Interactions of monoamine oxidase inhibitors, amines and foodstuffs. Adv. Pharmacol. Chemother. *8*:185–239.

Marshall, E. F., Mountjoy, C. Q., Campbell, I. C. et al (1978): The influence of acetylator phenotype on the outcome of treatment with phenelzine in a clinical trial. Br. J. Clin. Pharmacol. *6*:247–254.

Medina, J. L. and Diamond, S. (1977): Drug dependency in patients with chronic headaches. Headache *17*:12–14.

Medina, J. L. and Diamond, S. (1978): The role of diet in migraine. Headache *18*:31–34.

Meier, J. and Schreier, E. (1976): Human plasma levels of some antimigraine drugs. Headache *16*:96–104.

Mendelson, W. B., Jacobs, L. S., Reichman, J. D. et al (1975): Methysergide: suppression of sleep-related prolactin secretion and enhancement of sleep-related growth hormone secretion. J. Clin. Invest. *56*:690–697.

Merhoff, G. C. and Porter, J. M. (1974): Ergot intoxication: historical review and description of unusual clinical manifestations. Ann. Surg. *180*:773–779.

Mikropoulos, H. E. (1978): Toleration and effectiveness of pizotifen in migraine. Res. Clin. Stud. Headache *6*:167–172.

Miller, R. B., Leslie, S. T., Black, F. M., Boroda, C. (1978): A controlled release papaverine tablet (Papacontin): a study in normal volunteers. Br. J. Clin. Pharmacol. *5*:51–54.

Millichap, J. G. (1978): Recurrent headaches in 100 children. Child's Brain *4*:95–105.

Mondrup, K. and Møller, C. E. (1977): Prophylactic treatment of migraine with clonidine. Acta Neurol. Scand. *56*:405–412.

de Montigny, C. and Aghajanian, G. K. (1978): Tricyclic antidepressants: long-term treatment increases responsivity of rat forebrain neurons to serotonin. Science *202*:1303–1306.

Moore, R. Y., Halaris, A. E. and Jones, B. E. (1978): Serotonin neurons of the midbrain raphe: ascending projections. J. Comp. Neurol. *180*:417–438.

Morgane, P. J. and Stern. W. C. (1978): Serotonin in the regulation of sleep. *In* Serotonin in Health and Disease, Vol. 2, ed. W. B. Essman. Spectrum, New York, pp. 205–245.

Moyer, J. H., Tashnek, A. B., Miller, S. I., Snyder, H. and Bowman, R. O. (1952): The effect of theophylline and ethylene diamine (aminophylline) and caffeine on cerebral hemodynamics and cerebrospinal fluid pressure in patients with hypertension headaches. Am. J. Med. Sci. *224*:377–385.

Müller-Schweinitzer, E. (1978): Studies on the 5-HT receptor in vascular smooth muscle. Res. Clin. Stud. Headache *6*:6–12.

Müller-Schweinitzer, E. and Weidmann, H. (1978): Basic pharmacological properties. *In* Ergot Alkaloids and Related Compounds, Handbook of Experimental Pharmacology, Vol. 49, eds. B. Berde and H. O. Schild. Springer-Verlag, New York, pp. 87–232.

Mullinix, J. M., Norton, B. J., Hack, S. and Fishman, M. A. (1978): Skin temperature biofeedback and migraine. Headache *17*:242–244.

Murphy, D. L. (1978): Substrate-selective monoamine oxidases — inhibitor, tissue, species and functional differences. Biochem. Pharmacol. *27*:1889–1893.

Myers, R. D. and Waller, M. B. (1978): Thermoregulation and serotonin. *In* Serotonin in Health and Disease, Vol. 2, ed. W. B. Essman. Spectrum, New York, pp. 1–67.

Nanda, R. N., Johnson, R. H., Gray, J. et al (1978): A double blind trial of acebutolol for migraine prophylaxis. Headache *18*:20–22.

Nathanson, J. A. (1977): Cyclic nucleotides and nervous system function. Physiol. Rev. 57:157–256.

Natoff, I. L. (1965): Toxic reactions to foodstuffs during therapy with monoamine oxidase inhibitors. Med. Proc. 11:101–104.

Nattel, S., Rangno, R. E. and Van Loon, G. (1979): Mechanism of propranolol withdrawal phenomena. Circulation 59:1158–1164.

Nattero, G., Lisino, F., Brandi, G. et al (1976): Reserpine for migraine prophylaxis. Headache 15:279–281.

Neff, N. K. and Fuentes, J. A. (1976): The use of selective monoamine oxidase inhibitor drugs for evaluating pharmacological and physiological mechanisms. In Monoamine Oxidase and its Inhibition, Ciba Foundation Symposium 39. Elsevier, New York, pp. 163–179.

Nimmerfall, F. and Rosenthaler, J. (1976): Ergot alkaloids: hepatic distribution and estimation of absorption by measurement of total radioactivity in bile and urine. J. Pharmacokinet. Biopharm. 4:57–66.

Nimmo, W. S. (1976): Drugs, diseases, and altered gastric emptying. Clin. Pharmacokinet. 1:189–203.

Nybäck, H. V., Walters, J. R., Aghajanian, G. K. and Roth, R. H. (1975): Tricyclic antidepressants — effects on the firing rate of brain noradrenergic neurons. Eur. J. Pharmacol. 32:302–312.

Oleson, J., Hougard, K. and Hertz, M. (1978): Isoproteronol and propranolol: ability to cross the blood–brain barrier and effects on cerebral circulation in man. Stroke 9:344–349.

O'Neill, B. P. and Mann, J. D. (1978): Aspirin prophylaxis in migraine. Lancet 2:1179–1181.

Orlando, R. C., Moyer, P. and Barnett, T. B. (1978): Methysergide therapy and constrictive pericarditis. Ann. Intern. Med. 88:213–214.

Orton, D. and Richardson, R. J. (1978): Pharmacokinetics of ergotamine tartrate. Paper presented to the 2nd International Migraine Symposium, London, Sept. 1978.

Ostfeld, A. M. (1961): A study of migraine pharmacotherapy. Am. J. Med. Sci. 241:192–198.

Pare, C. M. B. (1976): Introduction to clinical aspects of monoamine oxidase inhibitors in the treatment of depression. In Monoamine Oxidase and its Inhibition, Ciba Foundation Symposium 39. Elsevier, New York, pp. 271–280.

Pearce, J. (1976): Hazards of ergotamine tartrate. Br. Med. J. 1:834–835.

Perkin, G. D. (1974): Ischaemic lateral popliteal nerve palsy due to ergot intoxication. J. Neurol. Neurosurg. Psychiatry 37:1389–1391.

Peters, G. A. and Horton, B. T. (1951): Headache: with special reference to the excessive use of ergotamine preparations and withdrawal effects. Mayo Clin. Proc 26:153–161.

Pettersson, G., Dahlström, A., Larsson, I. et al (1978): The release of serotonin from rat duodenal enterochromaffin cells by adrenoreceptor agonists studied in vitro. Acta Physiol. Scand. 103:219–224.

Pichler, E., Ostfeld, A. M., Goodell, H. and Wolff, H. G. (1956): Studies on headache: central versus peripheral action of ergotamine tartrate and its relevance to the therapy of migraine headache. Arch. Neurol. Psychiatry 76:571–577.

Pool, J. L., Storch, T. J. C. and Lennox, W. G. (1936): Effect of ergotamine tartrate on pressure of cerebrospinal fluid and blood during migraine headache. Arch. Intern. Med. 57:32–45.

Porter, C. C., Arison, B. H. Gruber, V. F. et al (1975): Human metabolism of cyproheptadine. Drug Metab. Disp. 3:189–197.

Poser, C. M. (1974): Papaverine in prophylactic treatment of migraine. Lancet 1:1290.

Price, K. P. and Tursky, B. (1976): Vascular reactivity of migraineurs and nonmigraineurs; a comparison of responses to self control procedures. Headache 16:210–217.

Pryor, J. G. and Kahn, O. (1979): Beta blockers and Peyronie's disease. Lancet 1:331.

Quattrone, A., Crunelli, V. and Samanin, R. (1978): Seizure susceptibility and anticonvulsant activity of carbamazepine, diphenylhydantoin and phenobarbital in rats with selective depletions of brain monoamines. Neuropharmacology 17:643–647.

Rabkin, R., Stables, D. P., Levin, N. W. and Suzman, M. (1966): The prophylactic value of propranolol in angina pectoris. Am. J. Cardiol. 18:370–383.

Raisfeld, I. H. (1972): Cardiovascular complications of antidepressant therapy. Am. Heart J. 83:129–133.

Regan, J. F. and Poletti, B. J. (1968): Vascular adventitial fibrosis in a patient taking methysergide maleate. J.A.M.A. 203:1069–1071.

Resnick, R. H., Adelardi, C. F. and Gray, S. J. (1962): Stimulation of gastric secretion in man by a serotonin antagonist. Gastroenterology 42:22–25.

Roberts, W. C. and Sjoerdsma, A. (1964): The cardiac disease associated with the carcinoid syndrome. Am. J. Med. 36:5–34.

Robinson, D. S., Nies, A., Ravaris, L. et al (1978): Clinical pharmacology of phenelzine. Arch. Gen. Psychiatry 35:629–635.

Rogers, H. J., Morrison, P. J. and Bradbrook, I. D. (1978): The half-life of amitriptyline. Br. J. Clin. Pharmacol. 6:181–183.

Rosen, T. S., Lin, M., Spector, S. and Rosen, M. R. (1979): Maternal, fetal, and neonatal effects of chronic propranolol administration in the rat. J. Pharmacol. Exp. Therap. 208:118–122.

Roth-Brandel, U., Bygdeman, M. and Wigvist, N. (1970): A comparative study on the influence of prostaglandin E, oxytocin, and ergometrin on the pregnant human uterus. Acta Obstet. Gynecol. Scand. (suppl.) 5:1–7.

Rothlin, E. (1955): Historical development of the ergot therapy of migraine. Int. Arch. Allergy Appl. Immunol. 7:205–209.

Routledge, P. A. and Shand, D. G. (1979): Clinical pharmacokinetics of propranolol. Clin. Pharmacokinet. 4:73–90.

Rowsell, A. R., Neylan, C. and Wilkinson, M. (1973): Ergotamine induced headache in migrainous patients. Headache 13:65–67.

Rutschmann, J. and Stadler, P. A. (1978): Chemical background. In Ergot Alkaloids and Related Compounds, Handbook of Experimental Pharmacology, Vol. 49, eds. B. Berde and H. O. Schild. Springer-Verlag, New York, pp. 29–85.

Saavedra, J. M. (1977): Distribution of serotonin and synthesizing enzymes in discrete areas of the brain. Fed. Proc. 36:2134–2141.

Sakai, F. and Meyer, J. S. (1978): Regional cerebral hemodynamics during migraine and cluster headaches measured by the ^{133}Xe inhalation method. Headache 18:122–132.

Saller, C-F. and Stricker, E. M. (1978): Gastrointestinal motility and body weight gain in rats after brain serotonin depletion by 5,7-dihydroxytryptamine. Neuropharmacology 17:499–506.

Sanders-Bush, E. and Massari, V. J. (1977): Actions of drugs that deplete serotonin. Fed. Proc. 36:2149–2153.

Saxena, P. R. (1972): The effects of antimigraine drugs on the vascular responses by 5-hydroxytryptamine and related biogenic substances on the external carotid bed of dogs: possible pharmacological implications to their antimigraine action. Headache 12:44–54.

Saxena, P. R. (1974): Selective vasoconstriction in carotid vascular bed by methysergide: possible relevance to its antimigraine effect. Eur. J. Pharmacol. 27:99–105.

Schiller, E. L. and Haese, W. H. (1973): Histologic processes of healing in hepatic injury due to eggs of Schistosoma mansoni in mice following curative chemotherapy. Am. J. Trop. Med. Hyg. 22:211–214.

Schmidt, R. and Fanchamps, A. (1974): Effect of caffeine on intestinal absorption of caffeine in man. Eur. J. Clin. Pharmacol. 7:213–216.

Schoenfeld, N., Epstein, O., Nemesh, L. et al (1978): Effects of propranolol during pregnancy and development of rats. I. Adverse effects during pregnancy. Pediatr. Res. 12:747–750.

Selby, G. and Lance, J. W. (1960): Observations on 500 cases of migraine and allied vascular headache. J. Neurol. Neurosurg. Psychiatry 23:23–32.

Senter, H. J., Lieberman, A. N. and Pinto, R. (1976): Cerebral manifestations of ergotism: report of a case and review of the literature. Stroke 7:88–92.

Shafar, J., Tallett, E. R. and Knowlson, P. A. (1972): Evaluation of clonidine in prophylaxis of migraine. Lancet 1:403–407.

Shand, D. G. (1974): Individualization of propranolol therapy. Med. Clin. North Am. 58:1063–1069.

Shand, D. G. and Wood, A. J. J. (1978): Propranolol withdrawal syndrome — why? Circulation 58:202–203.

Shane, J. M. and Naftolin, F. (1974): Effect of ergonovine maleate on puerperal prolactin. Am. J. Obstet. Gynecol. *120*:129–131.

Sharma, J. N., Sandrew, B. B. and Wang, S. C. (1979): CNS site of β-adrenergic blocker-induced hypotension in the cat: a microiontophoretic study of bulbar cardiovascular neurones. Neuropharmacology *18*:1–5.

Shelley, W. B. and Resnick, S. S. (1964): Methysergide induced degranulation of the basophil leukocyte in man. J. Invest. Dermatol. *43*:491–498.

Shuckit, M., Robins, E. and Feighner, J. (1971): Tricyclic antidepressants and monoamine oxidase inhibitors. Combined therapy in the treatment of depression. Arch. Gen. Psychiatry *24*:509–514.

Sicuteri, F. (1959): Prophylactic and therapeutic properties of 1-methyl-lysergic acid butanolamide in migraine: preliminary report. Int. Arch. Allergy Appl. Immunol. *15*:300–307.

Sicuteri, F., Anselmi, B. and Fanciullaci, M. (1974): The serotonin theory of migraine. *In* Advances in Neurology, Vol. 4, ed. J. J. Bonica. Raven Press, New York, pp. 383–394.

Sillanpää, M. and Koponen, M. (1978): Papaverine in the prophylaxis of migraine and other vascular headache in children. Acta Paediatr. Scand. *67*:209–212.

Sjaastad, O. and Stensrud, P. (1971): 2-(2,6-dichlorophenyl amino)-2-imidazoline hydrochloride (ST 155 or Catapresan) as a prophylactic remedy against migraine. Acta Neurol. Scand. *47*:120–122.

Sjaastad, O. and Stensrud, P. (1972): Clinical trial of a beta-receptor blocking agent (LB46) in migraine prophylaxis. Acta Neurol. Scand. *48*:124–128.

Sjöqvist, F. (1975): Assessment of antidepressants — pharmacokinetic aspects. *In* Advanced Medicine — Topics in Therapeutics I, ed. A. M. Breckenridge. Pitman Medical, Kent (U.K.), pp. 198–217.

Skinner, D. J. and Misbin, R. I. (1979): Uses of propranolol. N. Engl. J. Med. *293*:–1205.

Smits, J. F. and Struyker-Boudier, H. A. (1976): Intrahypothalamic serotonin and cardiovascular control in rats. Brain Res. *111*:422–427.

Sneddon, J. M. (1973): Blood platelets as a model for monoamine-containing neurones. Progr. Neurobiol. *1*:153–198.

Sofia, R. D. and Vassar, H. B. (1975): The effect of ergotamine and methysergide on serotonin metabolism in the rat brain. Arch. Int. Pharmacodyn. Ther. *216*:40–50.

Somerville, B. W. (1976): Treatment of migraine attacks with an analgesic combination (Mersyndol). Med. J. Aust. *1*:865–866.

Southwell, N., Williams, J. D. and MacKenzie, I. (1964): Methysergide in the prophylaxis of migraine. Lancet *1*:523–524.

Spatz, M. (1969): Tryptophan metabolism and cardiac disease. Ann. N.Y. Acad. Sci. *156*:152–163.

Speight, T. M. and Avery, G. S. (1972): Pizotifen (B.C.-105): a review of pharmacological properties and its therapeutic efficacy in vascular headaches. Drugs *3*:159–203.

Spiker, D. G. and Pugh, D. D. (1976): Combining tricyclic and monoamine oxidase inhibitor antidepressants. Arch. Gen. Psychiatry *33*:828–830.

Spira, P. J., Mylecharane, E. J. and Lance, J. W. (1976): The effects of humoral agents and antimigraine drugs on the cranial circulation of the monkey. Res. Clin. Stud. Headache *4*:37–75.

Steig, R. L. (1977): Double-blind study of belladonna–ergotamine–phenobarbital for interval treatment of recurrent throbbing headache. Headache *17*:120–124.

Stensrud, P. and Sjaastad, O. (1976): Short-term clinical trial of propranolol in racemic form (Inderal), d-propranolol, and placebo in migraine. Acta Neurol. Scand. *53*:229–232.

Stone, C. A., Wenger, H. C., Ludden, C. T. et al (1961): Antiserotonin-antihistaminic properties of cyproheptadine. J. Pharmacol. Exp. Ther. *131*:73–84.

Sutherland, J. M., Hooper, W. D., Eadie, M. J. and Tyrer, J. H. (1974): Buccal absorption of ergotamine. J. Neurol. Neurosurg. Psychiatry *37*:1116–1120.

Swanson, J. W. and Vick, N. A. (1978): Basilar artery migraine: 12 patients, with an attack recorded electroencephalographically. Neurology *28*:782–786.

Thompson, J. H. (1977): Serotonin and the alimentary system. *In* Serotonin in Health and Disease, Vol. 4, ed. W. B. Essman. Spectrum, New York, pp. 201–392.

Thomson, W. H. (1894): Ergot in the treatment of periodic neuralgias. J. Nerv. Ment. Dis. *19*:124–125.
Thonnard-Neumann, E. (1977): Migraine therapy with heparin: pathophysiologic basis. Headache *16*:284–292.
Tinker, J. H. and Michenfelder, J. D. (1976): Sodium nitroprusside: pharmacology, toxicology, and therapeutics. Anesthesiology *45*:340–354.
Tuttle, R. S. and McCleary, M. (1978): A mechanism to explain the anti-hypertensive action of propranolol. J. Pharmacol. Exp. Ther. *207*:56–63.
Valzelli, L. and Bernasconi, S. (1973): Behavioral and neurochemical effects of caffeine in normal and aggressive mice. Pharmacol. Biochem. Behav. *1*:251–254.
Vijayan, N. (1977): Brief therapeutic report: papaverine prophylaxis of complicated migraine. Headache *17*:159–162.
Volans, G. N. (1975): The effect of metoclopramide on the absorption of effervescent aspirin in migraine. Br. J. Clin. Pharmacol. *2*:57–63.
Volans, G. N. (1978): Migraine and drug absorption. Clin. Pharmacokinet. *3*:313–318.
von Storch, T. J. C. (1938): Complications following the use of ergotamine tartrate. J.A.M.A. *111*:293–300.
Wainscott, G., Sullivan, F. M., Volans, G. N. and Wilkinson, M. (1978): The outcome of pregnancy in women suffering from migraine. Postgrad. Med. J. *54*:98–102.
Walle, T. and Gaffney, T. E. (1972): Propranolol metabolism in man and dog; mass spectrometric identification of six new metabolites. J. Pharmacol. Exp. Ther. *182*:83–92.
Wang, H. S. and Obrist, W. D. (1976): Effect of oral papaverine on cerebral blood flow in normals: evaluation by the Xenon-133 inhalation method. Biol. Psychiatry *11*:217–225.
Warner, G. and Lance, J. W. (1975): Relaxation therapy in migraine and chronic tension headache. Med. J. Aust. *1*:298–301.
Waters, W. E. (1970): Controlled clinical trial of ergotamine tartrate. Br. Med. J. *2*:325–327.
Weber, R. B. and Reinmuth, O. M. (1972): The treatment of migraine with propranolol. Neurology *22*:366–369.
Welch, K. M. A., Spira, P. J., Knowles, L. and Lance, J. W. (1974): Simultaneous measurement of internal and external carotid blood flow in the monkey. Neurology *24*:450–457.
West, G. B. (1962): Drugs and rat pregnancy. J. Pharm. Pharmacol. *14*:828–830.
Wold, J. S. and Fischer, L. J. (1972): The tissue distribution of cyproheptadine and its metabolites in rats and mice. J. Pharmacol. Exp. Ther. *183*:188–196.
Wright, A. D., Barber, S. G., Kendall, M. J. and Poole, P. H. (1979): Beta-adrenoceptor-blocking drugs and blood sugar control in diabetes mellitus. Br. Med. J. *1*:159–161.
Wykes, P. (1968): The treatment of angina pectoris with coexistent migraine. Practitioner *200*:702–704.
Young, R. R., Growdon, J. H. and Shahani, B. T. (1975): Beta-adrenergic mechanisms in action tremor. N. Engl. J. Med. *293*:950–953.
Yuill, G. M., Swinburn, W. R. and Liversedge, L. A. (1972): A double-blind crossover trial of isometheptene mucate compound and ergotamine in migraine. Br. J. Clin. Pract. *26*:76–79.
Yuwiler, A. (1979): Serotonin and stress. *In* Serotonin in Health and Disease, Vol. 5, ed. W. B. Essman. Spectrum, New York, pp. 1–50.
Zatz, M., Kebabian, J. W. and O'Dea, R. F. (1978): Regulation of β-adrenergic function in the rat pineal gland. Receptors Horm. Act. *3*:195–219.
Ziegler, V. E., Clayton, P. J. and Biggs, J. T. (1977): A comparison study of amitriptyline and nortriptyline with plasma levels. Arch. Gen. Psychiatry *34*:607–612.

CHAPTER 5

TENSION HEADACHE

The prevalence of tension headache in the population at large is not clear; however, as an index of its frequency, over 40 per cent of 1,152 patients referred to an outpatient clinic were diagnosed as having tension headache (Lance et al, 1965). The traditional description of tension headache is much less clear than that of migraine. Features usually ascribed to this disorder are a bilateral, commonly occipitonuchal location; a tendency to wax and wane throughout the day; a heavy, pressing and tight quality of pain; an association with contracted muscles of the scalp and neck; and occurrence in relation to emotional conflict (Ziegler, 1978). However, it is evident from Table 5–1 that there are overlapping features between tension and migrainous headaches. Indeed, 56 patients who had been seen by neurologists, and of whom 24 were thought to have migraine, 11 combined tension and migraine and 20 tension headache, were re-evaluated by impartial investigators in a recent study (Bakal and Kaganov, 1977). Forty per cent of the migraine and tension headache patients reported throbbing headaches; 50 per cent of patients from each group reported associated visual disturbances; and almost 50 per cent of those in each group reported family members with recurring headache disorders. Nausea and vomiting occurred in 70 per cent of the patients diagnosed as migraine and in 36 per cent of those with tension headache.

A daily, constantly recurring headache, without associated focal neurologic symptoms or prominent vomiting, represents the clinical features that usually lead to the conclusion that a patient suffers from tension headaches. The lack of clear boundaries between migrainous and tension headaches unfortunately has led many physicians to assume that patients with headache disorders that occur without organic explanation, and lack the stereotypic features of migraine, are experiencing tension headache.

172

TABLE 5-1. *CHARACTERISTICS OF MIGRAINOUS AND TENSION HEADACHES* *

		PERCENTAGE	
		Migraine	Tension
Age at onset	< 20 years	55	30
	> 20 years	45	70
Premonitory symptoms		60	10
Frequency	daily	3	50
	< weekly	60	15
Duration	constant, daily	0	20
	1–3 days	35	10
Throbbing pain		80	30
Location	unilateral	80	10
	bilateral	20	90
Vomiting with attacks		50	10
Family history of headache		65	40

* Modified from Friedman et al, 1954.

Features formerly believed to be specific for tension headache, such as neck muscle contraction and its precipitation by stress and anxiety, are now known to occur just as often in migraine (see below); most patients with tension headache experience exacerbations of headache that are often accompanied by migrainous symptoms. Furthermore, the statistical aspects of tension headache regarding age at onset (Table 5–2), predominance in women (75 per cent), presence of recurring headache among family members and its natural history are not significantly different from those in migraine patients (Friedman et al, 1954). This lack of distinguishing features between migraine and tension headache suggests the possibility that these disorders are at two ends of a continuum. Recent evidence that platelet serotonin is low in patients subject to frequent tension headache supports this possibility (Rolf et al, 1977). Alterations of the cranial vasculature also occur in patients with ten-

TABLE 5-2. *AGE AT ONSET OF TENSION HEADACHE IN 466 PATIENTS* *

AGE (YEARS)	PERCENTAGE OF PATIENTS
0–10	16
10–20	24
20–30	19
30–40	17
40–50	15
50–60	6
60–70	2
70–80	1

* Data drawn from Lance et al, 1965.

sion headache, and in this chapter evidence will be reviewed regarding the possibility that tension headache and migraine are quantitatively different clinical manifestations of vasomotor instability.

MUSCLE CONTRACTION AND PAIN

Muscle contraction, formerly believed to be the mechanism of pain in tension headache, is probably a consequence, rather than a cause of headache (Poźniak-Patewicz, 1976; Bakal and Kaganov, 1977; Martin and Mathews, 1978).

Frontalis muscle contraction occurs to a greater degree in anxious subjects than in control subjects (Sainsbury and Gibson, 1954), an observation that is consistent with the not unreasonable hypothesis that emotionally disturbing situations, if sufficiently prolonged, may result in the contraction of scalp muscles, giving rise to pain. When muscle contraction is sustained, muscle tenderness and pain may become evident, probably because of compressed intramuscular arterioles and subsequent ischemia, the latter persisting for days after muscles relax (Simons et al, 1943). It is clear that contracted skeletal muscle may become a source of pain. Infiltration of procaine into contracted muscles may relieve a component of a patient's headache, but only rarely results in total removal of head pain.

Headache arising under many circumstances is known to be associated with contraction of the scalp and neck muscles. Electromyographic studies performed during headache attacks have shown that the neck muscles are more contracted than the temporal muscles, and that patients with migraine develop more intense contractions than those with tension headache (Poźniak-Patewicz, 1976; Bakal and Kaganov, 1977). During headache-free periods, more activity is found electromyographically in the temporal, frontal and neck muscles of migrainous subjects than in tension headache subjects.

VASCULAR FACTORS

Neck muscle contraction occurs not infrequently as a prodromal symptom in patients with migrainous attacks (Pearce, 1977), which raises the possibility that intramuscular arterial vasoconstriction, resulting in muscle ischemia, contraction and pain, may be an expression of vasomotor instability.

The view that intramuscular vasoconstriction is a correlate of tension headache is supported by the experimental diminution of headache resulting from the administration of vasodilators such as amyl nitrite, ethyl alcohol and nicotinic acid (Brazil and Friedman, 1956; Ostfeld et al, 1957). There also is evidence of more widespread vasoconstriction. The small conjunctival vessels have been photographed during tension headache and have been found to be constricted as long as the headache persisted (Ostfeld et al, 1957). Furthermore, temporal artery pulse amplitudes are lower in patients with tension headache than in control subjects (Tunis and Wolff, 1954).

An apparently paradoxical finding in patients during tension headache attacks is that the clearance of radioactive sodium after injection into the splenius capitis muscle is greater than in the same patients after the headache has subsided (Onel et al, 1961). The removal of Na^{24} measures the gross effective circulation to a tissue (Kety, 1949; Wisham and Yalow, 1952), and this appears to be increased during tension headaches. This may or may not reflect total arterial muscle blood flow, which would be predictably higher at a time when a muscle is active; whether muscle blood flow increases out of proportion to this increased metabolic activity has not yet been measured. It may be possible to explain the increased clearance of Na^{24} without involving increased arterial blood flow; alternative possibilities include the opening of closed capillaries, increased filtration and resorption, and an acceleration of the lymphatic circulation (Kety, 1949).

Cerebral blood flow is increased in the frontal and brain stem–cerebellar regions in some patients with tension headache, which is comparable to the cerebral circulatory alteration found in common migraine (Sakai and Meyer, 1978).

PSYCHOLOGIC FACTORS

Friedman et al (1953) reported that, in a series of 400 patients with tension headache, anxiety-provoking situations were contributory in all cases. Many similar experiential reports followed. Kolb (1963) contended that tension headaches were frequently the physical expression of a chronic anxiety state, and that the origins of anxiety resided in repressed resentment toward a loved one; the threat of underlying anger and hostility was believed to generate anxiety that was expressed in the form of a physical symptom. Others have come to similar conclusions (Martin et al, 1967; Martin, 1978). Martin (1972) in a series of 100 patients found that obvious tension was present in 74 per cent, depression was apparent in 35 per cent and secondary gain was evident in 56 per cent. The commonest psychologic problem areas were dependence, sexuality and control of urges. No control subjects have been studied in any series to date and the statistical significance of these data remains unclear. More-over, virtually all these data were derived from patients with histo-ries of longstanding headache, and much of the emotional turmoil described may have been the consequence of their living with chronic pain (Merskey and Boyd, 1978). In a random survey of a large population of headache patients, stress correlated poorly with the tension headache "pattern" (Ziegler et al, 1972).

Psychologic tests performed on patients with muscle-contraction headache are scarce. Davis et al (1976) found an associa-tion between types of headache and personality factors, using the California Personality Index. Martin et al (1967) administered the Minnesota Multiphasic Personality Inventory (MMPI) to 25 patients with tension headache and found that most showed responses characteristic of hypochondriasis, depression and hysteria; these re-sults are simlar to those derived from individuals with other chronic painful disorders.

Despite general agreement that stress and anxiety are important correlates of tension headache, no systematic studies of the outcome of treatment have been published. Indeed, intensive psychotherapy has been neither a practical nor a satisfactory approach for the large majority of these patients (Kudrow, 1976; Adams and Victor, 1977).

CLINICAL FEATURES

Symptoms begin before the age of 20 years in 40 per cent of patients with tension headache (Table 5–2). Headache is bilateral in about 90 per cent (Table 5–1); is usually described as dull, pressing or bandlike; waxes and wanes in intensity during the day; and has no predilection for any particular cranial location. The vast majority experience head pain daily and constantly, and their symptoms often date back 10 to 20 years (Table 5–3). Although the daily pain is rarely severe enough to confine patients to bed, exacerbations of headache occur with a variable frequency, are often accompanied by nausea and other symptoms characteristic of vascular headaches, and not uncommonly result in the patient going to bed. Headache is often present upon or shortly after awakening and persists throughout the day, without any obvious relationship to stress and anxiety (Ziegler et al, 1972). About 10 per cent of those with ten-sion headache are wakened by a throbbing headache between 1 and 4 a.m. (Lance, 1978). Neck pain accompanies tension headache no more often than in patients with other headache syndromes (Ziegler et al, 1972), contrary to a widely held view.

Photophobia, nausea and episodic lightheadedness occur with a variable frequency in these patients, and most have noted episodic and brief scintillating scotomata; however, very few, if any, have experienced the slowly evolving fortification spectrum that may characterize a classic migrainous attack. In a recent survey of patients in general practice, Philips (1977) noted the high frequency of "vascular" symptoms and severe headaches among those with tension headaches. Many patients begin their headache careers with clear-cut migraine headaches that become more and more frequent until the tension headache syndrome becomes evident. Sicuteri (1972) has found that 50 per cent of those with chronic tension headache experience exacerbation of their pain with head-jolting maneuvers or after the administration of histamine; these data are consistent with a labile cranial vasculature, and occur also in migrainous subjects.

In addition to these similarities to migraine, there appears to be an increased incidence of epilepsy among patients with tension headache. Lance and Anthony (1966) selected, from among 354 such patients, 100 who had never experienced an acute exacerbation of headache nor any migrainous symptoms; this group was to be as clearly representative of tension headache as possible, because its members were to serve as controls for comparison with 500 migrainous patients. The two groups were comparable in age, sex and duration of headache. In the assessment of the incidence of epilepsy among these patients, seizures occurring before the age of 5 years were excluded from consideration. The incidence of epilepsy in the migrainous population was 1.6 per cent, and in the tension headache group 2 per cent; in a comparable study Basser (1969) found the incidence of epilepsy to be 5.9 per cent in a population of 1,830 migrainous subjects and 1.1 per cent in 548 patients with tension headache. The incidence of epilepsy in both disorders is significantly higher than that estimated for the general population, 0.5 per cent (Hauser, 1978).

TABLE 5–3. DURATION OF TENSION HEADACHE
IN 430 PATIENTS[*]

DURATION (YEARS)	PERCENTAGE OF PATIENTS
0–5	25
5–10	18
10–15	11
15–20	10
20–30	16
30–40	7
40–50	9
50–65	4

[*] Data drawn from Lance et al, 1965.

TREATMENT

The physician's attitude toward headache patients will almost certainly influence the results he achieves. The communication of support and concern, at the very least, will help these individuals deal with the existing problem until effective treatment is arrived at; a careful, unhurried history and physical examination, and an explanation of the mechanism of headache including its trigger factors, are part of the process. In this setting, a patient is more likely to reveal his anxieties and unexpressed resentments when these factors are put into perspective as precipitants of headache. Many who are told that their problem is based on a "nervous"constitution or that they do not handle stress well eventually come to resent these implications. This is partly because of their operational inutility and, perhaps more importantly, also because the vast majority of these patients have at times suffered from headache during tranquil low-anxiety periods as well as during emotionally-charged intervals. None of us are free of anxiety and stress. It is almost simplistic to apply a universal attribute of human beings as the cause of someone's symptoms. Establishing a meaningful relationship with a patient based on trust and support must be more important than focusing on his vulnerabilities. The physician's responsibility in this relationship is to help the patient examine and comprehend the therapeutic options and goals, and to arrive at a mutual decision as to which mode appears to be most reasonable for him. Regarding the goals of therapy, it is important that the patient understand that recurring headache at present cannot be permanently cured; that the frequency and severity of headache attacks can often be reduced, at times dramatically so; and that chronic tension headache eventually runs its course via a mechanism that is not understood. Until this happens several therapeutic avenues are open that often help patients derive more pleasure from life.

In some instances, if the patient is going through a trying period in his life, formal psychotherapy is an option that should be exercised if the emotional problem *per se* warrants that approach, apart from the fact that headaches occur. Although controlled studies are lacking, there are abundant experiential data supporting the validity of psychotherapy in selected patients (Martin and Rome, 1967). The mainstay of therapy in tension headache, however, is pharmacotherapy, and techniques that induce relaxation are useful adjuncts.

RELAXATION METHODS

Just as stress and anxiety have been recognized as common precipitants of headache attacks, so also it appears to be true that relaxation may abort or lessen the severity of recurring headache (Warner and Lance, 1975). Some of the methods in use were originally proposed to directly relax contracted skeletal muscle, and thus improve on the putative source of pain in this condition. However, the bulk of the evidence points toward general relaxation as the common achievement of these methods, with the relaxation of contracted skeletal muscle as an index of a more generalized response (Haynes et al, 1975; Cohen, 1978). These methods appear to be as effective for patients with migraine as for those with tension headache (Bakal and Kaganov, 1977).

Simple measures, such as massage, manual stretching of the muscles of the neck and shoulder girdle, hot tub baths and application of local heat, should not be overlooked. Some patients relate more easily to other relaxation techniques such as meditation, hypnosis or yoga. It is worth exploring these options, although controlled studies are wanting.

The development of biofeedback conditioning techniques has received a great deal of publicity, but the instrumentation and expense of these procedures may not be necessary to achieve the same end result. Warner and Lance (1975) have described a simple, rapid method based on classic conditioning techniques that combines the muscular aspects of relaxation with mental relaxation (Jacobsen, 1938). Of 17 patients, 13 of whom were daily headache sufferers and four of whom had headache 12 to 14 days of the mouth, four were rendered headache-free by relaxation therapy; in another four headache was reduced to once a month, and in three headache was cut to two to four times per month. A marked reduction in medication accompanied this improvement, which was assessed six months after completion of relaxation training. These results are quite encouraging, albeit uncontrolled, in that placebo responses are seldom of this magnitude. Lance (1978) has reproduced a simple manual from which patients may learn to carry out relaxation exercises by themselves. For some this approach may be sufficient to alleviate tension headache, but for the vast majority pharmacologic support is necessary.

Biofeedback methods used in tension headache have usually employed feedback from the EMG of the frontalis or temporalis scalp muscles; the patient hears an EMG signal that varies in intensity in proportion to the degree of muscle contraction present. A controlled study of biofeedback in tension headache produced persuasive data (Budzynski et al, 1973). Six patients received 16 laboratory sessions aimed at reducing frontalis muscle contraction; six received a comparable number of sessions with false feedback (sounds that were not correlated with muscle activity); and there were six untreated control subjects. There was a substantially better outcome for the first group than for the two control groups; no differences were found between the control groups. Improvement was maintained for 18 months by three patients, as was slight improvement in one another; two patients were lost to follow-up. When the frontalis muscle EMG feedback method is compared to progressive relaxation training and a no-treatment control group, both types of treatment result in significant benefit and are equally effective (Cox et al, 1974; Haynes et al, 1975; Bruhn et al, 1979). There are no published data regarding the long-term follow-up of patients who have benefited from biofeedback procedures. In our experience, the benefits have been short-lived and, over-all, disappointing. Relaxation training appears to be more promising in that patients can continue to practice at home with occasional reinforcement from the physician, without instrumentation.

DRUGS

Whatever other methods are employed, pharmacologic intervention is almost always necessary in helping these patients through a difficult time in their lives. The treatment of individual attacks is mainly with analgesics. There is no evidence that any particular analgesic is generally better than any other for these patients, and the choice should be governed by the severity of pain. By the time an individual consults the physician about headache, the potential benefits of aspirin or acetaminophen usually have already been tested and found wanting. We find that the combination of acetaminophen, butalbital and caffeine is especially useful as a non-narcotic, non-phenacetin-containing analgesic for these patients. Codeine is a very useful analgesic and is unlikely to produce physical dependence at doses under 600 mg per day (Jaffe, 1975). Although more potent opiates with higher addictive potential should be discouraged for daily usage, it is sometimes important to support some patients temporarily through a particularly difficult headache siege. Meperidine is not likely to result in physical dependence at oral doses under 400 mg per day (Himmelsbach, 1943).

The most productive avenue of therapy for chronic tension headache sufferers is the daily use of prophylactic agents, whose mechanism of action in this condition is unknown. Amitriptyline has been shown in controlled studies to be the most effective of these agents, resulting in better than 50 per cent improvement in more than 65 per cent of cases (Lance and Curran, 1964); 25 per cent of patients become headache-free with the use of this drug (Table 5–4). The usual dosage range is 50 to 100 mg per day, but some may require considerably higher doses. A response is usually seen two to ten days after treatment is implemented. On occasion, we have used doses as high as 300 mg per day; some patients who achieve a satisfactory result initially may find that their headaches "break through" eventually. Elevation of the dosage for these indi-

TABLE 5-4. TREATMENT OF TENSION HEADACHE:
RESULTS WITH FIRST DRUGS ADMINISTERED*

| | NUMBER OF PATIENTS | | | |
	Headache-free	50% Improved	Unchanged	PERCENTAGE IMPROVED
Amitriptyline	22	38	21	73
Imipramine	6	8	15	47
Diazepam	1	5	4	60
Chlordiazepoxide	11	21	31	50
Ergotamine–phenobarbital–belladonna	9	13	22	49
Amobarbital	2	14	27	37
Placebo	1	5	12	30

*Modified from Lance et al, 1965.

viduals often results in renewed headache control. The results with this drug appear to be better in patients over 60 years of age and in those whose illness is of longer duration. The responsiveness of patients to amitriptyline is not contingent on the presence of concurrent depressive symptoms, which are found in about one-third of these cases (Lance and Curran, 1964). Moreover, other drugs with equivalent antidepressant actions, such as imipramine and tranylcypromine, appear to be less effective than amitriptyline (Table 5–5); it is unlikely, therefore, that the effectiveness of amitriptyline in tension headache is based on its mode of action in depression.

Other drugs that have been shown to be significantly better than placebo include diazepam, chlordiazepoxide, meprobamate (Friedman, 1957, 1962), imipramine, and a belladonna–ergotamine

TABLE 5-5. TREATMENT OF TENSION HEADACHE:
RESULTS WITH DRUGS GIVEN SEQUENTIALLY*

| | NUMBER OF PATIENTS | | | |
	Headache-free	50% Improved	Unchanged	PERCENTAGE IMPROVED
Amitriptyline	40	73	66	60
Imipramine	13	23	54	39
Tranylcypromine	3	3	14	29
Diazepam	9	13	17	56
Chlordiazepoxide	24	46	74	48
Ergotamine–phenobarbital–belladonna	10	27	49	42
Amobarbital	4	20	52	32
Placebo	2	9	34	22

These patients were assessed monthly. If no benefit was received from the first drug, another medication was prescribed for the next month. The results of all drugs are shown; those patients not responsive to medication are represented several times.

*Modified from Lance et al, 1965.

TABLE 5–6. *FACTORS SUPPORTING THE MECHANISTIC SIMILARITY OF TENSION HEADACHE TO MIGRAINE*

Clinically, many similarities and few differences; neck muscle contraction found in both disorders
Nuchal muscle contraction and pain a prodromal feature of migraine
Increased incidence of epilepsy in both disorders
Intramuscular vasoconstriction may be primary
Low platelet serotonin reported in both disorders
Psychologic data for both disorders are indistinguishable
Responsiveness of both disorders to amitriptyline and ergotamine–phenobarbital–belladonna

tartrate–phenobarbital combination. Responsiveness to the latter is not likely to be through the sedative effect of phenobarbital since sedation with amobarbital is not significantly better than placebo (Tables 5–4, 5–5). Ergotamine tartrate, used alone prophylactically, has not been studied in this condition, although Horton et al (1948) reported excellent results in five of 11 patients with tension headache when oral ergotamine was used for individual attacks. Other sedatives, vasodilators and methysergide have been found to be no better than placebo (Lance and Curran, 1964).

Despite our poor level of understanding of the mechanisms involved in tension headache, most of these patients can be substantially benefited by the therapeutic options now available. Those who receive benefit from drugs are advised to continue treatment for three to four months, then to taper the dosage slowly over three to four weeks. If headache increases in frequency or severity, the drug is reinstituted for another three- to four-month cycle.

In conclusion, the similarities between migraine and tension headache appear to be more striking than the differences (Table 5–6). One of the major operationally important differences appears to be differential pharmacologic responsiveness of these conditions, in that some drugs effective in migraine may be less so in tension headache. However, there are few data that bear on this point. Indeed, in one study, patients with tension headache were just as responsive to ergonovine, ergotamine and methysergide as were those with typical migrainous attacks (Barrie et al, 1968).

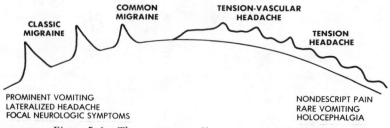

Figure 5–1. The continuum of benign recurring headache.

There is no compelling evidence to support a biologic mechanicam of tension headache that is qualitatively different from that of migraine. Moreover, there are lines of evidence that suggest that the varying clinical manifestations of recurring headaches are quantitatively different manifestations of labile vasomotor regulation. The clinical spectrum of benign, recurring headache may include classic migraine at one end; the variations of common migraine and tension migraine occupying the vast middle ground; and tension headache at the other end (Fig. 5-1).

REFERENCES

Adams, R. D. and Victor, M. (1977): Headache and other craniofacial pains. In Principles of Neurology, McGraw-Hill Book Co., New York, pp. 95–111.

Bakal, D. A. and Kaganov, J. A. (1977): Muscle contraction and migraine headache: psychophysiologic comparison. Headache 17:208–215.

Barrie, M. A., Fox, W. R., Weatherall, M. and Wilkinson, M. I. P. (1968): Analysis of symptoms of patients with headaches and their response to treatment with ergot derivatives. Q. J. Med. 37:319–336.

Basser, L. S. (1969): The relation of migraine and epilepsy. Brain 92:285–300.

Brazil, P. and Friedman, A. P. (1956): Craniovascular studies in headache. A report and analysis of pulse volume tracings. Neurology 6:96–102.

Bruhn, P., Olesen, J. and Melgaard, B. (1979): Controlled trial of EMG feedback in muscle contraction headache. Ann. Neurol. 6:34–36.

Budzynski, T. H., Stoyva, J. M., Adler, C. S. and Mullaney, D. J. (1973): EMG biofeedback and tension headache. A controlled outcome study. Psychosom. Med. 35:484–496.

Cohen, M. J. (1978): Psychophysiological studies of headache: is there similarity between migraine and muscle contraction headaches? Headache 18:189–196.

Cox, D. J., Freundlich, A. and Meyer, R. G. (1974): Differential expectiveness of electromyographic feedback, verbal relaxation instructions and medication placebo. J. Consult. Clin. Psychol. 43:892–898.

Davis, R. A., Wetzel, R. D., Kashiwag, M. D. et al (1976): Personality, depression and headache type. Headache 16:246–251.

Friedman, A. P. (1957): The treatment of chronic headache with meprobamate. Ann. N. Y. Acad. Sci. 67:822–827.

Friedman, A. P. (1962): Treatment of chronic headache. Int. J. Neurol. 3:388–397.

Friedman, A. P., de Sola Pool, N. and von Storch, T. J. C. (1953): Tension headache. J.A.M.A. 151:174–177.

Friedman, A. P., von Storch, T. J. C. and Merritt, H. H. (1954): Migraine and tension headaches. A clinical study of 2000 cases. Neurology 4:773–788.

Hauser, W. A. (1978): Epidemiology of epilepsy. In Advances in Neurology, Vol. 19, ed. B. S. Schoenberg. Raven Press, New York, pp. 313–339.

Haynes, S. M., Griffin, P., Mooney, D. and Parise, M. (1975): Electromyographic feedback and relaxation instructions in the treatment of muscle contraction headaches. Behav. Ther. 6:672–678.

Himmelsbach, C, K. (1943): Further studies of the addiction liability of Demerol. J. Pharmacol. Exp. Ther. 79:5–9.

Horton, B. T., Ryan, R. and Reynolds, J. L. (1948):Clinical observations on the use of E.C. 110, a new agent for the treatment of headache. Mayo Clin. Proc. 23:105–108.

Jacobsen, E. (1938): Progressive Relaxation. University of Chicago Press, Chicago.

Jaffe, J. H. (1975): Drug addiction and drug abuse. In The Pharmacological Basis of Therapeutics, 5th ed. eds. L. S. Goodman and A. Gilman. Macmillan, New York, pp. 284–324.

Kety, S. S. (1949): Measurement of regional circulation by the local clearance of radioactive sodium. Am. Heart J. 38:321–328.

184 TENSION HEADACHE

Kolb, L. C. (1963): Psychiatric aspects of the treatment of headache. Neurology 13:34–37.
Kudrow, L. (1976): Tension headache. *In* Pathogenesis and Treatment of Headache, ed. O. Appenzeller. Spectrum, New York, pp. 81–91.
Lance, J. W. (1978): Muscle contraction ("tension") headache. *In* Mechanism and Management of Headache, 3rd ed. Butterworths, London/Boston, pp. 104–129.
Lance, J. W. and Anthony, M. (1966): Some clinical aspects of migraine. Arch. Neurol. 15:356–361.
Lance, J. W. and Curran, D. A. (1964): Treatment of chronic tension headache. Lancet 1:1236–1239.
Lance, J. W., Curran, D. A. and Anthony, M. (1965): Investigations into the mechanism and treatment of chronic headache. Med. J. Aust. 2:909–914.
Martin, M. J. (1972): Muscle contraction headache. Psychosomatics 13:16–19.
Martin, M. J. (1978): Psychogenic factors in headache. Med. Clin. North Am. 62:559–570.
Martin, M. J. and Rome, H. P. (1967): Muscle-contraction headache: therapeutic aspects. Res. Clin. Stud. Headache 1:205–217.
Martin, M. J., Rome, H. P. and Swenson, W. M. (1967): Muscle-contraction headache: a psychiatric review. Res. Clin. Stud. Headache 1:184–204.
Martin, P. R. and Mathews, A. M. (1978): Tension headaches: psychophysiological investigation and treatment. J. Psychosom. Res. 22:389–399.
Merskey, H. and Boyd, D. (1978): Emotional adjustment and chronic pain. Pain 5:173–178.
Onel, Y., Friedman, A. P. and Grossman, J. (1961): Muscle blood flow studies in muscle contraction headaches. Neurology 11:935–939.
Ostfeld, A. M., Reis, D. J. and Wolff, H. G. (1957): Studies in headache. Bulbar conjunctival ischemia and muscle contraction headache. Arch. Neurol. Psychiatry 77:113–119.
Pearce, J. (1977): Migraine: a psychosomatic disorder. Headache 17:125–128.
Philips, C. (1977): Headache in general practice. Headache 16:322–329.
Poźniak-Patewicz, E. (1976): "Cephalgic" spasm of head and neck muscles. Headache 14:261–266.
Rolf, L. H., Wiele, G. and Brune, G. G. (1977): Serotonin in platelets of patients with migraine and muscle-contraction headache. Excerpta Med. 427:11–12.
Sainsbury, P. and Gibson, J. G. (1954): Symptoms of anxiety and tension and the accompanying physiological changes in the muscular system. J. Neurol. Neurosurg. Psychiatry 17:216–224.
Sakai, F. and Meyer, J. S. (1978): Regional cerebral hemodynamics during migraine and cluster headaches measured by the Xe[133] inhalation method. Headache 18:122–132.
Sicuteri, F. (1972): Dry and wet theory in headache. Res. Clin. Stud. Headache 3:159–165.
Simons, D. J., Day, E., Goodell, H. and Wolff, H. G. (1943): Experimental studies on headache: muscles of the scalp and neck as sources of pain. Assoc. Res. Nerv. Ment. Dis. 23:228–241.
Tunis, M. M. and Wolff, H. G. (1954): Studies in headache. Cranial artery vasoconstriction and muscle contraction headache. Arch. Neurol. Psychiatry 71:425–434.
Warner, G. and Lance, J. W. (1975): Relaxation therapy in migraine and chronic tension headache. Med. J. Aust. 1:298–301.
Wisham, L. H. and Yalow, R. S. (1952): Some factors affecting the clearance of Na[24] from human muscle. Am. Heart J. 43:67–76.
Ziegler, D. K. (1978): Tension headache. Med. Clin. North Am. 62:495–505.
Ziegler, D. K., Hassanein, R. and Hassanein, K. (1972): Headache syndromes suggested by factor analysis of symptom variables in a headache prone population. J. Chronic Dis. 25:353–363.

CHAPTER 6

CLUSTER HEADACHE

Although cluster headache ("migrainous neuralgia") had been recognized for over 100 years (von Möllendorff, 1867), it was Sir Charles Symonds' (1956) lucid account of this disorder that brought it into focus. Recognition of this clinical entity was almost certainly retarded by a variety of confusing names that were given to this condition, such as erythroprosopalgia, Raeder's syndrome, sphenopalatine neuralgia, ciliary neuralgia, vidian neuralgia and histamine cephalalgia (Sutherland and Eadie, 1972). Cluster headache is now firmly established as a distinctive syndrome (Table 6–1) whose recognition is important, since it is likely to be responsive to treatment. Although it is genetically, biochemically and clinically different from migraine, it is operationally useful to regard it as a migraine variant because of its vascular mechanism and its responsiveness to antimigrainous pharmacologic agents.

CLINICAL FEATURES

Cluster headache has an incidence approximately 2 to 9 per cent that of migraine (Friedman, 1969; Ekbom, 1970b). Males are

TABLE 6-1. CLINICAL STEREOTYPE OF THE
CLUSTER HEADACHE SYNDROME

Disorder of males; 20–50 peak age of onset
Paroxysmal, explosive, unilateral, periorbital pain
Frequently nocturnal
Cluster cycles (lasting weeks) with pain-free intervals (lasting weeks to months)
Ipsilateral nasal stuffiness, soft-tissue swelling, lacrimation, hyperemic eye, Horner's
  syndrome
Alcohol sensitivity during cluster cycles
No family history of migraine

---

affected more commonly than females in a proportion of 4 to 1. Although most patients begin experiencing headache between the ages of 20 and 50 years (mean of 35 years), the syndrome may begin as early as the first decade and as late as the eighth decade. Clearly, age alone is an insensitive diagnostic criterion.

CHARACTERISTICS OF PAIN

The pain commences abruptly, without warning, and reaches a crescendo within two to 15 minutes (Ekbom, 1975). It is often excruciating in intensity, and is deep, nonfluctuating and explosive in quality; only occasionally is it pulsatile. In addition, 10 to 20 per cent of patients report superimposed paroxysms of stabbing, icepick-like pains in the periorbital region that last for a few seconds and may occur once or several times in rapid succession; this paroxysmal pain usually heralds the end of an attack, the symptoms resolving rapidly in 1 to 2 minutes.

The pain usually begins in, around or above one eye or the temple; occasionally the face, neck, ear or hemicranium may be affected. It is always unilateral, and generally affects the same side in subsequent bouts; however, it occasionally may shift to the corresponding region of the opposite side.

PERIODICITY AND DURATION OF ATTACKS

Attacks last from 30 minutes to two hours (mean of 45 minutes) in about 80 per cent of cases. Occasionally, attacks — especially mild ones — may be as short as ten minutes, whereas others may be as long as several hours. They range in frequency from six per 24 hours to one per week, with a mean of one to two per day. Periodicity is a characteristic feature in about 85 per cent of patients, in that attacks of pain tend to recur at the same hour each day for the duration of the cluster bout; many individuals also experience additional attacks that occur randomly throughout the day. Attacks take place at night in about 50 per cent of cases (Hornabrook, 1964; Lance and Anthony, 1971), and in such circumstances pain characteristically awakens the patient within two hours of falling asleep.

CHARACTERISTICS OF BOUTS

The attacks of pain are clustered into cycles that usually last four to eight weeks, and are followed by a pain-free remission in about 90 per cent of patients. On occasion, bouts may be as short as a few days or as long as four months; infrequently, those with established cluster tempos enter a "chronic" phase wherein the attacks may persist for a year or more. Most patients experience one to two bouts per year; however, the interval between clusters ranges from three months to five years (Friedman and Mikropoulos, 1958), although in rare instances it may be as long as 25 years (Hornabrook, 1964). Eventually the bouts cease spontaneously, but more precise data on the natural history of the disorder are not yet available.

ASSOCIATED FEATURES

Lacrimation from the eye on the affected side is the most common associated symptom (Table 6–2). A blocked nasal passage, red eye, and flushing of the forehead and cheek are often found, but their absence does not exclude the diagnosis. A transitory, partial *Horner's syndrome* (pupillary miosis and/or lid ptosis) is a very useful sign in the differential diagnosis of facial pain, in that it is highly characteristic of the cluster headache syndrome, and after repeated occurrences it may become a permanent feature (Nieman and Hurwitz, 1961; Riley and Moyer, 1971). Involvement of the sympathetic plexus probably results from distention of the wall of the internal carotid artery in the carotid canal; this localization of the lesion in the sympathetic pathway is supported by three lines of evidence. The first is the observation that facial sweating is consistently spared in these patients. Since the sympathetic fibers subserving sweating part from the remainder of the sympathetic plexus at the bifurcation of the common carotid artery, and surround the external carotid artery and its branches, the injury must be cephalad to the carotid bifurcation. Second, supersensitivity of the miotic pupil to direct-acting sympathomimetic agents also places the lesion

TABLE 6–2. CLINICAL FEATURES OF CLUSTER HEADACHE: PERCENTAGE INCIDENCE*

Lacrimation	80
Conjunctival injection	50
Blocked nostril	50
Alcohol sensitivity	50
Running nostril	10
Partial Horner's syndrome	25
Nausea	40
Facial flushing	20
Prominent, tender temporal artery	20

*Data drawn from Friedman and Mikropoulos, 1958; Lance and Anthony, 1971; Sutherland and Eadie, 1972.

postganglionically (Riley and Moyer, 1971). Third, angiographic changes of the carotid siphon during a cluster headache attack (Ekbom and Greitz, 1970) also point to sympathetic plexus compression at this locus.

Focal neurologic symptoms of the type characteristic of migraine are very uncommon in the cluster headache syndrome; however, occasional patients experience typical photopsia, teichopsia, facial paresthesia or vertigo at the time of the attack.

Sensitivity to alcohol during a cluster bout occurs in approximately one-half of the patients, and ceases when the bout remits (Friedman and Mikropoulos, 1958); this alternating, on–off vulnerability is highly characteristic of the cluster headache syndrome. Patients who are sensitive to alcohol note that attacks are triggered within a five- to 45-minute period after the ingestion of modest amounts of alcohol — usually less than a single cocktail or glass of wine. The vast majority have noted that their sensitivity is less than total; i.e., alcohol triggers attacks in 70 to 80 per cent of exposures. This factor, together with many patients' misinterpretations regarding inquiries into their drinking habits, may account for the low incidence of alcohol sensitivity in several reported series (Symonds, 1956; Sutherland and Eadie, 1972).

A number of other *precipitating factors* have been noted in a smaller number of patients, including stress, exposure to heat or cold, glare, hay fever attacks, and occasionally the ingestion of a specific foodstuff (chocolate, eggs, dairy products). *Experimentally,* attacks can be triggered in nearly all patients *during a bout* by the administration of 1 mg of nitroglycerin sublingually (Ekbom, 1968), and in about 70 per cent of patients by subcutaneous histamine (Horton, 1961). There is generally a latent period of 30 to 50 minutes before headache is triggered, whereas the peak peripheral and central vascular effects of nitroglycerin occur within three to four minutes of its administration, and disappear in approximately 30 minutes (Sokoloff, 1959; Mason and Braunwald, 1965). Thus, the appearance of headache does not coincide with the maximal effect of nitroglycerin, and the mechanism by which nitroglycerin causes headache remains unclear. A period refractory to pharmacologic provocation occurs after spontaneous or pharmacologically-induced attacks, and may persist for two hours or more (Horton, 1961; Ekbom, 1968). Therefore, valid provocative tests must be administered during an active bout, several hours after the subsidence of an attack.

AMELIORATIVE FACTORS

Compression of the superficial temporal artery provides temporary relief for less than 10 per cent of patients (Lance and Anthony,

1971). Vigorous physical exertion at the earliest sign of an attack can be remarkably effective in ameliorating or even aborting it in some patients (Ekbom and Lindahl, 1970; Atkinson, 1977).

HEREDITARY DATA

Hereditary factors are significant in migraine and might be expected to be important in the cluster headache syndrome because of mechanistic and pharmacologic similarities. However, it is quite rare to find other examples of cluster headache in the family history; examples have been cited by Bickerstaff (1959), Balla and Walton (1964) and others. Bickerstaff (1959) carefully inquired about a previous history of migraine in a series of 20 consecutive patients with cluster headache, and found that 13 gave a history of migraine that had ceased at the onset of the cluster attacks. Others have found that migraine occurred previously in about 15 per cent of this patient population (Sutherland and Eadie, 1972). A family history of migraine is noted in about 20 per cent of patients with cluster headache, and this is no greater than in an age-matched control population (Lance and Anthony, 1971).

EXAMINATION FINDINGS

A carefully elicited history is the key to diagnosis. There are no abnormalities to be found upon physical or laboratory investigation other than occasional Horner's syndrome, and in approximately 70 per cent of patients with cluster headache the carotid artery is palpably tender at several points in the neck (Raskin and Prusiner, 1977). This phenomenon is discussed in detail in Chapter 2. The cluster headache syndrome is not associated with any underlying intracranial structural abnormalities (Russell et al, 1978).

PATHOPHYSIOLOGIC MECHANISMS

Evidence that paroxysmal instability of both intra- and extracerebral arteries is an important mechanism of cluster attacks will be reviewed in this section. However, how these vascular changes are initiated and the mechanism(s) that explain the periodicity and symptoms of parasympathetic discharge are largely unknown. One may speculate that paroxysmal excitability of vasomotor centers within the hypothalamus, for example, could explain the features of this disorder, as well as its responsiveness to agents that exert prominent effects on the central nervous system, such as lithium and the corticosteroids (see below). The drugs that are effective in the cluster headache syndrome bring about alterations of central serotonergic synapses similar to those that occur in the treatment of migraine (see Chapter 4), suggesting that defective modulation of neuronal release of serotonin may be common to both disorders.

VASOMOTOR INSTABILITY

Dilatation of extracerebral arteries appears to be the common denominator of both migraine and cluster headache; enhanced pulsation of the intraocular vascular bed occurs during cluster pain attacks but not during migraine attacks (Hørven et al, 1972, 1977), underlining the involvement of the internal carotid artery and its branches in the cluster headache syndrome. The frequency of paralysis of the ocular sympathetic supply, and the angiographic observation of narrowing of the extradural parasellar portion of the internal carotid artery (Ekbom and Greitz, 1970) (probably the result of edema of the wall of the artery), also point to the frequency of carotid involvement. Evidence that at least part of the pain of cluster headache is derived from dilatation of intracranial branches of the internal carotid artery stems from the observation of Thomas and Butler (1946) that the pain may be relieved in some patients by the intrathecal injection of saline, increasing the CSF pressure to 700 mm of water.

The importance of vascular dilatation in cluster headache is emphasized by the precipitation of headaches during a bout by vasodilators such as alcohol, histamine (Horton, 1941, 1952) and nitroglycerin (Ekbom, 1968); moreover, CBF is increased during an attack (Norris et al, 1976; Sakai and Meyer, 1978). Amelioration may be achieved by maneuvers that increase the cerebral resistance, such as the infusion of norepinephrine (Ekbom and Lindahl, 1970). However, these inferences regarding vasodilatation and vasoconstriction should be interpreted with caution; the lag period between the ingestion of alcohol or nitroglycerin and the resulting pain attack is not explicable by the known time-course of the effects of these drugs on the peripheral or central vasculature. There are diverse hemodynamic effects of norepinephrine that may be more to the point than the modification of CBF.

Friedman et al (1973), using facial thermography, have found in 85 per cent of patients with cluster headache multiple spotted areas of dense coolness ($1° C$) in the supraorbital region ipsilateral to the headache. These hypothermic islands are generally in the distribution of extracranial branches of the internal carotid artery, but are often distributed in the border zone that lies between the internal and external carotid circulation. In most patients the cool spots persist for several months after the bouts end. The mechanism of this presumably focal change in cutaneous circulation is not clear; it may simply be evidence of instability of vasomotor regulation. Reduction of the severity of angina pectoris and limb claudication has been noted during some cluster bouts (Ekbom, 1970a), so that, at least in some patients, an alteration of arterial tone outside the carotid circulation probably occurs.

BIOCHEMICAL MECHANISMS

A search for biochemical agents has been made on the presumption that the cluster headache syndrome may be mediated by a disorder of humoral control of blood vessels. The prominence of lacrimation, perspiration and suffusion of the conjunctivae are consistent with an excessive cholinergic discharge. This reasoning led Kunkle (1959) to examine CSF for acetylcholine-like activity, which he found in four out of 14 patients at the time of headache; it was not found in seven patients with classic migraine. Platelet serotonin does not change significantly during cluster headache attacks (Anthony and Lance, 1971).

The possibility that histamine may be involved is supported by the reportedly higher incidence of duodenal ulceration in patients with cluster headache (Ekbom, 1970a), as well as by the precipitation of attacks with small amounts of this substance. Anthony and Lance (1971, 1978a) have shown that there is a modest increase in whole blood histamine during an attack; furthermore, elevations of urinary histamine were found in four out of eight patients during cluster attacks (Sjaastad and Sjaastad, 1970). These reports are challenged by the lack of change in the catabolic pattern of intravenously administered C^{14} histamine in patients with cluster headache (Beall and Van Arsdel, 1960) and, since histamine is localized peripherally to basophilic leukocytes, caution is advisable in the interpretation of whole blood levels (Porter and Mitchell, 1972). Further, antihistaminic agents available in the past were disappointingly ineffective, as also has been histamine densensitization.

Although it has been apparent for some time that there are at least two histamine receptors, since some of the effects of histamine are not blocked by the usual antihistaminic agents (Ash and Schild, 1966), substantial evidence for two receptors, H_1 and H_2, has been provided recently by Black et al (1972). Since histamine-induced vasodilatation is only partly reversed by H_1 antagonists, and it now appears likely that both H_1 and H_2 receptors are present in the carotid vascular bed (Saxena, 1975), the recent availability of H_2 antagonists has renewed interest in testing the role of histamine in cluster headache. Appenzeller et al (1978) have noted that mast cells (the major repository of histamine in many tissues) are found in increased number in skin biopsies from the temples of cluster patients. Anthony et al (1978a,b) have used H_1 and H_2 antagonists in the therapy of cluster headache, without clear-cut success. It is possible that the elevation of blood histamine and the concentration of mast cells are the result of episodes of paroxysmal vascular instability, since histamine is but one of a group of diverse substances that includes the kinins, prostaglandins and others that are released from tissues during injury or inflammatory reactions (Beaven, 1976).

NEUROGENIC MECHANISMS

Stimulation of the greater superficial petrosal nerve evokes lacrimation and rhinorrhea (Robinson, 1958), but transection of this nerve has not been a useful therapeutic approach (Gardner et al, 1947). White and Sweet (1969) stimulated this nerve during craniotomy under local anesthesia, and produced periorbital or periaural pain in most of their patients. After section of the nerve, pain could be elicited by stimulation of only the central end, indicating that the effect was mediated through afferent fibers and not indirectly by peripheral vasodilatation. There are no reports of the consistent success of any surgical procedure in stopping bouts of cluster headache, although section of the trigeminal nerve may relieve the painful component of the attacks (Lance and Anthony, 1971). The recent demonstration of the clinical efficacy of lithium carbonate (a salt with diverse effects on the CNS and no known effects, direct or indirect, on blood vessels) has heightened interest in the possibility that the cluster syndrome is primarily central in origin.

PSYCHOLOGIC MECHANISMS

No compelling data have been presented to support the contention that a primary emotional disorder is important to the mechanism of cluster headache.

TREATMENT

The original rationale for therapy in this condition was to administer a vasoconstrictor such as ergotamine tartrate to antagonize the paroxysmal vasodilation that appears to be the cardinal mechanism of pain production. However, the efficacy of agents that have no direct vasoactivity, and have been arrived at empirically, has cast doubt on the vasoconstrictor hypothesis. It is possible that the different treatment modes discussed in this section are sucessful because of their effect on regulatory centers within the brain that initiate vascular instability.

The most satisfactory treatment is the administration of drugs to *prevent* cluster attacks until the bout is over. There are several effective pharmacologic options that may be pursued in this regard. However, whichever agent is used, there may be a lag period of days or, occasionally, weeks before effective suppression is achieved. For this reason, it is essential to attempt to treat the individual attacks until they can be prevented. Since the attacks are so brief and reach a crescendo so rapidly, orally administered, slowly absorbed drugs are generally ineffectual, but inhalational agents may be very useful. The ergotamine tartrate aerosol at a dosage of 0.36 to 0.72 mg (1 to 2 inhalations) is effective about 80 per cent of the time (Speed, 1960). Two important aspects of the use of the aerosol are often overlooked, and account for many apparent treatment failures:

(1) Because the drug is formulated as a suspension, it is essential that the canister be shaken vigorously before each administration.

(2) Patients should be instructed to administer the aerosol after a forced expiration, simultaneous with the onset of inspiration. The breath should then be held in deep inspiration for several seconds, and then slowly exhaled.

The inhalation of 100 per cent oxygen, a cerebral vasoconstrictor (Sokoloff, 1959), via a tight-fitting mask at a flow rate of 8 to 10 liters per minute for 5 to 10 minutes has been dramatically effective for most of those patients for whom this approach proved to be feasible; in our experience with 50 patients, 38 were markedly relieved by oxygen inhalation. This mode of therapy, although recommended by Horton (1952) almost 30 years ago, has never been substantiated by controlled trials. Dramatic anecdotes regarding oxygen use continue to be reported (Janks, 1978), and in view of its relative safety this appears to be a worthwhile approach. Sakai and Meyer (1979) have recently shown that marked cerebral vasoconstriction results from the administration of 100 per cent oxygen during cluster headache attacks.

Another option that is frequently useful is the inhalation of methoxyflurane, a rapid-acting analgesic. Patients are instructed to rapidly apply 10 to 15 drops to a handkerchief, pillow case or paper tissue, form a funnel with their hands and inhale for several seconds. They should be seated or reclining at this time, since light-headedness may ensue. The analgesia produced by this agent lasts but a few minutes, but if administered very early the attack may be aborted (Raskin, unpublished observations).

PROPHYLAXIS

Symonds (1956) was the first to describe the use and effectiveness of ergotamine tartrate in preventing attacks. Doses of 0.25 to 0.5 mg subcutaneously twice to three times daily for five days per week (the "off" days are to prevent cumulative effects and allow the patient to assess whether the bout had come to its natural conclusion) was the regimen that Bickerstaff (1959) found to be completely successful from the first full day of injections in 12 of 16 patients. The usual dosage was 0.25 mg three times daily. Others have found that 0.5 to 1.0 mg ergotamine tartrate in suppository form before retiring (for strictly nocturnal attacks) or twice daily is effective in a substantial proportion of patients, although precise data have not been published. The oral forms of this drug (2 to 4 mg daily) are less effective, and also offer less risk toward ergotism (Friedman et al, 1959). The advantage of ergotamine tartrate in this condition is that its clinical effect may be assessed within 24 hours, an obviously important consideration for patients experiencing several attacks of high-intensity pain every day. Long-term risk factors must be placed into the context of a relatively short exposure to whichever agent is chosen.

The beneficial effects of ergotamine tartrate identified the cluster headache syndrome as a condition responsive to this traditional antimigrainous drug; newer drugs that are effective in migraine have also been successful in treating cluster headache. Propranolol, amitriptyline and cyproheptadine are used widely, with anecdotal reports of success.

Three additional drugs, methysergide, prednisone and lithium, have recently been evaluated (Kudrow, 1978). Lithium carbonate appears to be especially promising in the treatment of chronic non-cyclic cluster attacks (Ekbom, 1974a,b; Kudrow, 1977, 1978; Mathew, 1978). The effective dosage has ranged from 600 to 1,500 mg per day, and favorable responses occur within the first week of treatment in approximately 80 per cent of these patients. The rationale for the introduction of lithium to cluster headache therapy was by a rather distant analogy drawn from manic-depressive psychosis, a cyclical lithium-responsive disorder (Ekbom, 1977). Lithium has no known peripheral vasoactive effects; at the neuronal level, within the CNS, intracellular sodium is displaced, the release of norepinephrine is inhibited and the turnover of serotonin is increased (Johnson and Johnson, 1978), to name a few of the effects of lithium on brain metabolism that may be relevant to cluster headache. The implication of lithium in the regulation of serotonin biosynthesis in brain (Mandell and Knapp, 1977) raises the possibility that the primary mechanism of cluster headache is closely related to that of migraine (see Chapter 4). However, its mode of action in both manic-depressive psychosis and cluster headache is unknown. The remarkably high success rate of this drug without known direct effects on blood vessels, but with prominent effects on the CNS supports the view that the cluster headache syndrome is central in origin.

Lithium is readily absorbed from the GI tract, and peak plasma levels are reached two to four hours after its ingestion. The drug should be given in three divided doses, initially 900 mg daily, which may be decreased if side-effects appear by breaking the tablet formulation of the drug into halves and adjusting the dosage downward. Since sodium depletion promotes the retention of lithium, the risk of intoxication is lessened by avoiding a low-salt diet and the use of natriuretic drugs (Jefferson and Kalin, 1979). Plasma levels obtained 12 hours after the last dose should be maintained below 1.2 meq per liter (Amdisen, 1978), and should be measured weekly during the first few weeks of therapy and monthly thereafter. Nausea, vomiting, diarrhea, tremor, blurred vision and gait unsteadiness are the commonest side-effects and are dose-related. A small proportion of patients with cluster headaches appear to be uniquely disposed to the development of occipital throbbing headaches due to lithium (Kudrow, 1977), which may preclude use of the drug. Higher plasma levels may produce myoclonic jerks, dysarthria, hypotension, convulsions and renal failure; rigidity of the limbs and fasciculations are characteristic features of moderate-to-severe degrees of intoxication. Hemodialysis is the most effective means of dealing with serious toxicity (Hansen and Amdisen, 1978).

A double-blind controlled study (Jammes, 1975) and other data (Kudrow, 1978) indicate that prednisone is highly successful (75 per cent) in the suppression of cluster cycles, although the mechanism for this is unclear. The dosage has varied from 20 mg every other day to 40 mg per day, and the drug is usually administered for two weeks and then tapered off. Dramatic improvement is seen most often within the first 24 hours of steroid administration. As with lithium, corticosteroids have prominent effects on the CNS (DeWied and Weijnen, 1970), including the regulation of neuronal serotonin synthesis (Costa and Meek, 1974) and little known vasoactivity.

Methysergide is effective in about 60 per cent of patients with cluster headache (Kudrow, 1978), in a dose range of 4 to 10 mg per day. The major (rare) hazard of methysergide therapy, retroperitoneal fibrosis, which may appear after several months of its use, is not an important consideration for a disorder that usually requires only four to six weeks of treatment. Improvement usually begins within the first few days of therapy; however, responses occasionally may be delayed for 10 to 14 days.

A variant of cluster headache, called chronic paroxysmal hemicrania, in which multiple, brief daily attacks of focal headache occur, has been found to be remarkably responsive to indomethacin, in doses of 25 to 150 mg daily, and not to the other drugs that are usually effective in cluster headache (Sjaastad and Dale, 1976; Price and Posner, 1978; Sjaastad et al, 1979).

Several pharmacologic agents are now available that are likely to provide substantial relief for patients with cluster headache. None are effective in all cases, so that perseverance and a systematic approach are important. The choice is arbitrary as to which agent should be employed first (except in the instance of chronic, noncyclic attacks in which lithium appears to be the drug of choice); many physicians prefer prednisone or ergotamine tartrate in order to gain an almost immediate effect. The frequency and intensity of the attacks, as well as the patient's other health problems, are the major factors that aid the physician in weighing the potential risks implicit in any pharmacologic program.

REFERENCES

Amdisen, A. (1978): Clinical and serum-level monitoring in lithium therapy and lithium intoxication. J. Anal. Toxicol. 2:193–202.

Anthony, M. and Lance, J. W. (1971): Histamine and serotonin in cluster headache. Arch. Neurol. 25:225–231.

Anthony, M., Lance, J. W. and Lord, G. (1978a): Migrainous neuralgia — blood histamine levels and clinical response to H_1 and H_2 receptor blockade. In Current Concepts in Migraine Research, ed. R. Greene. Raven Press, New York, pp. 149–151.

Anthony, M., Lord, G. D. A. and Lance, J. W. (1978b): Controlled trials of cimetidine in migraine and cluster headache. Headache 18:261–264.

Appenzeller, O., Becker, W. and Ragas, A. (1978): Cluster headache: ultrastructural aspects. Neurology 28:371.

Ash, A. S. F. and Schild, H. O. (1966): Receptors mediating some actions of histamine. Br. J. Pharmacol. 27:427–439.

Atkinson, R. (1977): Physical fitness and headache. Headache 17:189–195.

Balla, J. I. and Walton, J. N. (1964): Periodic migrainous neuralgia. Br. Med. J. 1:219–221.

Beall, G. N. and Van Arsdel, P. P. (1960): Histamine metabolism in human disease. J. Clin. Invest. 39:676–683.

Beaven, M. A. (1976): Histamine. N. Engl. J. Med. 294:30–36, 320–325.

Bickerstaff, E. R. (1959): The periodic migrainous neuralgia of Wilfred Harris. Lancet 1:1069–1071.

Black, J. W., Duncan, W. A. M., Durant, C. J. et al (1972): Definition and antagonism of histamine H_2 receptors. Nature 236:385–390.

Costa, E. and Meek, J. L. (1974): Regulation of the biosynthesis of catecholamines and serotonin in the CNS. Annu. Rev. Pharmacol. 14:491–511.

DeWied, D. and Weijnen, J.A.W.M. (1970): Pituitary, adrenal, and the brain. Progr. Brain Res. 32:1–357.

Ekbom, K. (1968): Nitroglycerin as a provocative agent in cluster headache. Arch. Neurol. 19:487–493.

Ekbom, K. (1970a): Patterns of cluster headache with a note on the relations to angina pectoris and peptic ulcer. Acta Neurol. Scand. 46:225–237.

Ekbom, K. (1970b): A clinical comparison of cluster headache and migraine. Acta Neurol. Scand. 46 (suppl.) 41:1–48.

Ekbom, K. (1974a): Clinical aspects of cluster headache. Headache 13:176–180.

Ekbom, K. (1974b): Litium vid kroniska symptom av cluster headache. Opusc. Med. 19:148–156.

Ekbom, K. (1975): Some observations on pain in cluster headache. Headache 14:219–225.

Ekbom, K. (1977): Lithium in the treatment of chronic cluster headache. Headache 17:39–40.

Ekbom, K. and Greitz, T. (1970): Carotid angiography in cluster headache. Acta Radiol. (Diagn.) (Stockh.) 10:1–10.

Ekbom, K. and Lindahl, J. (1970): Effect of induced rise in blood pressure on pain in cluster headache. Acta Neurol. Scand. 46:585–600.

Friedman, A. P. (1969): Atypical facial pain. Headache 9:27–30.

Friedman, A. P. and Mikropoulos, H. E. (1958): Cluster headaches. Neurology 8:653–663.

Friedman, A. P., von Storch, T. J. C. and Araki, S. (1959): Ergotamine tartrate: its history, action and proper use in the treatment of migraine. N. Y. State J. Med. 59:2359–2366.

Friedman, A. P., Wood, E. H., Rowan, A. J. and Frazier, S. H. (1973): Observations on vascular headache of the migraine type. In Background to Migraine, 5th Migraine Symposium, ed. J. N. Cumings. Springer-Verlag, New York, pp. 1–17.

Gardner, W. M., Stowell, A. and Dutlinger, R. (1947): Resection of the greater superficial petrosal nerve in the treatment of unilateral headache. J. Neurosurg. 4:105–114.

Hansen, H. E. and Amdisen, A. (1978): Lithium intoxication. Q. J. Med. 47:123–144.

Hornabrook, R. W. (1964): Migrainous neuralgia. N. Z. Med. J. 63:774–779.

Horton, B. T. (1941): The use of histamine in the treatment of specific types of headache. J.A.M.A. 116:377–383.

Horton, B. T. (1952): Histamine cephalgia. Journal-Lancet 72:92–98.

Horton, B. T. (1961): Histaminic cephalgia. Md. State Med. J. 10:178–203.

Hørven, I., Nornes, H. and Sjaastad, O. (1972): Different corneal indentation pulse patterns in cluster headache and migraine. Neurology 22:92–98.

Hørven, I. and Sjaastad, O. (1977): Cluster headache syndrome and migraine. Acta Ophthalmol. 55:35–51.

Jammes, J. J. (1975): The treatment of cluster headaches with prednisone. Dis. Nerv. Syst. 36:375–376.

Janks, J. F. (1978): Oxygen for cluster headaches. J.A.M.A. 239:191.

Jefferson, J. W. and Kalin, N. H. (1979): Serum lithium levels and long-term diuretic use. J.A.M.A. 241:1134–1136.

Johnson, F. N. and Johnson, S. (eds.) (1978): Lithium in Medical Practice, Proceedings of the 1st British Lithium Congress. University Park Press, Baltimore, 459 pp.

Kudrow, L. (1977): Lithium prophylaxis for chronic cluster headache. Headache 17:15–18.

Kudrow, L. (1978): Comparative results of prednisone, methysergide, and lithium therapy in cluster headache. In Current Concepts in Migraine Research, ed. R. Green. Raven Press, New York, pp. 159–163.

Kunkle, E. C. (1959): Acetylcholine in the mechanism of headaches of the migraine type. Arch. Neurol. Psychiatry 81:135–140.

Lance, J. W. and Anthony, M. (1971): Migrainous neuralgia or cluster headache? J. Neurol. Sci. 13:401–414.

Mandell, A. J. and Knapp, S. (1977): Regulation of serotonin biosynthesis in brain: role of the high affinity uptake of tryptophan into serotonergic neurons. Fed. Proc. 36:2142–2148

Mason, D. T. and Braunwald, E. (1965): The effects of nitroglycerin and amyl nitrite on arteriolar and venous tone in the human forearm. Circulation 32:755–766.

Mathew, N. T. (1978): Clinical subtypes of cluster headache and response to lithium therapy. Headache 18:26–30.

von Möllendorff (1867): Ueber Hemikranie. Virchows Arch. (Pathol. Anat.) 41:385–395.

Nieman, E. A. and Hurwitz, L. J. (1961): Ocular sympathetic palsy in periodic migrainous neuralgia. J. Neurol. Neurosurg. Psychiatry 24:369–373.

Norris, J. W., Hachinski, V. C. and Cooper, P. W. (1976): Cerebral blood flow changes in cluster headache. Acta Neurol. Scand. 54:371–374.

198

Porter, J. F. and Mitchell, R. G. (1972): Distribution of histamine in human blood. Physiol. Rev. 52:361–381.

Price, R. W. and Posner, J. B. (1978): Chronic paroxysmal hemicrania: a disabling headache syndrome responding to indomethacin. Ann. Neurol. 3:183–184.

Raskin, N. H. and Prusiner, S. (1977): Carotidynia. Neurology 27:43–46.

Riley, F.C. and Moyer, N. J. (1971): Oculosympathetic paresis associated with cluster headaches. Am. J. Ophthalmol. 72:763–768.

Robinson, B. W. (1958): Histaminic cephalgia. Medicine 37:161–180.

Russell, D., Nakstad, P. and Sjaastad, O. (1978): Cluster headache — pneumoencephalographic and cerebral computerized axial tomography findings. Headache 18:272–273.

Sakai, F. and Meyer, J. S. (1978): Regional cerebral hemodynamics during migraine and cluster headaches measured by the Xe^{133} inhalation method. Headache 18:122–132.

Sakai, F. and Meyer, J. S. (1979): Abnormal cerebrovascular reactivity in patients with migraine and cluster headache. Headache 19:257–266.

Saxena, P. R. (1975): The significance of histamine H_1 and H_2 receptors on the carotid vascular bed in the dog. Neurology 25:681–687.

Sjaastad, O. and Dale, I. (1976): A new clinical headache entity "chronic paroxysmal hemicrania" 2. Acta Neurol. Scand. 54:140–159.

Sjaastad, O., Egge, K., Hørven, I. et al (1979): Chronic paroxysmal hemicrania: mechanical precipitation of attacks.Headache 19:31–36.

Sjaastad, O. and Sjaastad, O. V. (1970): The histaminuria in vascular headache. Acta Neurol. Scand. 46:331–342.

Sokoloff, L. (1959): The action of drugs on the cerebral circulation. Pharmacol. Rev. 11:1–85.

Speed, W. G. (1960): Ergotamine tartrate inhalation: a new approach to the management of recurrent vascular headaches. Am. J. Med. Sci. 240:327–331.

Sutherland, J. M. and Eadie, M. J. (1972): Cluster headache. Res. Clin. Stud. Headache 3:92–125.

Symonds, C. P. (1956): A particular variety of headache. Brain 79:217–232.

Thomas, W. A. and Butler, S. (1946): Treatment of migraine by intravenous histamine. Am. J. Med. 1:39–44.

White, J.C. and Sweet, W. H. (1969): Pain and the Neurosurgeon. Charles C Thomas, Springfield, Ill, pp. 345–372.

CHAPTER 7

POST-TRAUMATIC HEADACHE

In 1975 there were 1.4 million seriously head-injured people in the United States, at a cost to the community of over 2 billion dollars (Caveness, 1977). A substantial number of these individuals complain of headache, vertigo, impairment of memory and concentration, and emotional instability for weeks, months or even years after the injury. This syndrome is not known to be associated with anatomic lesions of the central nervous system and may occur whether or not a person was rendered unconscious by head trauma. Since the designation "concussion" is customarily restricted to a syndrome of head injury associated with loss of consciousness, the term "post-traumatic syndrome" will be used here descriptively, although others have used "post-concussive" to describe an identical syndrome.

Headache persisting for more than two months occurs in 40 to 60 per cent of patients hospitalized after closed head injury (Brenner et al, 1944). Although intense post-traumatic symptoms may arise following major head injury, severe and protracted headache disorders also are found after seemingly trivial head trauma. The development of headache does not correlate with the duration of unconsciousness or post-traumatic amnesia when these occur, nor with electroencephalographic abnormalities, presence of skull fracture or the finding of blood in the CSF (Brenner et al, 1944; Kay et al, 1971). The appearance of severe symptoms in the absence of neurologic signs or evidence of external head injury has led to divergent views regarding psychologic and organic factors that may bear on the mechanism of the post-traumatic syndrome.

It can be difficult to disentangle the symptoms occurring after head trauma from those that relate more directly to the initiation of

199

a claim for compensation. Although the recognition of the post-traumatic syndrome preceded the inauguration of compensation payments (Taylor, 1967), over the years, as financial settlements have been more vigorously pursued, the incidence of complaints following head injury has increased. Moreover, early settlement of an outstanding claim may be the single most significant factor contributing to ultimate recovery (Miller, 1961). Nevertheless, there is substantial evidence that an organic mechanism is operative in a large proportion of these patients. The problem confronting the physician is to assign the correct proportion of organic and psychologic factors in each particular instance. It is our intention in this chapter to characterize the clinical syndrome so that this distinction may be made more easily; furthermore, we will examine the putative mechanism(s) of this syndrome as well as avenues of therapy.

CLINICAL SYNDROME

Headache is the dominant symptom of the post-traumatic syndrome. It usually appears within 24 hours of the occurrence of head injury, although about 6 per cent of patients do not experience headache until some days or even weeks afterward (Jacobson, 1963). It usually worsens over a period of days to weeks, and then gradually improves over a similar time-course. Occasionally it exhibits a waxing and waning course, and dramatic worsening of headache may occur several months after it had subsided to a considerable extent. The large majority of patients experience a dull, aching, constant, generalized discomfort, with exacerbations that may be polar (i.e., bifrontal, bitemporal or bioccipital) (45 per cent), generalized (35 per cent) or unilateral (20 per cent), and usually persist for several hours. At such times the pain is usually throbbing in quality (Symonds, 1974; Behrman, 1977) and in about 10 per cent of patients is accompanied by scintillating scotomata (Simons and Wolff, 1946). Headache is commonly worsened by effort, stooping, coughing or rapid movement of the head, and alleviated by reclining and/or sleep — features characteristic of vascular headaches. Nausea often accompanies intense headache episodes and vomiting occurs in about 15 per cent of cases (Jacobson, 1963). Ergotamine tartrate can abort the intense throbbing component of the syndrome in a minority of patients (Simons and Wolff, 1946).

Vertigo, lightheadedness or giddiness occur almost as often as headache (Denny-Brown, 1945), and although such symptoms most often appear during severe headache bouts, they may arise quite independently of headache, as is true for the other symptoms that comprise this syndrome. Vertigo is usually experienced as a rotary illusion, although sensations of rocking, falling, tilting and rising off the ground have also been noted. It is often accentuated or produced by movement of the head or rapid change in body position. When syncope takes place as it does in about 10 per cent of cases, it is almost invariably in vertiginous patients (Jacobson, 1963). Occasionally, patients experience episodic paresthesia of the limbs or ataxia. Syncopal episodes following the onset of a paroxysmal headache sometimes occur and should not be confused with seizures (Osler and Fusillo, 1965).

Impaired concentration and memory, easy fatigability and irritability occur with remarkable uniformity in most patients with other post-traumatic symptoms, and occasionally in the absence of vertigo or headache. It has recently become clear that virtually all of those who have suffered concussion for a period are unable to process information at a normal rate (Gronwall and Wrightson, 1974), and also manifest impaired visual reaction times (Van Zomeren and Deelman, 1978). Clinical recovery parallels improvement in these relatively objective tests. The occurrence of additional symptoms when cognitive abilities are reduced is explicable by straightforward psychologic mechanisms. A patient who has made a good physical recovery after concussion may feel well enough to return to work; his apparent intelligence is unaffected. However, jobs that he previously could have completed easily now require his entire attention, and soon tire him. Simultaneous attention to multiple tasks may be beyond his capacity. The anxiety generated from this circumstance, aggravated by doubting and nonsupportive physicians, may result in hypochondriasis, depression, obsessional trends and conversion reactions (Merskey and Woodforde, 1972). These secondary psychologic reactions arise independent of pending claims for compensation, and tend to improve over a time-course that does not appear to be altered if a financial settlement is made (Merskey and Woodforde, 1972; Kelly, 1975). The development of these symptoms into a disease in its own right ("accident neurosis") probably depends to a large measure on the patient's reaction to a disabling condition that he cannot understand. How he responds will depend on his emotional stability as well as the explanation and support that he receives.

Children who sustain head injuries and develop post-traumatic symptoms respond differently from adults. Hyperkinesia, poor anger control, impaired attention and enuresis occur as the dominant symptoms of the syndrome; headache is a less severe symptom and vertigo is rare (Dillon and Leopold, 1961; Black et al, 1969).

Post-traumatic migraine. Recurring attacks of migraine have been recorded as sequelae of closed head injury (Michael and Williams, 1952; Burke and Peters, 1956; Behrman, 1977). Moreover, attacks indistinguishable from classic migraine may repeatedly occur immediately after blows to the head and in no other circumstances

(Haas and Sovner, 1969; Matthews, 1972; Greenblatt, 1973). Whether the mechanism involved in these instances is identical to that of the post-traumatic syndrome is not clear. The responsiveness of at least some patients with post-traumatic headache to propranolol (Vijayan and Dreyfus, 1975) raises the possibility that vasomotor instability may be common to both.

NATURAL HISTORY

Most published reports of the outcome of patients with post-traumatic symptoms consider those with penetrating brain wounds, cerebral contusions and lacerations, as well as those with simple concussion, so that there is a paucity of data regarding the natural history of the latter circumstance, which is the commonest problem confronted by physicians. Denker's (1944) series of 100 selected patients with the post-traumatic syndrome is one that includes only those who had sustained a simple closed head injury, who were followed for at least three years to establish the course of the syndrome. For none of these patients was there any pending litigation or compensation. In no case was there focal neurologic abnormality, evidence of skull fracture or blood in the CSF. Eighty of these patients were unconscious for varying periods after head injury, but none for longer than one hour. Of the remainder, there was no alteration of awareness whatever in 12 and only momentary stunning in eight. Neither the severity nor the duration of post-traumatic symptoms correlated with the duration of unconsciousness in this or in other series of cases (Russell, 1932). Only about ten of these patients were symptom-free in a month (Table 7–1), and at the end of a year about 30 continued to complain of headache, dizziness and cerebration difficulties. About 15 patients continued to be symptomatic after three years. Russell (1932) found that 60 per cent of those in his series continued with symptoms after six months. In a study of over 300 males, many of whom sustained penetrating wounds of the brain during World War II, Walker and Erculei (1969) found that 60 per cent continued to complain of headache,

TABLE 7–1. DURATION OF THE POST-TRAUMATIC SYNDROME
IN 100 PATIENTS*

Less than 30 days	10%
Less than 1 year	70%
Less than 2 years	80%
Less than 3 years	85%

*Data drawn from Denker, 1944.

vertigo and impaired concentration *15 years* after the injury. Thus, the *duration*, but not the incidence nor the intensity, of the post-traumatic syndrome appears to correlate with the severity of brain injury. Anosmia is significantly more common in patients who develop post-traumatic symptoms than in those who do not (Kay et al, 1971). Individuals over 40 years of age are more likely to have persisting symptoms than those under 30 (Denker, 1944).

The duration of *disability* following the appearance of post-traumatic symptoms appears to be based on the persistence of symptoms of impaired concentrating ability, difficulty in thinking, and anxiety (Denny-Brown, 1945; Miller, 1961). Kelly (1975) has suggested that originally organically-determined symptoms may become perpetuated as an anxiety reaction or depressive illness because physicians' nonsupportive or skeptical attitudes generate these manifestations of fear, hopelessness and helplessness. Using a positive, supportive approach he was able to show that 84 of 110 patients with post-traumatic symptoms returned to work, completely recovered, *before* a financial settlement was made.

PATHOPHYSIOLOGIC MECHANISMS

The sequelae of head injury with which we are concerned may be related to the mechanism of concussion *per se*, a brief review of which follows. Other lines of biologic evidence that point to prolonged vascular and neuronal dysfunction following concussion, some of which correlate with post-traumatic symptoms, will also be reviewed.

CONCUSSION

The clinical effects of concussion are well-known. Ommaya and Gennarelli (1974) have reviewed the evidence that concussion may occur without loss of consciousness; nevertheless, there is almost always an immediate depression of consciousness (lasting seconds to hours) which is accompanied by a brief period of respiratory arrest, bradycardia, hypotension and extensor plantar responses. After a variable period, the superficial reflexes return and the patient begins to stir and open his eyes, but cannot see. Gradually he returns to a level of alertness wherein perceptions may be made accurately but may not be remembered. Finally, there is full recovery and memory storage is again possible. The amnestic period often includes a period prior to the occurrence of injury. The duration of the post-traumatic amnestic period correlates fairly well with the severity of cerebral injury (Russell, 1935; Kay et al, 1971).

Experimental models of concussion have shown that an animal is rendered unconscious by a much lesser blow if the head is freely movable; the stationary head is more likely to be fractured, in which case energy is absorbed and diverted from the production of shearing stresses in cerebral tissue that appear to be important to the genesis of concussion (Denny-Brown and Russell, 1941). Moreover, head rotation during impact has been shown to be a critical factor in producing the diffuse shear strains (Ommaya and Gennarelli, 1974) that ultimately result in a rotary motion of brain; such motions probably underlie the syndrome of concussion. Ommaya and his colleagues (1968) have shown that cerebral concussion may be produced by rotational displacement of the head on the neck without significant direct head impact, i.e., a whiplash injury. Ommaya and Gennarelli (1976) contend that cortical and subcortical injury occurs initially, and that the rostral brain stem is affected when the degree of strain is large enough. It is not surprising that diffuse microscopic lesions of brain may result from such physical force, and this has been documented in human patients as well as in experimental animals (Oppenheimer, 1968; Gurdjian, 1972). Whether these lesions are causally related to the sequelae of concussion (Symonds, 1962) or whether they are epiphenomena (Ward, 1966) is not entirely clear. The bulk of the evidence supports the latter view.

In animal models of concussion, a biphasic cerebrovascular response occurs following brain trauma (Dila et al, 1976). In the injured region of brain, there is an early increase in the rate of arterial filling and perfusion flow which is probably the result of dilatation of precapillary arteries and arterioles. About one hour after trauma, there is either restitution of the pattern and rate of regional CBF to normal, or reduction to subnormal levels. These data imply that either the caliber of precapillary arteries returns to normal or that vasoconstriction occurs. This latter vascular response is accompanied by venous dilatation and stasis (Smith et al, 1969). Cerebral autoregulation is lost since these vascular responses to trauma are not modified by changes in arterial pCO_2. These observations, taken together with data demonstrating that the cerebral circulation is slowed in the post-traumatic syndrome, (Taylor and Bell, 1966; Oldendorf and Kitano, 1967), suggest the possibility that prolongation of vasoconstriction and vasomotor dysregulation occurs in some patients following head trauma, and may bear on the mechanism of the post-traumatic syndrome (see below).

Biochemical correlates of concussion are few. Acetylcholine-like activity, not normally present in CSF, appears in relatively high concentrations in the CSF following head injury (Bornstein, 1946); these elevations of acetylcholine levels may last for days or weeks, and parallel the profundity and duration of coma. With clinical improvement, CSF acetylcholine levels fall. Since acetylcholine in high concentrations can block synaptic transmission by depolarization of the postsynaptic membrane, elevated CSF levels are consistent with a theory of blockade of neural transmission in circuits known to be important for the maintenance of wakefulness (Ward, 1966). How neural membranes are altered to release acetylcholine is not clear. Anticholinergic drug therapy has not been shown to be effective in concussed patients.

POST-TRAUMATIC SYNDROME

No pathologic studies have been performed comparing brains of patients who manifested post-traumatic symptoms with those of individuals who were concussed and were soon thereafter asymptomatic. Both Taylor and Bell (1966) and Oldendorf and Kitano (1967) have shown that cerebral circulation time is significantly increased in patients with post-traumatic symptoms. Improvement of symptoms correlated with a return of the circulation time to normal. Skinhøj (1966), in seven patients with post-traumatic symptoms, found that CBF was reduced in one and the cerebral oxidative metabolic rate was reduced in two. It has been suggested (Taylor, 1967) that these findings support the concept that vasomotor instability is an important mechanism of the post-traumatic syndrome. This is supported by some of the clinical data described above, viz, vascular qualities of the headache disorder, "migrainous" phenomena in some patients, orthostatic and exertional aggravation of headache in many cases, and responsiveness to ergotamine tartrate and other vasoactive drugs in some patients. Furthermore, Friedman and Brenner (1944) showed that, in 13 of 22 patients with focal post-traumatic headache, injections of histamine, a dilator of intracerebral arteries, reproduced their characteristic headache, which was qualitatively different from the usual headache produced by histamine. This sensitivity to histamine is consistent with defective vasomotor regulation in these patients.

Two lines of evidence support the contention that diffuse cerebral dysfunction occurs in association with, and possibily is causally related to, the post-traumatic syndrome. In patients with persisting post-traumatic symptoms, the *visual evoked response* (VER) to light flashes of varying frequency is abnormal in that there is an inability for the VER to follow an increasing rate of stimulation. As the patient recovers, the VER (which receives contributions from cortical activity) is then able to follow higher rates of stimulation (Ommaya and Gennarelli, 1976). These findings may be analogous to those of Gronwall and Wrightson (1974), who studied concussed patients soon after head injury and found a delay in information rate-processing that usually returned to normal within 35 days. Individuals with post-traumatic symptoms required a significantly longer time than the concussed patient control group before being able to process information at a normal rate. Their symptoms receded as this test of cognition became normal. The possibility that a concurrent depression could have contributed to these results however, was not completely excluded in this study.

Electroencephalograms are abnormal in 55 per cent of patients with symptoms that follow closed head injury; focal slow waves account for over one-half of the abnormalities, with the remainder diffusely abnormal (Denker and Perry, 1954). Some of the most striking abnormalities have been seen in those who, clinically, were believed to be neurotic. The same frequency of EEG abnormalitiy occurs in those patients with either no loss of consciousness or only momentary dazing, as in those who have been unconscious for periods up to one hour. Similar changes are found in patients with recent head injuries of less than three months' duration as compared with those whose head injury had taken place one or two years previously.

Vestibular function has been assessed in large numbers of patients who complained of post-traumatic vertigo. Using electronystagmography, Toglia et al (1970), in over 100 patients, found 61 per cent to have abnormal caloric tests, 36 per cent to have latent vestibular nystagmus and 44 per cent to have abnormal rotary tests. Only a few of these patients were normal. The precise localization of the injury that explains these findings is not clear; in some of these individuals the vestibular end-organ apparatus had clearly been injured (Harrison, 1956), whereas in others a central disturbance was more likely.

Although much has been written regarding the *psychiatric aspects* of this syndrome (Miller, 1961), very few data have been collected systematically. At present, there are no data that allow one to approximate what proportion of patients channel the anxiety generated by a serious accident into a neurotic symptom complex of depression, hysteria, phobias or free anxiety. Merskey and Woodforde (1972) followed for two to four years 27 patients who were referred for psychiatric treatment, in none of whom was financial compensation an issue. The outcome of this group approximated the natural history of the disorder. These authors make the point that depression and anxiety are often valid sequelae of a frightening accident, and often occur independent of post-traumatic symptoms, although the two sets of symptoms may be superimposed. Depressive symptoms most often supervened after a lapse of one to three months, and were best explained as a response to head injury and its sequelae. No evidence for a primary psychiatric illness was found.

TREATMENT

Because the mechanisms of this syndrome are not understood, substantiated therapeutic programs have not yet been formulated. The following remarks regarding therapy are a summary of our point of view as well as the opinions of others, drawn from a large experience with patients with this disorder.

More important, perhaps, than in the treatment of any other group of those who complain of headache is the physician's attitude. Caring for and having an interest in these patients is essential for any therapeutic program. Communicating enthusiasm, support and a positive approach are certainly helpful in helping someone through what is very likely to be a self-limited problem. A careful explanation of the cause, mechanism and natural history of the symptoms, underlining the high probability of complete subsidence of symptoms within a relatively short period, is the first step; continued reassurance of the likelihood of remission on subsequent visits is also useful. A program of planned and graduated rehabilitation according to the patient's occupation and degree of disability, together with pharmacologic support, outlines the format used by Kelley (1975) in succeeding with 84 of 110 patients, all of whom returned to work before settlement of their claim, completely recovered.

The ergot alkaloids have been useful (Friedman, 1969), especially when used prophylactically, perhaps because of the evidence that the regulation of cranial arteries is altered and that the vessels are more susceptible to painful dilatation. Amitriptyline and propranolol are useful in an additional segment of these patients. Employing these three classes of drugs sequentially, alone or in combination in 100 consecutive patients with posttraumatic headache, 19 were markedly improved, 24 were moderately improved, and the remainder were either slightly better or unchanged (Raskin, unpublished observations). Additional analgesic support is usually necessary, and limits to the daily use of analgesics must be firmly drawn.

As with virtually all patients with chronic head pain, secondary neck muscle contraction may aggravate the over-all pain problem. Heat, massage, neck traction, a collar, a neck pillow and injection of trigger points with 1 per cent procaine are temporarily useful at times, and are worth pursuing (Friedman, 1969).

Over-all, the physician's impact in markedly modifying these patients' complaints is far less than in treating migraine, for example. Nevertheless, the large majority of these patients can and do return to work and experience eventual remission of symptoms.

REFERENCES

Behrman, S. (1977): Migraine as a sequela of blunt head injury. Injury 9:74–76.
Black, P., Jeffries, J. J., Blumer, D., Wellner, A. and Walker, A. E. (1969): The post-

traumatic syndrome in children. *In* The Late Effects of Head Injury, eds. A. E. Walker, W. F. Caveness and M. Critchley. Charles C Thomas, Springfield, Ill. pp. 142–149.

Bornstein, M. B. (1946): Presence and action of acetylcholine in experimental brain trauma. J. Neurophysiol. 9:349–366.

Brenner, C., Friedman, A. P., Merritt, H. H. and Denny-Brown, D. E. (1944): Post-traumatic headache. J. Neurosurg. 1:379–391.

Burke, E. C. and Peters, G. A. (1956): Migraine in childhood. Am. J. Dis. Child. 92:330–336.

Caveness, W. F. (1977): Incidence of craniocerebral trauma in the United States, 1970–1975. Trans. Am. Neurol. Assoc. 102:136–138.

Denker, P. G. (1944): The post concussion syndrome: prognosis and evaluation of the organic factors. N. Y. State J. Med. 44:379–384.

Denker, P. G. and Perry, G. F. (1954): Post concussion syndrome in compensation and litigation. Neurology 4:912–918.

Denny-Brown, D. (1945): Disability arising from closed head injury. J.A.M.A. 127:429–436.

Denny-Brown, D. and Russell, W. R. (1941): Experimental cerebral concussion. Brain 64:93–164.

Dila, C., Bouchard, L., Myer, E., Yamamoto, L. and Feindel, W. (1976): Microvascular response to minimal brain trauma. *In* Head Injuries, ed. R. McLaurin. Grune and Stratton, New York, pp. 213–215.

Dillon, H. and Leopold, R. L. (1961): Children and the post-concussion syndrome. J.A.M.A. 175:86–92.

Friedman, A. P. (1969): The so-called post-traumatic headache. *In* The Late Effects of Head Injury, eds. A. E. Walker, W. F. Caveness and M. Critchley. Charles C Thomas, Springfield, Ill., pp. 55–71.

Friedman, A. P. and Brenner, C. (1944): Post-traumatic and histamine headache. Arch. Neurol. Psychiatry 52:126–130.

Greenblatt, S. H. (1973): Post-traumatic transient cerebral blindness. J.A.M.A. 225:1073–1076.

Gronwall, D. and Wrightson, P. (1974): Delayed recovery of intellectual function after minor head injury. Lancet 2:605–609.

Gurdjian, E. S. (1972): Recent advances in the study of the mechanism of impact injury of the head. Clin. Neurosurg. 19:1–42.

Haas, D. C. and Sovner, R. D. (1969): Migraine attacks triggered by mild head trauma and their relation to certain post-traumatic disorders of childhood. J. Neurol. Neurosurg. Psychiatry 32:548–554.

Harrison, M.S. (1956): Notes on the clinical features and pathology of post-concussional vertigo with especial reference to positional nystagmus. Brain 79:474–482.

Jacobson, S. A. (1963): The Post-Traumatic Syndrome Following Head Injury. Charles C Thomas, Springfield, Ill.

Kay, D. W. K., Kerr, T. A. and Lassman, L. P. (1971): Brain trauma and the postconcussional syndrome. Lancet 2:1052–1055.

Kelly, R. (1975): The post-traumatic syndrome: an iatrogenic disease. Forensic Sci. 6:17–24.

Matthews, W. B. (1972): Footballer's migraine. Br. Med. J. 2:326–327.

Merskey, H. and Woodforde, J. M. (1972): Psychiatric sequelae of minor head injury. Brain 95:521–528.

Michael, M. I. and Williams, J. M. (1952): Migraine in children. J. Pediatr. 41:18–24.

Miller, H. (1961): Accident neurosis. Br. Med.J. 1:919–925, 992–998.

Oldendorf, W. H. and Kitano, M. (1967): Radioisotope measurement of brain blood turnover time as a clinical index of brain circulation. J. Nucl. Med. 8:570–587.

Ommaya, A. K., Faas, F. and Yarnell, P. (1968): Whiplash injury and brain damage. J.A.M.A. 204:285–289.

Ommaya, A. K. and Gennarelli, T. A. (1974): Cerebral concussion and traumatic unconsciousness. Brain 97:633–654.

Ommaya, A. K. and Gennarelli, T. A. (1976): A physiopathologic basis for noninvasive diagnosis and prognosis of head injury severity. *In* Head Injuries, ed. R. L. McLaurin. Grune and Stratton, New York, pp. 49–75.

Oppenheimer, D. R. (1968): Microscopic lesions in the brain following head injury. J. Neurol. Neurosurg. Psychiatry 31:299–306.
Osler, L. D. and Fusillo, M. G. (1965): A peculiar type of post-concussive "blackout." J. Neurol. Neurosurg. Psychiatry 28:344–349.
Russell, W. R. (1932): Cerebral involvement in head injury. Brain 55:549–603.
Russell, W.R. (1935): Amnesia following head injuries. Lancet 2:762–763.
Simons, D. J. and Wolff, H. G. (1946): Studies on headache: mechanisms of chronic post-traumatic headache. Psychosom. Med. 8:227–242.
Skinhøj, E. (1966): Determination of regional cerebral blood flow in man. In Head Injury, eds. W. F. Caveness and A. E. Walker. J. Lippincott, Philadelphia, pp. 431–438.
Smith, D. R., Ducker, T. B. and Kempe, L. G. (1969): Experimental in vivo microcirculatory dynamics in brain trauma. J. Neurosurg. 30:664–672.
Symonds, C. P. (1962): Concussion and its sequelae. Lancet 1:1–5.
Symonds, C. P. (1974): Concussion and contusion of the brain and their sequelae. In Brock's Injuries of the Brain and Spinal Cord and Their Coverings, 5th ed., ed. E. H. Feiring. Springer, New York, pp. 100–161.
Taylor, A. R. (1967): Post-concussional sequelae. Br. Med. J. 3:67–71.
Taylor, A. R. and Bell, T. K. (1966): Slowing of cerebral circulation after concussional head injury. Lancet 2:178–180.
Toglia, J. U., Rosenberg, P. E. and Ronis, M. L. (1970): Post-traumatic dizziness. Arch. Otolaryngol. 92:485–492.
Vijayan, N. and Dreyfus, P. M. (1975): Posttraumatic dysautonomic cephalgia. Arch. Neurol. 32:649–652.
Walker, A. E. and Erculei, F. (1969): Head Injured Men. Charles C Thomas, Springfield, Ill., pp. 44–57.
Ward, A. A., Jr. (1966): The physiology of concussion. In Head Injury, eds. W. F. Caveness and A. E. Walker. J. B. Lippincott, Philadelphia, pp. 203–208.
Van Zomeren, A. H. and Deelman, B. G. (1978): Long-term recovery of visual reaction time after closed head injury. J. Neurol. Neurosurg. Psychiatry 41:452–457.

CHAPTER 8:

HEADACHES WITH PRIMARY DISORDERS OF THE CENTRAL NERVOUS SYSTEM

The large majority of patients who complain of headache do not have a structural intracranial abnormality; those few who do have lesions usually have serious disorders that should be recognized and dealt with promptly. There are patterns of headache that shift the diagnostic probabilities toward an underlying structural disorder, and often aid the physician in sorting out which of these patients should be subjected to costly, time-consuming and sometimes uncomfortable or potentially dangerous laboratory examinations. It is our intention in this chapter to examine those aspects of headache disorders that may be helpful in making this distinction.

GENERAL CLINICAL PRINCIPLES

The brain, its ependymal linings and much of its meningeal coverings are pain-insensitive (Ray and Wolff, 1940). The most important intracranial structures that are pain-sensitive are vascular, especially the proximal portions of the cerebral and dural arteries and the large veins and dural sinuses. An intracranial mass lesion produces headache by displacing vessels; the headache may have a throbbing quality and may be worsened by exertion, sudden movements of the head or the Valsalva maneuver. Headache of similar type may also occur in other conditions that dispose to vascular headaches such as fever, giant cell arteritis and migraine, to name

210

but a few. Therefore, it is unwise to assume that a vascular headache of recent onset is idiopathic (migraine) in origin. The provocation of headache by the ingestion of certain foods (alcohol, chocolate, dairy products, etc.) (Henderson and Raskin, 1972); a previous history of dramatic ice cream headache or orthostatic symptoms (vertigo, visual obscuration or scintillating scotomata) (Raskin and Knittle, 1976); the presence of a tender carotid artery (Raskin and Prusiner, 1977); and an association with the menstrual cycle all point, however, toward the likelihood of migraine. Responsiveness to a therapeutic trial of vasoactive drugs is also corroborative, but there have been instances in which patients with proved brain tumors have undergone dramatic remission of headache upon the institution of these agents (Raskin, unpublished observations).

Contraction of skeletal muscles is a common, apparently reflex mechanism with which the body responds to pain (Lewis and Kellgren, 1939). Thus, a contracted ("rigid") abdominal wall is a common finding in patients with appendicitis, as are spastic paravertebral muscles in those with herniated intervertebral discs. Painful intracranial lesions of all varieties similarly have the capacity to produce cervical muscle spasm; furthermore, contracted skeletal muscles may become a source of pain and tenderness (probably because of muscle ischemia) that sometimes outlasts the original contraction by hours or days (Simons et al, 1943). It is not at all uncommon for patients with episodic headache caused by intracranial mass lesions to manifest cervical muscle spasm and tenderness; the intensity of head pain need not correlate with the degree of neck tenderness. In fact, the chief complaint may well be neck pain if the concurrent headache problem is of mild-to-moderate intensity. Therefore, the mere presence of neck discomfort and the finding of cervical muscle spasm does not warrant a diagnosis of tension headache.

Of all the features of visceral pain that have diagnostic value in uncovering the source of pain, the intensity of pain has the least value. Thus, myocardial infarction may result in little or no pain, and dissection of an aortic aneurysm is sometimes painless. It is certainly true that, in general, the head pain of cluster headache, migraine, ruptured saccular aneurysm and meningitis is of high intensity; however, the confidence limits of this observation are narrow, and should be applied cautiously to an individual patient. On the other hand, this is the single most important pain attribute to consider when deciding on the analgesic to prescribe for symptomatic relief.

It is a commonly held view among physicians that incessant headache *per se* warrants a psychiatric diagnosis. This contention is not supported by data. A substantial incidence of continuous, unremitting headache has been recorded in patients with brain neo-

TABLE 8-1. CHARACTERISTICS OF BRAIN TUMOR HEADACHES
IN 132 PATIENTS*

Intensity:	40% severe; 40% moderate; 20% mild
Rhythmicity:	85% intermittent; 15% constant
Quality:	25% throbbing; 75% dull and steady
Aggravating Factors:	stooping or lying down–20%; exertion, coughing –25%
Timing:	nocturnal–5%; awakened earlier than usual–5%; upon arising, 15%
Associated Features:	increased intracranial pressure–40%; nausea and vomiting–50%

*Data from Rushton and Rooke, 1962.

plasms, subdural hematoma and migraine (Rushton and Rooke, 1962). It appears to be especially common in those who experience very intense headache episodically and never return to a completely pain-free baseline. In eliciting the headache history in such patients, it is important to focus on the features of the paroxysmal, severe exacerbations rather than the baseline headache, which is often nondescript.

INTRACEREBRAL NEOPLASMS

At least 60 per cent of patients with brain tumors complain of headache; one-half of these consider headache to be their primary complaint (Northfield, 1938; Rushton and Rooke, 1962). The typical brain tumor headache has a dull (nonthrobbing) quality, is of moderate intensity, occurs intermittently, is worsened by exertion or change in posture, and is associated with nausea and vomiting (Rushton and Rooke, 1962). Thus, the headache presented by brain tumor patients is not distinctive; the same pattern of symptoms results more often from migraine than from brain tumor. However, there are several features of head pain which, although of infrequent occurrence, have diagnostic value. In addition to considering these, it would be well to examine more closely the incidence of the features of headaches in patients with tumors (Table 8–1).

Although headaches that disturb sleep occur in only 10 per cent of patients with brain tumor, this fact is notable. Sleep also may be disturbed in those with cluster headache or glaucoma, but it is a headache feature that should alert one to the possibility of a neoplasm.

HEADACHE SYNDROMES DISTINCTIVE OF NEOPLASM

The patterns to be described are not common; however, when they appear, brain tumor should be excluded with certainty.

Paroxysmal headache. This syndrome (Harris, 1944) begins quite suddenly in a patient previously free of headache. In the course of one or two seconds, pain reaches maximal intensity that may persist for minutes to an hour or two, and then disappears as quickly as it came. The pain is most often bifrontal or generalized, of quite high intensity, and may be associated with loss of consciousness, vomiting, transient amaurosis or sudden weakness of the legs ("drop attacks"); the presence of one or more of these latter features considerably raises the probability of brain tumor. Certain positions or rapid movement of the head may precipitate a paroxysm; conversely, changing the position of the head or lying supine may dramatically relieve the headache. The full-blown syndrome is seen most often with colloid cysts of the third ventricle, but has also been recorded with tumors of the lateral ventricle (Gassel and Davies, 1961), hemispheres and cerebellum, as well as with craniopharyngomas and pinealomas (Kelly, 1951). Approximately one-third of patients with paroxysmal headaches who eventually prove to harbor tumors have colloid cysts of the third ventricle. In the absence of localizing signs, paroxysmal headaches associated with obtundation or a drop attack are most likely to be the result of a colloid cyst. Intermittent obstruction of flow of CSF from the lateral ventricles through the foramina of Monro, resulting in abrupt increases of intracranial pressure, has been put forth as a possible mechanism of this intriguing syndrome. Precipitation and amelioration of headache by an alteration in the position of the head has raised the possibility that cysts may move in response to gravitational forces to occlude the interventricular foramina in a ball-valve fashion. However, autopsy studies do not support this view. Colloid cysts appear to be fixed too securely in the third ventricle to move an appreciable distance, and their shape precludes the likelihood of their obstructing the interventricular foramina in a ball-valve manner (Yenerman et al, 1958). Furthermore, tumors distant to the foramina of Monro produce an identical syndrome. Vasomotor alterations secondary to abrupt increases in intracranial pressure (Forbes and Wolff, 1928) appear to be a more likely explanation for these phenomena.

Cough (exertional) headache. When transient pain in the head is precipitated by coughing, other actions such as sneezing, straining at stool, laughing, bending or lifting often have the same effect. For the large majority of patients who experience this symptom, there are no serious inferences and the condition is self-limited. However, about 10 per cent of such individuals harbor intracranial lesions, and these are usually located in the posterior fossa (Rooke, 1968). Arnold-Chiari malformation and basilar impression are the commonest abnormalities found, but subdural hematoma, hemispheric, brain stem and cerebellar tumors also may be responsible (Table 8–2).

TABLE 8–2. COUGH (EXERTIONAL) HEADACHE
CHARACTERISTICS*

Precipitants:	cough, sneezing, bending, straining at stool, laughing
Male:Female Ratio:	4:1
Mean Age:	55 years
Course:	benign in 90%
Causes:	idiopathic; structural lesions, usually in the posterior fossa
Localization:	Unilateral in one-third of patients with benign disorder
Treatment:	Dental extractions, lumbar puncture occasionally therapeutically dramatic; indomethacin may relieve dramatically

*Data from Rooke, 1968.

The course of the benign form of this disorder is favorable; about 30 per cent of patients are symptom-free within five years, and over 70 per cent are improved or headache-free within ten years (Rooke, 1968). Since benign exertional headache is an uncommon disorder (brain tumors are far more common), patients who present with this symptom should be thoroughly investigated. If the initial studies are negative, computerized tomography should be repeated at least annually, since there are many examples of patients later proved to have brain tumors whose initial studies were negative.

There have been several cases of dramatic cessation of exertional headache following extraction of abscessed teeth, and occasionally following lumbar puncture (Symonds, 1956; Rooke, 1968). Diamond and Medina (1979) have reported that indomethacin at a dosage of 75 mg per day has often been very helpful for patients with benign exertional headaches. The mechanism of this headache has not been delineated.

HEADACHE LOCALIZATION AND BRAIN TUMORS

The pain-sensitive structures located supratentorially are innervated by the trigeminal nerve (Ray and Wolff, 1940). Stimulation of these structures produces pain in the anterior portion of the head. Stimulation of the infratentorial pain-sensitive structures results in pain in the posterior portion of the head; innervation is via the ninth and tenth cranial nerves and the upper three cervical nerves. It follows, then, that posterior fossa tumors often result in occipital headache, and supratentorial tumors often produce frontal headache; however, whereas the large majority (80 per cent) of cerebellar tumors result in occipital headache, about one-half of the patients with supratentorial tumors also experience occipital headache (Northfield, 1938). Headache is more likely to be the first symptom of a tumor located below the tentorium than of one above it. Moreover, when headache is lateralized it is often (80 per cent) homolateral to the tumor (Kunkle et al, 1942). These statistics are often useful clinically, but do not provide high enough levels of certainty to allow for precise localization in the absence of other clinical data.

PITUITARY TUMORS

Headache is the presenting complaint in approximately 20 per cent of patients with pituitary adenomas (Nurnberger and Korey, 1953), and is a common symptom (70 per cent) of acromegaly (Lawrence et al, 1970). Because these tumors are often indolent, a headache history of 5 to 10 years with features indistinguishable from migraine may result. The sella turcica, at present, is not completely visualized by CAT scanning (Volpe et al, 1978); a lateral plain film of the skull and tomography of the sella (Kricheff, 1979) are, therefore, important diagnostic procedures in the evaluation of patients with recurring headache.

NON-NEOPLASTIC INTRACRANIAL MASS LESIONS

Since displacement of intracranial vascular structures is probably the common mechanism of headache, the characteristics of headache resulting from neoplasms are generally true of all intracranial mass lesions; the nature of the mass may be revealed clinically by its other features, e.g., fever with brain abscess, and obtundation with subdural hematoma.

INCREASED INTRACRANIAL PRESSURE

The frequency and severity of headaches that accompany intracranial lesions correlate poorly with the presence or degree of intracranial hypertension (Northfield, 1938; Pickering, 1939); the latter, therefore, is unlikely to be an important mechanism of headache in these settings. Whether intracranial hypertension, per se, can result in headache at all is unresolved. Kunkle et al (1943) found, in four subjects, that elevation of the CSF pressure to between 680 and 850 mm of water for two minutes did not result in headache, and concluded that intracranial hypertension does not produce headache. However, Fay (1940) performed a similar experiment and found CSF pressure thresholds for headache production that varied greatly among people. It has been suggested that the *rate* at which the CSF pressure increases is critical to headache production. There are no data, however, to support this contention.

The syndrome of *benign intracranial hypertension* (pseudotumor cerebri) is associated with headache in the large majority of patients (Weisberg, 1975). The lateral ventricles are not enlarged in this disorder, so that traction and displacement of periventricular pain-sensitive structures is not likely to be a mechanism of headache as it might be in obstructive hydrocephalus. Headache is sometimes, but inconsistently, relieved by lumbar puncture in this disorder, despite the restoration of CSF pressure to normal levels. Intracranial hypertension in the laboratory animal results in a compensatory dilatation of pial arteries (Forbes and Wolff, 1928), vasomotor instability and a loss of cerebral vasomotor regulation (Langfitt et al, 1965), and it is possible that the magnitude and persistence of these vasomotor responses are important to the mechanism of headache. Studies of cerebral hemodynamics in patients with benign intracranial hypertension have shown that cerebral blood volume is increased, but have led to differing conclusions regarding the impairment of autoregulation in this condition (Mathew et al, 1975; Raichle et al, 1978).

RUPTURED INTRACRANIAL ANEURYSMS

Congenital, arterial, saccular (berry) aneurysms that are prone to rupture most commonly originate from the circle of Willis. The aneurysmal sac lies in the subarachnoid space, so that the resulting hemorrhage almost always produces grossly bloodstained CSF. Focal neurologic signs generally are not in evidence, since hemorrhage into brain parenchyma is not a common consequence of rupture. The dramatically abrupt onset of often excruciating headache ("like a sledgehammer"), accompanied by stiff neck, vomiting and obtundation, is the clinical stereotype for this condition. Headache is certainly the most common presenting symptom, and its cataclysmic and devastating nature is unmatched. Excruciating, blinding, bursting, explosive, violent, etc., are the usual terms used by patients to describe it. Inexplicably, 1 to 2 per cent experience no headache at all. For about 50 per cent the headache is a continuous, steady, high-level pain; only 5 per cent note a throbbing quality. Twenty per cent note exacerbation with head motion and 10 per cent note worsening with coughing or stooping. Five per cent experience headache as paroxysmal or shooting in quality.

Because of the subtentorial trajectory of the hemorrhage, most patients experience occipitonuchal pain; however, one-third suffer frontal, temporal, vertex or generalized headache which is occasionally lateralized. Lumbar puncture often dramatically alleviates this headache.

About one-half of these patients lose consciousness at the onset of the hemorrhage, another 25 per cent become obtunded within 15 minutes, and most of the remainder do so within 12 hours. For the majority, loss of consciousness is relatively brief (up to one hour in most cases and up to 24 hours in a few) (Walton, 1956).

Ruptured arteriovenous malformations of the brain produce a syndrome often indistinguishable from that of ruptured aneurysms. The presence of a cranial bruit or a history of recurring seizures should shift the diagnostic probabilities toward an A–V malformation.

UNRUPTURED INTRACRANIAL VASCULAR ANOMALIES

Periodic headache, usually ipsilateral to the angioma, occurs in 5 to 25 per cent of patients with arteriovenous malformations (MacKenzie, 1953; Lees, 1962; Troost and Newton, 1975). These headaches appear to be vascular in mechanism, and may cease after rupture or surgical resection. Because the incidence of idiopathic vascular headaches in the general population is substantial, it has remained uncertain whether the headaches that are associated with vascular anomalies are coincidentally or etiologically related. In large series of patients with migraine, diagnostic studies do not disclose angiomas or aneurysms, whether the headache pattern is strictly unilateral or not (Lees, 1962). From the data currently at hand, the contention that intracranial vascular anomalies result in recurring headache disorders cannot be supported with compelling evidence.

MULTIPLE SCLEROSIS

Initial bouts of multiple sclerosis are accompanied by headache in about 15 per cent of patients (Kurtzke, 1970). Little descriptive data exist regarding the features of the headache; however, in the authors' experience the pattern is usually vascular. Acute demyelination is known to produce focal edema that may behave as an intracranial mass lesion. The mechanism of headache may well be traction and displacement.

BACTERIAL AND VIRAL MENINGITIS

A distinctive feature of headaches seen in these infectious disorders is a prominent retro-orbital component which is markedly exacerbated by the slightest motion of the eyes (Raskin, unpublished observations). This phenomenon is also seen in optic neuritis and idiopathic vascular headaches; however, its presence in a setting of a headache disorder of recent onset should alert the physician to the possibility of meningitis.

REFERENCES

Diamond, S. and Medina, J. L. (1979): Benign exertional headache: successful treatment with indomethacin. Headache 19:249.

Fay, T. (1940): A new test for the diagnosis of certain headaches, the cephalgiogram. Dis. Nerv Syst. 1:312–315.

Forbes, H. S. and Wolff, H. G. (1928): The vasomotor control of the cerebral vessels. Arch. Neurol. Psychiatry 19:1057–1086.

Gassel, M. M. and Davies, H. (1961): Meningiomas in the lateral ventricles. Brain 84:605–627.

Harris, W. (1944): Paroxysmal and postural headaches from intraventricular cysts and tumours. Lancet 2:654–655.

Henderson, W. R. and Raskin, N. H. (1972): "Hot dog" headache: individual susceptibility to nitrite. Lancet 2:1162–1163.

Kelly, R. (1951): Colloid cysts of the third ventricle. Brain 74:23–65.

Kricheff, I. I. (1979): The radiologic diagnosis of pituitary adenoma. Radiology 131: 263–265.

Kunkle, E. C., Ray, B. S. and Wolff, H. G. (1942): Studies on headache: the mechanisms and significance of the headache associated with brain tumor. Bull. N. Y. Acad. Med. 18:400–422.

Kunkle, E. C., Ray, B. S. and Wolff, H. G. (1943): Experimental studies on headache: analysis of the headache associated with changes in intracranial pressure. Arch. Neurol. Psychiatry 49:323–358.

Kurtzke, J. F. (1970): Clinical manifestations of multiple sclerosis. In Handbook of Clinical Neurology, Vol. 9, eds. P. J. Vinken and G. W. Bruyn. American Elsevier Publishing Co., New York, pp. 161–216.

Langfitt, T. W., Weinstein, J. D. and Kassell, N. F. (1965): Cerebral vasomotor paralysis produced by intracranial hypertension. Neurology 15:622–641.

Lawrence, J. H., Tobias, C. A., Linfoot, J. A., Born, J. L., Lyman, J. T., Chong, C. Y., Manougian, E. and Wei, W. C. (1970): Successful treatment of acromegaly: metabolic and clinical studies in 145 patients. J. Clin. Endocrinol. Metab. 31:180–198.

Lees, F. (1962): The migrainous symptoms of cerebral angiomata. J. Neurol. Neurosurg. Psychiatry 25:45–50.

Lewis, T. and Kellgren, J. H. (1939): Observations relating to referred pain, visceromotor reflexes and other associated phenomena. Clin. Sci. 4:47–71.

MacKenzie, I. (1953): The clinical presentation of the cerebral angioma. Brain 76:184–214.

Mathew, N. T., Meyer, J. S. and Ott, E. O. (1975): Increased cerebral blood volume in benign intracranial hypertension. Neurology 25:646–649.

Northfield, D. W. C. (1938): Some observations on headache. Brain 61:133–162.

Nurnberger, J. I. and Korey, S. R. (1953): Pituitary Chromophobe Adenomas. Springer Publishing Co., New York.

Pickering, G. W. (1939): Experimental observations on headache. Br. Med. J. 1:907–912.

Raichle, M. E., Grubb, R. L., Jr., Phelps, M. E., Gado, M. H. and Caronna J. J. (1978): Cerebral hemodynamics and metabolism in pseudotumor cerebri. Ann. Neurol. 4:104–111.

Raskin, N. H. and Knittle, S. C. (1976): Ice cream headache and orthostatic symptoms in patients with migraine. Headache 16:222–225.

Raskin, N. H. and Prusiner, S. B. (1977): Carotidynia. Neurology 27:43–46.

Ray, B. S. and Wolff, H. G. (1940): Experimental studies on headache. Pain sensitive structures of the head and their significance in headache. Arch. Surg. 41:813–856.

Rooke, E. D. (1968): Benign exertional headache. Med. Clin. North Am. 52:801–808.

Rushton, J. G. and Rooke, E. D. (1962): Brain tumor headache. Headache 2:147–152.

Simons, D. J., Day E., Goodell, H. and Wolff, H. G. (1943): Experimental studies on headache: muscles of the scalp and neck as sources of pain. Assoc. Res. Nerv. Ment. Dis. 23:228–241.

Symonds, C. (1956): Cough headache. Brain 79:557–568.

Troost, B. T. and Newton, T. H. (1975): Occipital lobe arteriovenous malformations. Arch. Ophthalmol. 93:250–256.

Volpe, B. T., Foley, K. M. and Howieson, J. (1978): Normal CAT scans in craniopharyngioma. Ann. Neurol. 3:87–89.

Walton, J. N. (1956): Subarachnoid Hemorrhage. E. and S. Livingstone, London, pp. 48–64.

Weisberg, L. A. (1975): Benign intracranial hypertension. Medicine 54:197–207.

Yenerman, M. H., Bowerman, C. I. and Haymaker, W. (1958): Colloid cysts of the third ventrical. Acta Neuroveg. 17:211–277.

CHAPTER 9

GIANT CELL ARTERITIS

The most dramatic and characteristic clinical features of giant cell arteritis (GCA) are caused by inflammatory and obliterative alterations of branches of the external carotid and ophthalmic arteries. These features led to its discovery by Hutchison (1890), its elucidation by Horton et al (1932) and its designation for several years as *temporal arteritis.* It has become clear that GCA is a generalized disorder of medium- and large-sized arteries that is not restricted to the cranial arteries — in fact, they may be spared. It is characterized morphologically by an arterial inflammation, containing histiocytes, lymphocytes and giant cells, that fragments and distorts the arterial internal elastic lamina. However, the designation *giant cell arteritis* has proved to be less than optimal since it appears that the alterations of arterial elastic tissue are more characteristic, constant features of the illness than is the presence of giant cells (Parker et al, 1975).

The spectrum of this disorder of unknown cause has been expanded in recent years by the recognition that the underlying etiologic mechanism may also be expressed by a syndrome that has come to be known as *polymyalgia rheumatica* (PR) (Barber, 1957), in which inflammation of synovial membranes is at least one important pathogenetic factor (Ettlinger et al, 1978). The major clinical manifestation of PR is pain and stiffness of the limb girdles, and this occurs in about 50 per cent of patients with cranial arteritis that is clinically evident and proved by temporal artery biopsy (Huston et al, 1978). Moreover, a substantial proportion (40 to 50 per cent) of those patients with the PR syndrome without clinical involvement of the cranial arteries have been reported to have GCA in temporal artery biopsy specimens (Hamrin, 1972; Fauchald et al, 1972).

It is thus clear that these two disorders are closely related; whether they represent different pathologic responses, arteritis and synovitis, to a common etiologic mechanism is not certain. The clinical course of either syndrome is self-limited to one to two years, but the clinical involvement of cranial arteries may result in permanent bilateral blindness in 20 to 30 per cent of patients if treatment with corticosteroids is not instituted (Birkhead et al, 1957; Ladas, 1973). Although the risk of blindness is considerably less in those with PR alone without clinically evident cranial arteritis, especially if the temporal artery biopsy is negative, blindness nevertheless does occur (Fessel and Pearson, 1967). The ischemic optic neuropathy produced by GCA is the major cause of rapidly developing bilateral blindness in the patient over 60 years of age (Walsh and Hoyt, 1969). The preservation of the visual function of patients is the single most important reason for all physicians to become familiar with the protean manifestations of GCA.

DEMOGRAPHY

Women account for about 65 per cent of the reported cases of GCA, and the average age at onset is 65 years, with a range of 50 to 85 years (Hamilton et al, 1971; Hamrin, 1972; Fauchald et al, 1972). It is decidedly rare for GCA to begin before the age of 50 years, but biopsy-proved cases have been described in patients who were 35 (Bethlenfalvay and Nusynowitz, 1964) and 22 years of age (Meyers and Lord, 1948) respectively. Recently, a disorder called *juvenile temporal arteritis* (Lie et al, 1975) has been reported, but is probably unrelated to GCA because of substantial clinical and histopathologic differences. The racial backgrounds of the GCA individuals described have been overwhelmingly Caucasian; however, several black patients with the disease have recently been reported, and its frequency in the black population may be more common than has been appreciated previously (Ballou et al, 1978).

Giant cell arteritis is a common disorder of the elderly; its frequency characteristics have been determined in the population aged 50 and older in Olmstead County, Minnesota, between 1970 and 1974. The average annual incidence was 17.4 per 100,000 people, and the prevalence of patients with a diagnosis of GCA on 1 January 1975 was 133 per 100,000 (Huston et al, 1978). A prospective autopsy study suggests that GCA is considerably more common than is clinically evident; Östberg (1973) found GCA in 1.7 per cent of almost 900 deceased patients from whom multiple sections of the temporal artery and of the aorta were studied.

TABLE 9-1. CLINICAL FEATURES OF GIANT CELL ARTERITIS*

PERCENTAGE INCIDENCE OF COMMON FEATURES AT INITIAL EVALUATION	%	LESS COMMON BUT CHARACTERISTIC FEATURES
Headache	85	Raynaud's phenomenon of limbs
Temporal artery tenderness	70	or tongue**
Jaw claudication**	65	Tender scalp nodules
Lingual**, limb or swallowing claudication	20	Thick, tender occipital arteries
Brachiocephalic bruits	50	Necrotic lesions of scalp, tongue
Thickened or nodular temporal artery	45	Carotid artery tenderness
Pulseless temporal artery	40	Swelling of the hands
Visual symptoms	40	Taste, smell disturbances
Fixed blindness, partial or complete	15	Distended, beaded retinal veins
Polymyalgia rheumatica	40	Diminished or absent radial
Weight loss > 6 kg	35	artery pulses
ESR > 50 mm/hr	95	Mononeuropathy — median,
> 100 mm/hr	60	peroneal, cervical root
Fever (> 37.7°C)	20	
Abnormal liver function	50	
Anemia (hct < 35%)	50	

*Data drawn from Hamrin, 1972; Healey and Wilske, 1977; Huston et al, 1978.
** Pathognomonic symptoms.

CLINICAL SYNDROME

The most common initial symptoms of GCA are headache and polymyalgia rheumatica. Fever (Ghose et al, 1976), jaw claudication, weight loss, blindness (Simmons and Cogan, 1962), anemia, and limb or tongue claudication were other frequent presenting complaints in two recent large series of patients (Healey and Wilske, 1977; Huston et al., 1978). The clinical data from Hamrin's (1972) group of patients were also culled, and Table 9-1 presents an approximation of the incidence of the common features of the disorder that were present before the establishment of the diagnosis. Jaw or lingual claudication and lingual Raynaud's phenomenon are probably pathognomonic of GCA (Ettlinger et al, 1978). The symptoms of GCA generally are rapidly and remarkably improved by corticosteroid administration, with the exception of visual failure; once fixed loss of vision has occurred steroids are not likely to improve matters, except to prevent further visual loss (Cohen, 1973). Certain aspects of the clinical features of GCA are worth discussing in some detail.

HEADACHE

If the dominant symptom of GCA, headache of varying intensity, is not present initially, it usually develops later in the course

TABLE 9–2. LOCATION OF HEADACHE IN 44 PATIENTS
WITH GIANT CELL ARTERITIS*

Pain Location	No. Patients**
Temporal	24
Frontal	11
Occipital	11
Parietal	9
Nuchal	7
Maxillary	5
Holocephalic	5
Temporomandibular	3

*Data drawn from Mumenthaler, 1978.
**Some patients reported more than one locus.

of the disorder. Retrospectively, many patients note vague malaise and muscle aches prior to the appearance of headache which may be unilateral or bilateral, and commonly located temporally, but may involve any and all aspects of the cranium (Table 9–2). Pain usually appears gradually over a few hours before its peak intensity is reached; occasionally it is explosive in onset. The quality of pain is seldom throbbing; rather, it almost invariably is described as sharp and boring, with superimposed episodic icepick-like, lancinating pains (Russell, 1959; Hamilton et al, 1971), similar to the sharp pains that occur in migraine and cluster headache. Most patients can recognize that the origin of their headache is superficial, external to the skull, rather than from within the cranium. Scalp tenderness is present, often to a marked degree, in most of those who report headache; brushing the hair or resting the head on a pillow may be impossible because of pain. Headache is usually worse at night and is often *aggravated by exposure to cold* (Hollenhorst et al, 1960). This latter feature is highly characteristic of GCA; migraine patients at times note precipitation or worsening of headache upon exposure to low ambient temperatures, but rarely to the degree and with the consistency reported by those with GCA. Reddened, tender nodules or red-streaking of the skin overlying the temporal arteries are found in highest frequency in patients with headache, as is tenderness of the temporal or, less commonly, the occipital arteries. The pulsations of the temporal artery are usually diminished on the painful side but not completely absent. Curiously, and inexplicably, temporal artery biopsy not infrequently coincides with cessation of headache (Dantes, 1946; Harrison, 1948); similarly, the appearance of symptoms of visual failure is sometimes simultaneous with improvement or cessation of headache (Russell, 1959).

Polymyalgia Rheumatica

Pain and stiffness of the proximal limbs usually evolves insidiously over weeks to months, but in about 40 per cent of patients the onset is acute and resembles viremia in the setting of myalgia and fever. The occurrence of painful swallowing may render the correct diagnosis even more difficult (Healey and Wilske, 1977). Fatigue, anorexia, weight loss, low-grade fever and shivering appear roughly at the same time as the myalgic symptoms. In most patients the periarticular areas of the neck and shoulder girdle are the first to become painful; in the rest, the hips and thighs become involved first. Pain usually is not specifically referred to the joints themselves, but to the areas around the joints. Pain may appear unilaterally, but over the succeeding weeks it invariably becomes bilateral; this successive involvement of muscle groups is characteristic, and may continue until most of the proximal and axial musculature and tendinous insertions are painful. Morning stiffness of the proximal joints is a prominent and characteristic feature of PR. Patients frequently have difficulty in rising from bed in the morning; their spouse may have to pull them out of bed. Some may have to roll out of bed to achieve a position on the floor on hands and knees, and then push themselves up to an erect position. Muscle strength is usually unimpaired, and electromyography and serum enzyme levels generally are not abnormal.

Swelling of the hands is reported by 25 per cent of patients, and knee effusions have been noted in about 10 per cent. Tenderness of tendon insertions is commonly found (Hamrin, 1972). Biopsies of muscle are usually negative; the occasional presence of inflammatory infiltrates in muscle septae or perivascular areas has been reported (Gordon et al, 1964), as well as nonspecific type II muscle atrophy (Brooke and Kaplan, 1972). Synovitis, although not clinically apparent, probably produces most if not all of the painful symptoms of PR; it has been documented by radioisotopic joint scan and biopsy (Ettlinger et al, 1978).

The symptoms of polymyalgia are exceptionally responsive to steroid therapy, and complete resolution of symptoms often takes place in one to two days with as little as 10 to 15 mg of prednisone. If symptoms of cranial arteritis such as headache, jaw claudication or visual symptoms are not adjoined to the symptoms of PR for six months or longer, and temporal artery biopsy is negative, the vast majority of patients do not develop blindness. Rather than subject such individuals to the substantial risks of long-term high-dosage steroid therapy, it is reasonable to use anti-inflammatory drugs or low-dosage steroids so long as they are vigilantly followed.

Vision

Diplopia occurs in 10 per cent of patients with GCA (Huston et al, 1978); it may be horizontal or vertical, since one-half of the patients manifest sixth nerve palsies and the other half third nerve palsies with sparing of the pupil. Extraocular muscle paresis is demonstrable in only one-half of those who report diplopia, and the symptom is sometimes expressed as blurred vision. Diplopia usually appears shortly after the onset of headache, suddenly and painlessly, and recovery generally takes place slowly over several weeks. Diplopia heralds the onset of visual failure in about 50 per cent of untreated patients, and thus is a symptom to be taken very seriously. The temporal sequence of ophthalmoparesis preceding or, less commonly, appearing concurrently with ischemic optic neuropathy appears to be inviolate. The mechanism of ophthalmoparesis in GCA is likely to be occlusion of the vasa nervorum, analogous to diabetic ophthalmoplegia (Asbury et al, 1970), but direct pathologic proof is lacking (Hollenhorst et al, 1960; Meadows, 1966).

Visual loss is by far the most common and the most dreaded ocular symptom. The first symptom of visual failure usually occurs four to seven weeks after the onset of headache, and may arise sooner in the presence of tender, indurated temporal arteries·(Birkhead et al, 1957); visual loss is rare if headache has been present for six months or more (Meadows, 1966). Visual failure generally is monocular initially and is abrupt in onset in over 50 per cent of patients; it is often noted on awakening in the morning. It is commonly described as a mist or dark veil over all or part of the field of vision on the involved side, which becomes denser over the ensuing several hours. Others report a gradual deterioration of visual acuity over several days, and about 10 per cent of those with visual symptoms describe recurring episodes of visual loss that recover completely in the course of minutes to hours; the episodes may be reported as sensations of gray patches or colors before the affected eye. About one-half of those with transitory visual loss progress to permanent visual loss if untreated. When visual loss occurs unilaterally, the second eye is affected in 75 per cent of patients one day to three weeks later (Wagener and Hollenhorst, 1958; Jonasson et al, 1979). If the second eye is not involved within two months of the first eye, it probably will not be affected at all (Hollenhorst et al, 1960).

Ischemic optic neuropathy is the pathologic mechanism that accounts for the visual failure in 90 per cent of the patients who experience this complication, because the blood supply of the optic nerve is derived from the ophthalmic artery and its posterior ciliary branches, which are most consistently and profoundly involved in GCA (Henkind et al, 1970; Wilkinson and Russell, 1972). The visual field defects produced by this disturbance may or may not be associated with decreased visual acuity. One of the most frequently encountered is an altitudinal defect, particularly an inferior one. A large central scotoma breaking into the periphery is also commonly found. If a patient has been experiencing transient visual obscurations he may have a completely normal eye examination; if he arrives soon after the onset of visual acuity and field loss, the ophthalmoscopic examination may still be normal, since the signs of ischemic optic neuropathy develop over a 24- to 36-hour interval (Hayreh, 1969). Eventually, edema of the optic disc appears in association with narrowing of the retinal arterioles and small, peripapillary nerve fiber layer hemorrhages. In many instances, there also are spottily distributed cotton wool retinal infarcts. The retinal veins sometimes appear to be distended, beaded and irregular (Russell, 1959). The disc edema increases over a few days and usually resolves by the tenth day, leaving in its wake a pale, atrophic optic disc.

Central retinal artery occlusion accounts for most of the remaining patients who sustain loss of vision. Profoundly decreased visual acuity almost always results from these lesions, and the ophthalmoscopic examination usually reveals massive retinal edema, a foveal cherry-red spot and arteriolar "boxcarring." Within days to weeks the retina regains its normal color and texture and the cherry-red spot fades.

NEUROLOGIC DISORDERS

Involvement of the internal carotid artery and its intracranial branches, with the exception of the ophthalmic artery, is decidedly unusual in GCA, so that the frequency of hemiplegia, seizures, aphasia or other symptoms related to cerebral ischemia is relatively low (Hollenhorst et al, 1960). Several patients have been reported with mononeuropathies involving the median or peroneal nerves or a cervical nerve root (Russell, 1959; Meadows, 1966; Fryer and Singer, 1971; Healey and Wilske, 1977). The prognosis for recovery of peripheral neural (but not CNS) involvement with corticosteroids is good.

Hamrin (1972) found that almost one-half of 85 patients with GCA noted impaired taste or smell that usually began during the first month of the illness. Parageusia and parosmia were common complaints; many patients stopped drinking coffee which had begun to taste bitter, and some no longer smoked cigarettes because of their disagreeable odor. These symptoms responded promptly to steroid therapy.

The CSF is usually normal, but occasionally there are mild elevations in total protein and pleocytosis; rarely, cell counts of 650 lymphocytes or polymorphonuclear leukocytes have been found (Hamilton et al, 1971; Hamrin, 1972).

LARGE ARTERY INVOLVEMENT

Hamrin (1972) and Bruk (1967) reported bruits over the carotid, subclavian, axillary, brachial and temporal arteries in over one-half of the patients in whom auscultation was carefully performed. Östberg (1973) showed that GCA frequently involves the aorta and its branches pathologically, and this is expressed clinically in about 15 per cent of the patients. The aortic arch syndrome, comprising claudication of the limbs, Raynaud's phenomenon, or unequal pulses or blood pressure measurements was reported to occur in 34 of 248 patients (Klein et al, 1975). Three of the latter patients died of aortic rupture. Tenderness of the cervical carotid artery occasionally arises (Hamrin, 1972; Huston et al, 1978).

GCA is confined to arteries that contain an internal elastic lamina, and does not involve small arterioles (Wilkinson and Russell, 1972). Therefore, the kidney is only rarely damaged, and patients with GCA do not sustain more cerebral or myocardial infarctions than an age-matched population (Huston et al, 1978).

ERYTHROCYTE SEDIMENTATION RATE AND OTHER LABORATORY ABNORMALITIES

The most striking and consistent laboratory finding in GCA is an elevation of the erythrocyte sedimentation rate (ESR) to a mean of 100 mm/hr. The major factor accounting for this phenomenon is probably the marked elevation of plasma fibrinogen that accompanies the disease (Hamrin, 1972). The ESR almost always becomes elevated as the disease progresses, but there are now numerous examples of normal ESRs in well-documented GCA (Kansu et al, 1977); indeed, Whitfield et al (1963) discovered a normal ESR in six of 72 patients. An important issue that pertains to GCA is that there is now substantial evidence that the ESR increases with age, and for patients over 60 years of age the upper limit of normal is probably at least 40 mm/hr by either the Wintrobe or the Westergren method (Table 9–3). In a study of patients about to undergo elective surgery, without evidence of inflammatory disorders, 19 per cent of those over the age of 50 years had an ESR greater than 30 mm/hr and 6 per cent had an ESR greater than 40 mm/hr by the Wintrobe method (Hayes and Stinson, 1976). Kulvin (1972) came to the same

TABLE 9–3. ERYTHROCYTE SEDIMENTATION RATES
(Wintrobe Method) RELATED TO AGE*

AGE (YRS)	NO. PATIENTS	MEAN (mm/hr)	S.D.	PERCENTAGE >20 mm/hr
<30	23	9	6	0
30–39	26	12	8	12
40–49	24	15	8	21
50–59	25	15	12	24
60–69	32	19	9	47
70–79	22	23	13	46
80–89	12	27	14	47

*Data drawn from Hayes and Stinson, 1976.

conclusions using the Westergren method in a study of 105 patients 50 years of age and older.

There is ample documentation to negate the clinical axiom that a normal ESR excludes GCA. To put the matter in perspective, in three large series of patients with GCA, comprised of a total of 185 patients, 12 had an ESR below 50 mm/hr at their initial presentation (Hamrin, 1972; Healey and Wilske, 1977; Huston et al, 1978); in five of Hamrin's patients, the ESR ranged from 15 to 30 mm/hr. An important practical point regarding the ESR is that the determination should be made soon after venopuncture is performed. If there is a delay of more than two to three hours, spuriously low results may be obtained (Miale, 1972).

Abnormal liver function tests — alkaline phosphatase, SGOT, prothrombin time or BSP retention — are found commonly (Dickson et al, 1973) for reasons that are not clear. Liver biopsies have usually shown no abnormalities, and hepatitis-associated antigen has not been detected. These serologic abnormalities are quite responsive to steroid therapy.

The anemia that commonly occurs in association with GCA is usually mild and normochromic or hypochromic in type (Wilske and Healey, 1967); the range of hemoglobin levels is 8 to 14 g/dl with a median of 11.5 g/dl (Huston et al, 1978). The serum protein electrophoretic pattern is characterized by decreased albumin and increased α-2 globulin fractions.

TEMPORAL ARTERY BIOPSY

The arteritis occurs in a patchy distribution, skipping segments of arteries, and involving part of the circumference of a vessel but not completely surrounding it (Klein et al, 1976). Histologically, the inflammatory cells appear on either side of the internal elastic lamina, disrupting it, and are often spread throughout all the layers of the vessel wall (Fig. 9–1). Fibrous proliferation takes place at the intimal layer, and giant cells, when present, occur at the intima-medial junction. Fibrinoid necrosis is absent. The lumen of the vessel is often markedly narrowed by the edematous intima and is sometimes occluded by thrombus. The presence or absence of giant cells or the intensity of the inflammatory reaction in biopsy specimens does not correlate well with the clinical severity, nor with the course of the disease (Huston et al, 1978).

A clinically involved portion of the temporal artery should be biopsied if possible; when there are no findings referable to the cranial arteries, a 4- to 6-cm portion of one temporal artery should be obtained and examined at multiple levels. The contralateral temporal artery should be biopsied if frozen sections show no disease in the first specimen, since GCA is strictly unilateral in 5 per cent of patients (Klein et al, 1976). Because of the possibility of impending blindness in those with clinically evident cranial arteritis, steroids should not be deferred to obtain a temporal artery biopsy; if biopsy is performed within 48 hours of the commencement of steroid therapy it is unlikely that the histopathologic features of arteritis will be obscured.

Establishing the diagnosis of GCA unambiguously is an important matter, since very often there are therapeutic and prognostic

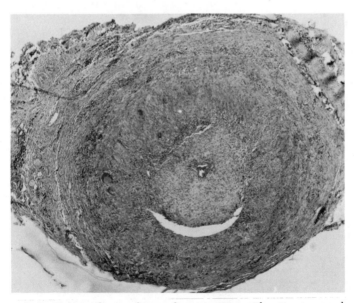

Figure 9–1. Temporal artery biopsy from a patient with active temporal arteritis. The vessel wall is thickened and the lumen is almost totally occluded. Inflammatory cells have infiltrated all layers of the vessel wall. Giant cells are present. (Hematoxylin and eosin stain, magnification of 580×.)

risk factors that are not trivial. For most patients temporal artery biopsy is an important diagnostic procedure in this regard; however, biopsies have been negative in otherwise unequivocal instances of GCA, and in some cases a biopsy may not be necessary. The physician must judge each case on its merits, and evaluate in advance the information that might be gained from temporal artery biopsy. If a positive biopsy is obtained in a patient with PR without the clinical manifestations of arteritis such as headache, jaw or limb claudication, arterial bruits or visual symptoms, it is not as yet clear whether all such cases should be treated with a high-dosage, long-term steroid regimen. If, after review of the data, the physician's view is that biopsy evidence of cranial arteritis is sufficient to warrant aggressive treatment, it follows that temporal artery biopsy will be performed very often, if not in all patients.

PATHOGENESIS

The prevailing theory that most of the vasculitides are caused by, or closely associated with, the deposition of immune complexes in blood vessel walls (Fauci, 1978) has caused attention to be focused on immune mechanisms in GCA. Increased numbers of circulating immunoblasts (Eghtedari et al, 1976), anti-IgG activity in temporal artery biopsy specimens (Waaler et al, 1976) and immunoglobulin deposition within the walls of involved temporal arteries (Liang et al, 1974) support the hypothesis of an immune complex-mediated vasculopathy. Cell-mediated immune reactivity, a less common mechanism of vasculitis, may be reflected histopathologically; the electron-microscopic appearance of involved temporal arteries in GCA is consistent with that of a cell-mediated immune response (Parker et al, 1975). Antigenic determinants of the internal elastic lamina may be altered by some aspect of aging to serve as the stimulus for a cell-mediated immune inflammatory response in the wall of arteries; however, little evidence thus far supports this possibility.

TREATMENT

Giant cell arteritis is a self-limited disease that usually persists for one to two years (Hamilton et al, 1971; Beevers et al, 1973); spontaneous remission may occur as soon as six months, and occasionally the illness may persist for more than three years. There is no evidence that corticosteroid therapy shortens its duration. The purpose of high-dosage long-term steroid therapy is to prevent the catastrophic complications of arteritis, blindness and aortic rupture, by suppressing the inflammatory arterial component of the disease until it spontaneously enters its quiescent stage.

All patients with clinical evidence of arteritis, and perhaps all those with biopsy evidence of arteritis also, should be treated initially with 60 to 80 mg of prednisone per day. There is evidence that an alternate-day 90-mg regimen is not as effective in suppressing the arteritis (Hunder et al, 1975). Within four to 72 hours after treatment is begun, there almost always is improvement in malaise, fever, anorexia, PR and headache (Birkhead et al, 1957). There may be some visual acuity improvement, probably because of a decrease in optic nerve or retinal edema, and not by a reversal of the process of optic nerve infarction. Patients who are totally blind rarely regain vision with steroid therapy.

High doses of prednisone should be continued for at least four to six weeks, and an assessment of progress made at that time. If the patient has become asymptomatic and the ESR has returned to normal levels, a gradual tapering of the steroid dosage to the lowest necessary maintenance level should be implemented by reducing the daily dosage by 10 per cent at weekly intervals. The ESR may become slightly elevated as dosage reduction proceeds, but if the patient remains asymptomatic this does not usually indicate a relapse. The symptoms of PR appear in 25 per cent of patients during the tapering of steroids, and probably do not constitute an indication to re-elevate the dosage (Huston et al, 1978). If a recrudescence of symptoms occurs, higher doses should be resumed and the tapering dosage schedule may have to be executed more slowly. If treatment is discontinued in less than two years, relapse takes place within one year in about 20 per cent of GCA patients (Fauchald et al, 1972). Therefore, all patients should be treated for at least one year, and many for at least two years to prevent this possibility. A repeat temporal artery biopsy may offer assurance that it is safe to stop steroids (Cohen, 1973).

It appears to be reasonably clear that impairment of vision is prevented by steroid therapy, based on retrospective matching analyses, although a prospective controlled study has never been done and probably never will be. In a study carried out at the Mayo Clinic (Birkhead et al, 1957) comparing the outcome of patients treated with steroids with that of those of the pre-steroid era, a threefold increase in bilateral blindness was evident in those who did not receive steroids. Of those GCA patients who presented with visual symptoms and were not treated with steroids, approximately 50 per cent developed bilateral blindness. In those who have presented with monocular amblyopia, preservation of vision in the other eye and cessation of slowly progressive visual deterioration appears to have been achieved in the vast majority of treated patients (Hamilton et al, 1971; Cohen, 1973). An occasional individual has become totally blind despite steroid therapy (Boghen and Glaser, 1975).

As noted above, it is not yet clear whether PR is always a manifestation of GCA; there appear to be PR patients without clinically evident cranial arteritis who can be managed with 10 to 15 mg of prednisone daily and appear to run a low risk of blindness. However, the risk is not zero (Fessel and Pearson, 1967), and a definitive answer to this problem is not yet available. This uncertainty is balanced by the risk of adverse side-effects from steroid therapy in an elderly patient population. Symptomatic vertebral compression fractures occur in one-quarter of the patients, steroid myopathy in 15 per cent and subcapsular cataracts in 5 per cent (Huston et al, 1978). A low-dosage steroid regimen with vigilant follow-up is a reasonable course of action in such patients.

REFERENCES

Asbury, A. K., Aldredge, H., Hershberg, R. et al (1970): Oculomotor palsy in diabetes mellitus: a clinico-pathological study. Brain 93:555–566.
Ballou, S. P., Khan, M. A. and Kushner, I. (1978): Giant cell arteritis in a black patient. Ann. Intern. Med. 88:659–660.
Barber, H. S. (1957): Myalgic syndrome with constitutional effects: polymyalgia rheumatica. Ann. Rheum. Dis. 16:230–237.
Beevers, D. G., Harpur, J. E. and Turk, K. A. D (1973): Giant cell arteritis — the need for prolonged treatment. J. Chronic Dis. 26:571–584.
Bethlenfalvay, N. C. and Nusynowitz, N. L. (1964): Temporal arteritis: a rarity in the young adult. Arch. Intern. Med. 114:487–489.
Birkhead, N. C., Wagener, H. P. and Schick, R. M. (1957): Treatment of temporal arteritis with adrenal corticosteroids: results of 55 cases in which lesions were proven at biopsy. J.A.M.A. 163:821–827.
Boghen, D. R. and Glaser, J. S. (1975): Ischaemic optic neuropathy: the clinical profile and natural history. Brain 98:689–708.
Brooke, M. H. and Kaplan, H. (1972): Muscle pathology in rheumatoid arteritis, polymyalgia rheumatica, and polymyositis. Arch. Pathol. 94:101–118.
Bruk, M. I. (1967): Articular and vascular manifestations of polymyalgia rheumatica. Ann. Rheum. Dis. 26:103–116.
Cohen, D. N. (1973): Temporal arteritis: improvement in visual prognosis and management with repeat biopsies. Trans. Am. Acad. Ophthalmol. Otolaryngol. 77:74–85.
Dantes, D. A. (1946): Temporal arteritis. J.A.M.A. 131:1265–1269.
Dickson, E. R., Maldonado, J. E., Sheps, S. G. et al (1973): Systemic giant-cell arteritis with polymyalgia rheumatica. Reversible abnormalities of liver function. J.A.M.A. 224:1496–1498.
Eghtedari, A. A., Esselinckx, W. and Bacon, P. A. (1976): Circulating immunoblasts in polymyalgia rheumatica. Ann. Rheum. Dis. 35:158–162.
Ettlinger, R. E., Hunder, G. G. and Ward, L. E. (1978): Polymyalgia rheumatica and giant cell arteritis. Annu. Rev. Med. 29:15–22.
Fauchald, P., Rygvold, O. and Øystese, B. (1972): Temporal arteritis and polymyalgia rheumatica: clinical and biopsy findings. Ann. Intern. Med. 77:845–852.
Fauci, A. S., Haynes, B. F. and Katz, P. (1978): The spectrum of vasculitis. Ann. Intern. Med. 89(Part I):660–676.
Fessel, W. J. and Pearson, C. M. (1967): Polymyalgia rheumatica and blindness. N. Engl. J. Med. 276:1403–1405.
Fryer, D. G. and Singer, R. S. (1971): Giant cell arteritis with cervical radiculopathy. Bull. Mason Clin. 25:143–151.
Ghose, M. K., Shensa, S. and Lerner, P. I. (1976): Arteritis of the aged (giant cell arteritis) and fever of unexplained origin. Am. J. Med. 60:429–439.

Gordon, I., Rennie, A. M., and Branwood, A. W. (1964): Polymyalgia rheumatica: biopsy studies. Ann. Rheum. Dis. 23:447–455.

Hamilton, C. R., Jr., Shelley, W. M. and Tumulty, P. A. (1971): Giant cell arteritis: including temporal arteritis and polymyalgia rheumatica. Medicine 50:1–27.

Hamrin, B. (1972): Polymyalgia arteritica. Acta Med. Scand. (Suppl.) 533:1–131.

Harrison, C. V. (1948): Giant-cell or temporal arteritis: a review. J. Clin. Pathol. 1:197–211.

Hayes, G. S. and Stinson, I. N. (1976): Erythrocyte sedimentation rate and age. Arch. Ophthalmol. 94:939–940.

Hayreh, S. S. (1969): Blood supply of the optic nerve head and its role in optic atrophy, glaucoma, and oedema of the optic disc. Br. J. Ophthalmol. 53:721–747.

Healey, L. A. and Wilske, K. R. (1977): Manifestations of giant cell arteritis. Med. Clin. North Am. 61:261–270.

Henkind, P., Charles, N. C. and Pearson, J. (1970): Histopathology of ischemic optic neuropathy. Am. J. Ophthalmol. 69:78–90.

Hollenhorst, R. W., Brown, J. R., Wagener, H. P. and Schick, R. M. (1960): Neurologic aspects of temporal arteritis. Neurology 10:490–498.

Horton, B. T., Magath, T. B. and Brown, G. E. (1932): An undescribed form of arteritis of temporal vessels. Mayo Clin. Proc. 7:700–701.

Hunder, G. G., Sheps, S. G., Allen, G. L. and Joyce, J. W. (1975): Daily and alternate-day corticosteroid regimens in treatment of giant-cell arteritis: comparison in a prospective study. Ann. Intern. Med. 82:613–618.

Huston, K. A., Hunder, G. G., Lie, J. T., Kennedy, R. H. and Elveback, L. R. (1978): Temporal arteritis: a 25 year epidemiologic, clinical and pathologic study. Ann. Intern. Med. 88:162–167.

Hutchison, J. (1890): Disease of the arteries. I. On a peculiar form of thrombotic arteritis of the aged which is sometimes productive of gangrene. Arch Surg. 1:323–329.

Jonasson, F., Cullen, J. F. and Elton, R. A. (1979): Temporal arteritis: a 14-year epidemiological, clinical and prognostic study. Scott. Med. J. 24:111–117.

Kansu, T., Corbett, J. J., Savino, P. and Schatz, N. J. (1977): Giant cell arteritis with normal sedimentation rate. Arch. Neurol. 34:624–625.

Klein, R. G., Campbell, R. J., Hunder, G. G. and Carney, J. A. (1976): Skip lesions in temporal arteritis. Mayo Clin. Proc. 51:504–510.

Klein, R. G., Hunder, G. G., Stanson, A. W. and Sheps, S. G. (1975): Large artery involvement in giant cell (temporal) arteritis. Ann. Intern. Med. 83:806–812.

Kulvin, S. M. (1972): Erythrocyte sedimentation rates in the elderly. Arch. Ophthalmol. 88:617–618.

Ladas, G. J. (1973): Temporal arteritis: A review of the Washington Hospital Center experience with comparison of the literature. Med. Ann. D.C. 42:273–276.

Liang, G. C., Simkin, P. A. and Mannik, M. (1974): Immunoglobulins in temporal arteries: an immunofluorescent study. Ann. Intern. Med. 81:19–24.

Lie, J. T., Gordon, L. P. and Titus, J. L. (1975): Juvenile temporal arteritis: biopsy study of four cases. J.A.M.A. 234:496–499.

Meadows, S. P. (1966): Temporal or giant cell arteritis. Proc. R. Soc. Med. 59:329–333.

Meyers, L. and Lord, J. W., Jr. (1948): Cranial arteritis; report of its occurrence in a young woman. J.A.M.A. 136:169–171.

Miale, J. B. (1972): Laboratory Medicine: Hematology, 4th ed. C. V. Mosby Co., St. Louis, pp. 469–475.

Mumenthaler, M. (1978): Giant cell arteritis (cranial arteritis, polymyalgia rheumatica). J. Neurol. 218:219–236.

Östberg, G. (1973): On arteritis with special reference to polymyalgia arteritica. Acta Pathol. Microbiol. Scand. 237(Suppl. A):1–59.

Parker, F., Healey, L. A., Wilske, K. R. and Odland, G. F. (1975): Light and electron microscopic studies on human temporal arteries with special reference to alterations related to senescence, atherosclerosis and giant cell arteritis. Am. J. Pathol. 79:57–80.

Russell, R. W. R. (1959): Giant-cell arteritis: a review of 35 cases. Q. J. Med. 28:471–489.

Simmons, R. J. and Cogan, D. G. (1962): Occult temporal arteritis. Arch. Ophthalmol. 68:8–18.

Waaler, E., Tönder, O. and Milde, E. J. (1976): Immunological and histological studies of temporal arteries from patients with temporal arteritis and/or polymyalgia rheumatica. Acta Pathol. Microbiol. Scand. (Sect. A) 84A:55–63.

Wagener, H. P. and Hollenhorst, R. W. (1958): The ocular lesions of temporal arteritis. Am. J. Ophthalmol. 45:617–630.

Walsh, F. and Hoyt, W. (1969): Clinical Neuro-Ophthalmology, Vol. II. Williams and Wilkins Co., Baltimore, pp. 1878–1886.

Whitfield, A. G. W., Bateman, M. and Cooke, T. W. (1963): Temporal arteritis. Br. J. Ophthalmol. 47:555–566.

Wilkinson, I. M. and Russell, R. W. (1972): Arteries of the head and neck in giant cell arteritis: a pathological study to show the pattern of arterial involvement. Arch. Neurol. 27:378–391.

Wilske, K. R. and Healey, L. A. (1967): Polymyalgia rheumatica: a manifestation of systemic giant-cell arteritis. Ann. Intern. Med. 66:77–86.

INDEX

Edema, cerebral, high altitude, 15
pulmonary, high altitude, 15
Electroencephalography, in migraine, 73
in post-traumatic syndrome, 206
Endarterectomy, headache following,
10–11
Endocardial fibrosis, as side-effect of
methysergide, 142
Endorphins, distribution of, analgesic
effect, 4
Epilepsy, migraine and, 39, 66, 177
abdominal pain in, 70–71
tension headache and, 177
Ergonovine, contraindications, 147
dosage, 130, 146–147
effect on serotonin, 146
in migraine, 118, 146–147
putative action at serotonergic
synapses, 135, 137
side-effects, 130
structure, 146, 146
vs. ergotamine and methysergide, 146
Ergotamine, caffeine and, 119–120, 120
clinical use, 122–125
dosage, 122–125, 128, 130
early history, 117–118
effect on serotonin turnover, 121
in cluster headache, 193–194, 196
in migraine, 117–128, 117
in tension headache, 181–182
mechanisms of action, 120–122
parenteral vs. oral, 118–119
patient tolerance of, 125–127
pregnancy and, 127–128
putative action at serotonergic
synapses, 135, 137
side-effects, 125–126, 130
gangrene of limbs, 126
in pregnancy, 127–128
toxicity, 125–127
tritiated, distribution, 119
vasoconstrictive effect of, 120–121
Ergot-containing drugs, 123
Ergotism, 126
Erythrocyte sedimentation rate,
elevation of, in giant cell arteritis,
227–228
Ethanol. See Alcohol.
Ethyl alcohol, metabolism of, 17. See
also Alcohol.
Exercise, migraine and, 43, 51
Exertional headache, 213–214
Eye disorders, percentage occurrence, 9

Facial migraine, 30
Fasting, as migraine precipitant, 99–100
Fatty acid metabolism, migraine and,
99–100
Fever, migraine and, 41

Fibrosis, as side-effect of methysergide,
endocardial, 142
pleuropulmonary, 142
retroperitoneal, 141–142
Fibrotic disorders, as side-effect of
methysergide, 141–144
mechanisms, 143–144
Focal neurologic symptoms, migraine
and, 39
Fluid retention, migraine and, 40
Flushing, facial, in cluster headache, 187
Food, as trigger for headache, 20–22
Fortification spectra, 31
migraine and, 38, 59–62, 61

Gangrene of limbs, as side-effect of
ergotamine, 126
Gastrointestinal disturbances, migraine
and, 37–38
Gastrointestinal motility, during drug
treatment, 116–117
Gate-control theory, of pain, 2
Giant cell arteritis, 220–234
central retinal artery occlusion and,
226
clinical features, 222–227
headache, 222–223
large artery involvement, 227
neurologic disorders, 226–227
polymyalgia rheumatica, 221, 224
visual, 225–226
demography, 221
diplopia and, 225
duration, 230–231
elevation of ESR in, 227–228
ischemic optic neuropathy and,
225–226
laboratory abnormalities in, 227–228
anemia, 228
liver function tests, 228
pathogenesis, 230
polymyalgia rheumatica and,
relationship, 221, 224, 231–232
temporal artery biopsy in, 228–230
treatment, 230–232
prednisone, 231
side-effects, 232
visual improvement, 231
Glutamate, monosodium, as precipitant
for Chinese restaurant syndrome,
20–21

Hallucinations, migraine and, 59, 60, 65
Hangover, mechanism of, 17–18
vascular headache and, 16–18
Head trauma. See Post-traumatic
headache.